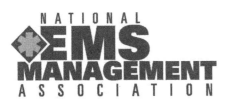

NATIONAL
EMS
MANAGEMENT
ASSOCIATION

EMS
SUPERVISOR

PRINCIPLES AND PRACTICE

ORLANDO J. DOMINGUEZ, JR., RPM, MBA
Division Chief of EMS
Brevard County Fire Rescue
Brevard County, Florida

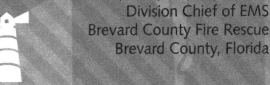

JONES & BARTLETT
LEARNING

World Headquarters
Jones & Bartlett Learning
5 Wall Street
Burlington, MA 01803
978-443-5000
info@jblearning.com
www.jblearning.com

Jones & Bartlett Learning books and products are available through most bookstores and online booksellers. To contact Jones & Bartlett Learning directly, call 800-832-0034, fax 978-443-8000, or visit our website, www.jblearning.com.

Substantial discounts on bulk quantities of Jones & Bartlett Learning publications are available to corporations, professional associations, and other qualified organizations. For details and specific discount information, contact the special sales department at Jones & Bartlett Learning via the above contact information or send an email to specialsales@jblearning.com.

Production Credits
Chief Executive Officer: Ty Field
President: James Homer
Chief Product Officer: Eduardo Moura
VP, Executive Publisher: Kimberly Brophy
Executive Editor: Christine Emerton
Associate Managing Editor: Amanda Brandt
Production Editor: Nora Menzi
Vice President of Sales, Public Safety Group: Matthew Maniscalco
Director of Sales, Public Safety Group: Patricia Einstein

Director of Marketing: Alisha Weisman
VP, Manufacturing and Inventory Control: Therese Connell
Composition: Cenveo Publisher Services
Cover Design: Kristin E. Parker
Rights and Media Research Coordinator: Laura Piasio
Media Development Assistant: Shannon Sheehan
Cover Background Pattern: © Eky Studio/ShutterStock, Inc.
Printing and Binding: Strategic Content Imaging (SCI)
Cover Printing: Strategic Content Imaging (SCI)

Library of Congress Cataloging-in-Publication Data
Dominguez, Orlando J., author.
  EMS supervisor : principles and practice / Orlando Dominguez.
  p. ; cm.
  ISBN 978-0-7637-7643-5 (pbk.)
  I. Title.
  [DNLM: 1. Administrative Personnel. 2. Emergency Medical Services–organization & administration. 3. Emergency Medical Technicians—organization & administration. 4. Leadership.   WX 215]
  RA975.5.E5
  616.02'5092—dc23
                                                                                2014036063
6048

Printed in the United States of America
27 26 25 24 23   10 9 8 7 6 5 4

Contents

Acknowledgments

Jones & Bartlett Learning would like to thank the National EMS Management Association (NEMSMA) for its partnership in this project, and Troy Hagen for his dedicated review of each chapter.

The author, Orlando J. Dominguez, Jr., would like to thank:

My Lord for making this project possible and for all blessings.

My family for your unwavering support and love.

Mom for your wisdom and teaching me that anything is possible.

All public safety personnel, for doing what you do and putting others first every day. You make this world a better place.

Christine and Amanda, thank you for the journey.

And my best friend Rafael, this is for you.

Reviewers

Leaugeay C. Barnes, MS, NRP
Tulsa Community College
Tulsa, Oklahoma

Christopher Black, MA Ed
Program Director
Estrella Mountain Community College
Avondale, Arizona

Stephen Blackburn, AAS, EMT-P
Clinical Education Coordinator
Lenoir Community College
Kinston, North Carolina

Chad Bluschke, CCP, EMS-I
Station Manager
Midwest Medical Transport
Grand Island, Nebraska

Wesley Carter, BS, NREMT-P
Lenoir Community College
Kinston, North Carolina

Matthew Drake, EMT-P, I/C
Clinical Coordinator
Mobile Medical Response
Saginaw, Michigan

James B. Eubanks, NREMT-P, CCEMT-P, PNCCT, FP-C
Carolinas Healthcare System—MedCenter Air/Event Medicine
Critical Care Paramedic/Base Lead/Base Clinical Educator
Novant Health—Critical Care Transport
Charlotte Hornets NBA Paramedic
Charlotte, North Carolina
Piedmont Medical Center EMS Paramedic
Rock Hill, South Carolina
Palmetto Health/USC School of Medicine Simulation Center Educator
Columbia, South Carolina

Ron Feller, Sr., MBA, NRP
Director, Emergency Medical Sciences
Oklahoma City Community College
Oklahoma City, Oklahoma

SBPA Edward M. Fowler, NRP
Medical Section Chief
US Customs & Border Protection
Advanced Training Center
Harpers Ferry, West Virginia

Troy Hagen
Chief Executive Officer
Care Ambulance Service
Orange, California

Marc Holyfield
Arizona Western College
Yuma, Arizona

Paul Honeywell, CEP, NRP
Paramedic Educator
Flagstaff Medical Center
Flagstaff, Arizona

Justin Hunter, MPA, NRP, FP-C
Oklahoma State University
Oklahoma City, Oklahoma
EMSStat
Norman, Oklahoma

Amy Marsh, BA, NRP
EMS Educator
Sioux Falls Fire Rescue
Sioux Falls, South Dakota

Jacob Offerman EMT-P, I/C
QI/Education Supervisor
Livingston County EMS
Howell, Michigan

Tim Petreit, NRP
Montgomery Fire/Rescue-Division of
    Training
Montgomery, Alabama

Michael Price, BS, NRP
Director of EMS Education
Central Piedmont Community College
Charlotte, North Carolina

Shaun P. Pochik, BS, EMT-P, IC
Director of EMS Education
Huron Valley Ambulance
Ann Arbor, Michigan

John Reed, MPH, BSN, RN, NRP
Birmingham Regional EMS System
Birmingham, Alabama

John Russell, AAS, Paramedic
Sinclair Community College
Dayton, Ohio

Peter Struble, MPA, NRP
Fire Chief (Ret.)
Lecturer, University of New Haven
West Haven, Connecticut

Derrick Swanson, MSM, NR-Paramedic
Fire Chief (Fmr)
Training Group Supervisor (Fire & EMS)
Alabama Fire College & Personnel
    Standards Commission
Tuscaloosa, Alabama

**David M Tauber, BS, NR-P, CCEMT-P,
FP-C, NCEE**
EMS Education Coordinator, Yale-New
    Haven Sponsor Hospital Program
New Haven, Connecticut
Executive Director, Advanced Life Support
    Institute
Conway, New Hampshire

Justin G. Tilghman, MS, CEM, EMT-P
Director of Public Safety Education
Lenoir Community College
Kinston, North Carolina

John Todaro, BA, NRP, RN, TNS, NCEE
EMS/CME Academic Department
    Coordinator
St. Petersburg College
Pinellas Park, Florida

Michael Torino, EMT-P/EMS-I
Paramedic Programs Coordinator
Yale New Haven Sponsor Hospital
   Program
New Haven, Connecticut

Gary S. Walter, BA, NREMT-P, EMSI
Union College, International Rescue &
   Relief
Lincoln, Nebraska

Ken Walters, BS, NRP, CCEMT-P
American Medical Response
Jackson, Mississippi

Bruce J. Walz, PhD
Professor and Chair
Department of Emergency Health Services
University of Maryland, Baltimore County
Baltimore, Maryland

James J. (J.J.) Wohlers
Grand Island Fire Department
Grand Island, Nebraska

**Thomas Worthington, BAS, EMT-P,
   EMSIC**
EMT/Paramedic Program Coordinator
Schoolcraft College
Garden City, Michigan

1

Dynamics of EMS Leadership and Organizational Structure

Learning Objectives

After studying this chapter, you should be able to:

- Identify the general levels of emergency medical service (EMS) officers and discuss their roles and responsibilities.

- Describe how to get a big-picture overview of the EMS organization and explain why doing so is an important step as an EMS officer.

- Identify and describe the five business priorities (5 BPs).

- Discuss the use of organizational spokes in keeping the various organizational components on track.

- Discuss the role of organizational culture in the success of the EMS officer and the organization.

- Identify ways that the EMS officer can become a market leader.

- Describe the steps the EMS officer should take immediately after promotion.

Introduction

The field of emergency medical services (EMS) is continuously evolving to keep up with advances in prehospital patient care, exceed customer expectations, ensure that the EMS organization is well positioned to manage operational and administrative issues, and improve how officers manage and lead personnel. EMS officers must stay informed within this continuously changing landscape and must remain well positioned to make any necessary adjustments. It is critical that, once promoted, the EMS officer begin to understand that he or she will need to become very familiar with not only the prehospital aspect of EMS, but what is needed to ensure that the organization or division will remain viable in offering its services. EMS officers must be prepared to execute their management and leadership abilities within all levels of the organization. Although the emphasis of this text is on the newly promoted EMS manager, it can also benefit other front-line EMS officers, and can even serve as a template for any organizational leader in a non-EMS business environment.

Although it is important to embrace the traditions of public safety and their origins, organizational leaders must not overlook the importance of promoting a business-culture mindset within their EMS organization. Today's EMS leaders must realize that fire and EMS organizations are in the service delivery business—yes, *business*. Therefore, the goal for every organizational leader and the members of the EMS organization must be to embrace a business-culture mindset that will maximize positive organizational outcomes, both operationally and administratively.

Levels of EMS Officers

Just as each fire and EMS organization is structured differently, so it is likely that the rank structure and the roles assigned to members will differ among these organizations. Certain general terms to describe EMS officers have been identified by the National EMS Management Association (NEMSMA):

- Supervising EMS Officer: The primary responsibility of this entry-level EMS officer is supervising EMS personnel in the field. Secondary responsibilities may include EMS administrative duties. The role of the supervising EMS officer may entail on-scene patient care supervision; quality assurance; EMS training; issuing discipline; and completing supervisors' reports pertaining to personnel injuries, hazard exposure, or equipment damage. The rank structure of an organization is typically tailored to the size of the organization, which may result in many of the same duties being assigned to both a managing EMS officer and a supervising EMS officer.

- Managing EMS Officer: This position is commonly held by a mid-level EMS officer who manages the EMS division or bureau. Responsibilities may include managing and leading functional working groups; analyzing and monitoring the EMS division budget; strategic planning; identifying performance measure goals; developing strategic objectives, performance benchmarks, and targets pertaining to the EMS division's performance measures; and ensuring the support of a continuous quality improvement plan. The managing EMS officer may participate in collective bargaining negotiations and hospital/EMS consortia as well. Depending on the size of the organization and budget constraints, the duties of an EMS manager may sometimes be assigned to front-line EMS supervisors or vice versa.

- Executive EMS Officer: This EMS officer provides top-level leadership and management for the entire organization, typically through a director or chief executive officer (CEO) position.

At the supervising officer level, individuals may hold the rank of EMS lieutenant, EMS captain, EMS district supervisor, or EMS battalion supervisor, or the officer may simply be referred to as an EMS supervisor. Similarly, a managing EMS officer may hold the rank of EMS division chief or EMS bureau chief, and an executive EMS officer may also be the fire chief, CEO, commander, or director of the organization. Even as the titles differ among organizations, the duties at these three basic levels are likely to be similar. Depending on the size and structure of the organization, some of these officer levels could overlap.

Depending on the level of responsibilities assigned to you as an EMS officer, you may be responsible not just for completing the tasks assigned to you, but also for ensuring that the tasks you have assigned to your team members are completed correctly and in a timely manner. You must therefore seek ways of ensuring your team remains motivated and performs at a high level.

The information in this text centers on the front-line supervising and managing EMS officer, who will be referred to as "EMS officer." The goal of this text is to provide the new EMS officer with the information needed to support and add value to the day-to-day operational and administrative duties now assigned to him or her. Regardless of his or her rank title, an EMS officer must be able to manage and lead personnel and also handle the day-to-day operational and administrative demands placed on the officer and the division. The ultimate goal of any EMS officer is to be a good managerial leader. In turn, managers at all levels must understand the importance of the interworking components that support an organization.

Understanding the Big Picture

Once promoted to an EMS officer, you have additional responsibilities that will have a significant impact on the organization's overall service delivery performance. Your primary focus must be to ensure that the organization—and not just your division—is moving in the right direction and achieving positive outcomes. However, you will not be able to accomplish these new responsibilities without a plan and without the people who will help you execute the plan. Therefore, as part of a business-culture mindset, a new EMS officer must review a **vertical snapshot** of the organization to become familiar with its make-up. The vertical snapshot includes the organizational chart of divisions within the organization and assists the new EMS officer in getting to know the division leaders, personnel, process workflow, and layout of the EMS buildings and stations. Moreover, as you review the sections/departments, you will begin to detect which organizational spokes (discussed later in this chapter) are in place that directly impact your area of responsibility versus the entire organization.

With the vertical snapshot, you will start to understand the **big picture** of how the organization conducts business on a daily basis. Although you cannot immediately become intimately familiar with every process within each division, it is important for an EMS officer to understand the day-to-day administrative and operational workflow and personnel within the organization. For example, you may be assigned to purchase EMS equipment. To fulfill this responsibility, you would need to become familiar with budgeting, requests for proposals (RFP), the vendor selection process, material requisition forms, and logistics (including storing, maintaining, and disseminating equipment). All of these specific processes contribute to the organization's purchasing system. Although every organization will be different, as a new EMS officer you will need to be familiar with the processes that affect your scope of responsibility.

The big picture will help the EMS officer understand the direction in which the organization is currently moving, and whether that is in accordance with the organization's vision, mission, and goals. The big picture can shed light on which sections are adding value to the organization, what is preventing the organization from delivering quality outcomes, and other overarching concerns.

In addition, the big picture is important because you must understand the composition of the organization before you implement changes. Managers sometimes make the mistake of coming into an organization or division and immediately making changes. If change needs to be made, you certainly should not wait to make it; at the same time, you should try to avoid making uninformed and hasty changes. If you were missing key information when you rushed into the change, you might subsequently find that change to have been a mistake, in which case both your leadership and your organization will suffer.

The big picture will be easier to understand if you are promoted from within an organization, but there may still be certain areas of the organization with which you are unfamiliar, and those areas may impact your area of responsibility. If you are coming into a new organization in a management role, find out to whom you will be reporting and ask whether you can spend some time shadowing that individual or a senior employee prior to your first day on the job. This observation period will give you an opportunity to see some of the systems and processes and the functional units in place and will allow you to meet some of your colleagues before taking your post, thereby facilitating a smooth transition into the organization. In addition, you should take some time to understand the current state of the organization; its vision, mission, and goals; means by which the organization measures its outputs and performance; its financial stability; and the ways (both good and bad) in which internal and external customers are being treated.

Five Business Priorities

Regardless of rank title, every EMS officer needs to become familiar with **five business priorities** (**5 BPs**) that must be at the core of every organization and must be continuously supported:

1. People: The most important asset, this includes customers and all members of the organization.
2. Strategic objectives: Such objectives may include improving current and future services, processes, and systems; developing a continuous improvement plan; monitoring competitors regularly; ensuring the most qualified people are doing the right jobs; and measuring systems and processes.

3. Financial management objectives: These objectives include understanding the division's budget, knowing how much money is available to keep your section viable, planning for capital improvement expenditures, and forecasting.

4. Learning objectives: These objectives include making sure your team is well informed and knowledgeable about the service being delivered, keeping up with new trends, and supporting team members as they learn and grow with the organization.

5. Culture of quality: This element focuses on analyzing and improving performance outcomes, setting benchmarks, and seeking ways to exceed customer expectations.

In assessing the organization's big picture and determining whether the 5 BPs are in place, the EMS officer will also need to identify how well these priorities are being supported by the organization. The 5 BPs provide a template for issues that the EMS officer can begin addressing on day 1. If they are not already in place, the new EMS officer can use them as an action plan in improving the organization. After evaluating the 5 BPs, the EMS officer can then determine which organizational spokes (discussed later in this chapter) are in place to support the 5 BPs. This template should be revisited and adjusted regularly to ensure it continues to meet the needs of the organization.

The 5 BPs must be at the very core of the organization and will need organizational spokes in place to support them. Once you begin to understand, implement, and support the 5 BPs through key organizational spokes, you will be on your way to leading for success and ensuring that the organization or division is equipped for business. It will be impossible to address every business concept in this text; however, by narrowing the focus to some of the most critical elements of basic business practices, you can begin to lay a strong business foundation and be successful in your new role.

If you are wondering how you are supposed to implement these 5 BPs on the first day, or if you are thinking this is too much information for an organization that is reluctant to change, keep in mind that the 5 BPs do not have to be implemented immediately. In fact, they should not be implemented until you have a thorough understanding of the organization and its culture. Each of the 5 BPs is referenced in later chapters, and they are briefly outlined here to serve as a foundation for later discussion.

People

The first business priority is all about the people, external and internal, whom you will now serve as an EMS officer. One of the biggest mistakes EMS officers make when they are initially promoted is getting so involved with the day-to-day processes (micromanaging) that they overlook the people who run the processes. A new officer must learn quickly that he or she cannot do everything alone and must depend on a good team. Assuming the role of an officer encompasses much more than giving orders. Working alongside and encouraging your team members to stay engaged is also vital for the success of the organization. You and your service delivery will be only as good as your team allows you to be.

Team members like to feel valued, and including them in your operational decisions is a good step in establishing trust and fostering collaboration. How well do you think your team members will perform their duties if they are unhappy with their current roles or they do not feel that what they say matters? How well do you think they will perform their duties if they are being micromanaged? How well do you think they will perform if they are blamed for all failures? The more engaged a team member is, the more productive he or she will be.

Strategic Objectives

The second business priority is establishing the organization's strategic objectives. This is where you put together a specific organizational roadmap that will guide the organization in the appropriate direction. As an EMS officer, it is important to implement a vision, mission, goals, performance measures, and objectives to set your organization on the right path for achieving the desired outcomes for the EMS division or the entire EMS organization. The formulation of a plan will help you and your team members stay focused and outline a path that everyone can follow. In contrast, attempting to lead an organization without a plan is a recipe for failure.

Financial Management Objectives

Although strategic objectives are a must, financial management objectives occupy an equally important place in the organization. As a new officer, you will be asked to attend budget meetings and workshops, work with capital improvement projects, begin putting your section's budget together for approval, and get involved with other aspects of the organization's finances. You will need to understand enough financial terminology and accounting practices to help you make the appropriate decisions. Although most organizations have a finance section/department, you should not depend on those personnel to answer all your budget questions. Becoming familiar with some basic financial terminology, understanding basic accounting principles, forecasting, and understanding the financial parameters within your new role will help you be better prepared to make informed decisions.

Having a plan is essential and must be a top priority for all decision makers, especially when dealing with financial management objectives. If you do not plan appropriately, your project may end up being more expensive than anticipated and going over budget; if the organization does not have enough money to cover the additional expense, the result may be an incomplete project.

Conversely, if you are not familiar with the process or the interpretation of budget allocation, you may have funds at your disposal that you did not realize existed. In many organizations, if a section's budgeted funds are not used by a certain time, the perception is that the section does not need the requested item or the money. Someone in another section within the organization may need money for a new project, and the money you had been counting on could be reallocated to that section's budget, leaving your own section short on dollars. Developing financial management objectives is critical to the organization and your section to keep systems aligned and improve day-to-day service delivery.

"Budget time" may be the most grueling period during your new assignment. During this period, you must meet with your supervisor and explain why the organization or your division should purchase the items you requested. If you have targeted key financial management objectives prior to engaging in this process, and if these objectives are aligned with your strategic objectives, it will be easier to explain the need and you will be more likely to experience a positive outcome. If you have not kept up in monitoring your budget and have not included financial management objectives as part of the organizational spoke system, however, it will be difficult to remain viable and to keep up with your competitors.

Learning Objectives

As an EMS officer, you must promote a learning environment and establish learning objectives for your team members. One key point to keep in mind early in your new role is that you do not have all the answers—and you never will. You should be as prepared and well informed as you possibly can be. A fundamental principle in ensuring that you and your team are successful in meeting the challenges of day-to-day operation is to have the right team members doing the right job. It is then your responsibility as an officer to encourage your team to learn and grow. The team's positive evolution will help the organization by improving the quality of production and will lead to a more engaged workforce. If employees feel that they are contributing to the outcome of the plan, product, or process, they will be more engaged and productive. It is important for you to encourage your team members to become as proficient as they can be within their current roles.

Set learning objectives that you would like your team to accomplish. As technology continues to advance and new products enter your business market, it is critical that your employees remain focused and knowledgeable within their field of expertise.

Culture of Quality

The last business priority centers on ensuring that your organization creates a culture of delivering quality products and service. Numerous methodologies exist that focus on quality improvement, including total quality management (TQM), continuous quality improvement (CQI), and Lean and Six Sigma. You may have all the right people on your team, they may all be knowledgeable with the process, you and your team may have designed good strategic and financial management objectives, and your team may be eager to stay on the cutting edge by learning more current and future processes. But how do you make sure the work being done truly adds value for the organization? This is where implementing a quality improvement program within your organization—and, more specifically, within your section—will prove to be extremely valuable. Whatever quality improvement program your organization chooses to use will most likely work, as long as it is followed correctly.

One example of a quality management program is Six Sigma, which focuses on identifying variations (changes from the norm). Six Sigma is a method of improving processes, ensuring a continuous analysis of processes, keeping customers happy, and identifying variations in processes. The goal is to make sure that what you are doing is adding value to the organization and its customers. The Six Sigma quality initiatives use the DMAIC methodology (discussed further in the "Creating a Culture of Quality" chapter):

- **D**efine the project that you would like to address.
- **M**easure the current situation.
- **A**nalyze the current process so that you can identify the possible defects.
- **I**mprove the current process.
- **C**ontrol the new process to ensure that you maintain the level of efficiency and effectiveness with the processes at hand.

Six Sigma can be a very powerful tool, as can other quality methodologies. A basic understanding will help you review and improve some of your current processes, and stress the importance of having a quality program within your organization. Regardless of whether you select Six Sigma or another quality management program for implementation, every organization must include a quality management system as part of its quality management initiative. Early detection of underperforming processes or variations from the expected outcomes is critical for any EMS organization. For example, a quality management system can detect and correct deviations from protocols, lengthy response times, and poor patient care. Quality management must be a priority for anyone in a leadership role and must be part of the organization's culture.

Organizational Spokes

As an EMS officer, you must become familiar with the components that support, add value, and keep the organization moving on the right path. In this text, we refer to these components as **organizational spokes**. Leading an organization or division without a business-culture mindset will have a negative impact on the organization and on you as an EMS officer. What makes a business-culture mindset so important is that it embraces the importance of organizational spokes, which support the organization's sustainability. Organizational spokes are operational or administrative sections, processes, culture, or anything else within an organization that is responsible for contributing valuable support to the overall mission of the organization. For example, if an organization has a training division, the training division would be considered a key organizational spoke that adds value to the organization. The training division is responsible for the continued training of the employees, and the employees then provide a service by using the skills taught or reinforced during a training session.

The organizational spokes can be determined from a "macro" or "micro" level. For example, a fleet division of an EMS organization is responsible for repairing vehicles and ensuring that the ambulance units are operational and ready for service. The fleet division is an organizational spoke because it adds value to the mission of the organization. From a "macro" (wide angle) view, the organization must determine whether it is more cost-effective to employ mechanics, financially support a shop where the units can be repaired, and purchase all the necessary tools needed to repair the ambulance units or to outsource the responsibilities related to the fleet division. Which option will add the most value to the organization? The EMS officer can also review the fleet services from a "micro" (more specific) view. For example, is the current process of repairing ambulance units adding value to the organization? How long does it take to get an ambulance unit back in service after it has been delivered to the fleet division for repair? If returning an ambulance to service is taking too long, then this organizational spoke must be addressed because it is not adding value to the organization. The time that it takes to repair the ambulance unit affects how effective the organization is in providing EMS to the community. If there are no units available to respond to emergencies, not only will the service not be provided, but there will also be a liability issue. Therefore, the EMS officer must evaluate anything that impacts the organization, understand its role as an organizational spoke, and determine whether it is worth keeping.

The size of the organization will often determine the number and specific types of organizational spokes needed to support the organization's business operation. Nevertheless, there are some organizational spokes that, regardless of the size of the organization, must be in place to ensure that the organization is equipped for business. These are shown in **Figure 1-1**.

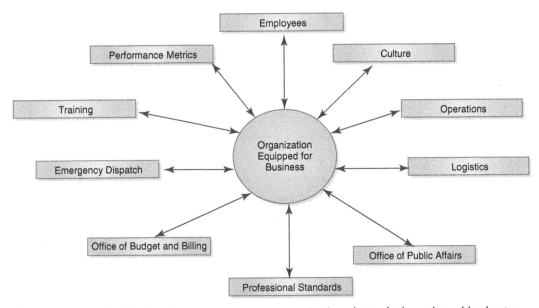

Figure 1-1 Organizational spokes may vary among organizations, but only those that add value to the organization should be left in place.

An organizational spoke can also be a nontangible component, such as culture, collaboration, or communication. For example, if the organization has a positive working culture, then the likelihood of the organization achieving positive outcomes will be much greater than it would be in a negative working culture. Therefore, a positive working culture is a value-added spoke. Value-added spokes must be in place to meet the daily organizational demands and to ensure the organization is **equipped for business** and ready to deliver positive results. An organizational leader, in turn, must keep an eye out for non–value-added spokes, which cause the organization to be unproductive and to stagnate. When identified, these negative organizational spokes must be reviewed immediately and either revised or eliminated. The key is to make sure that the organizational spokes are effective in adding value to the organization as a whole.

Although the number of organizational spokes will vary according to the size of the organization, every EMS organization should have as one of its organizational spokes a positive working culture that includes effective communication and collaboration among all members of the organization. Other necessary organizational spokes and the roles they serve to support the organization include the following:

- Finance section: Supports and monitors the organization's financial activities to ensure EMS service delivery.

- Training section: Provides continuous EMS training to employees and oversees new-hire orientation.

- Human resources section: Provides employees support through insurance benefits, employee assistance programs, retirement planning, new recruitment, and other personnel-related aspects.

- Logistics section: Responsible for inventory, purchase, and maintenance of EMS equipment.

- Fleet section: Ensures that the EMS units are working properly and are ready for service.

- Operations section: Oversees all aspects of direct EMS service delivery.

- Dispatch section: Processes emergent requests for EMS service and dispatches the calls to awaiting EMS units. In addition, this section provides ongoing communication support for crews while they are actively involved on a call.

- Information systems section: Provides continued support for computer platform applications such as patient care report writing, mobile data terminals, and administrative computer support.

Organizational spokes are also interdependent. For example, a problem with the finance section could easily affect the fleet section if the issue involves insufficient funds or poor distribution of funds. This would in turn impact the operations section if emergency vehicles are not able to respond to emergencies. Similarly, if the training section is inadequate, repercussions may be seen in the human resources section if there is high employee turnover, in the dispatch section if dispatch employees are insufficiently trained, and in the operations section if response skills are not practiced and updated.

Organizational spokes can be either operational or administrative. As an EMS officer, you will need to become familiar with many organizational spokes within the department, especially the spokes that directly impact the EMS officer's area of responsibility. Once you determine which spokes directly affect EMS service delivery, it would be prudent to determine whether each spoke is adding value. An entry-level officer may be responsible for just a few spokes that directly impact his or her section; a higher level officer, by comparison, may be responsible for ensuring all essential positive organizational spokes are in place. Regardless of your title, it is important that you make every attempt to become familiar with the organizational spokes that support your organization. This will help you adjust accordingly when making decisions.

Organizational Spoke Example: Training

Suppose you are planning to implement a new medical protocol. Before you can release that protocol, however, a set amount of EMS protocol training will need to be completed. Does your organization have a training spoke in place to support the organization's education needs? If the organization does not have a dedicated training section to address the training needs of the organization, you will need to adjust your implementation plans for the new protocol. You cannot roll out the protocol without the personnel having been trained in how to execute that specific protocol. Therefore, you will need to find an alternative method of ensuring that the necessary training is accomplished. Knowing which spokes are present and adding value within your organization will certainly impact your decision making and operational directives. Similarly, knowing which spokes are not present or do not add value is just as important.

Managerial Leadership **BRIEFCASE**

Adding Value

It is up to each EMS officer to assess, implement, and support organizational spokes that add value to the EMS division and the organization. As an EMS officer, you must begin assessing the organizational spokes that add value to your area of responsibility. In addition, many other spokes within the organization will either directly or indirectly impact your ability to get the job done. Do not focus all of your attention on your area of responsibility and ignore the many organizational spokes that contribute to the organization's ability to move forward. Although it would be impossible to keep tabs on every process being conducted by each functional unit within the organization, much can be gained from taking a periodic vertical snapshot of the organization, assessing the big picture, and determining how well the organizational spokes currently in place are adding value to your division.

Organizational Spoke Example: Public Relations

Suppose the media are requesting an interview and additional information about an incident that occurred earlier in the day. Does the organization have an organizational spoke in place to address the request from the media? If your organization does not have a public information officer or an official spokesperson, then it will be important to recommend a strategy to address the current media request as well as those that might occur in the future. An organizational spoke dedicated to public relations is very important because it promotes the brand of the organization. If the organization does have a department spokesperson, does that person represent the organization well during both good and challenging times? The issue here is not simply having an organizational spoke in place to address the daily demands placed on the organization; instead, as an EMS officer, you must determine whether it is a value-adding spoke and whether it requires updating.

Organizational Spoke Example: Equipment

One of the many tasks assigned to you as an EMS officer is to ensure that your personnel have the necessary equipment to do their jobs. Two organizational spokes will directly impact your ability to make the decisions related to equipment availability. First, does the organization have a capital improvement plan to replace older equipment before the current equipment stops working? Second, are you familiar with the organization's purchasing process? These two key organizational spokes—a capital improvement plan and an efficient purchasing process—add value not just to your section, but to the department as a whole.

Organizational Spoke Example: Performance

How, as an EMS officer, will you know if your organization or division is meeting or exceeding expectations? Performance metrics and benchmarks are organizational spokes that are essential to the organization because they provide baseline information as to how well the organization is performing. It is the responsibility of every organizational leader to have metrics in place and to benchmark the organization with industry leaders to ensure that the organization is providing the best service possible.

Organizational Culture

One of the many reasons for reviewing the organization's big picture is to determine the organization's culture. Does the organization have a positive or negative culture? What is organizational culture? Understanding organizational culture—a set of norms, beliefs, and attitudes that have permeated an organization—is an important step for every organizational leader. An organization's beliefs may be formal (directed by senior management) or informal (displayed by senior employees). As an EMS officer, you must get to know your organization's culture before implementing any operational or administrative initiative. The culture within the organization can either impede or accelerate the success of the organization. Seek to understand why your organization's culture is the way it is. Consider the following questions when assessing your organization's culture:

- How did the current organizational culture come to exist?
- Why does this culture continue?
- Why do employees buy into it?
- What do you need to do to ensure that your message can penetrate this culture?
- How can you change this culture if needed?

These are all tough questions, and unless a plan is in place to address them, you run the risk of overlooking some key indicators that may prevent the organization from achieving its maximum potential.

Culture within an organization typically arises from a set of norms and values within the organization. **Norms** are attitudes and behaviors that the organization or individuals within the organization see as normal. **Values** are ideas that reflect what the organization or individuals believe is right or wrong, good or bad. Having employee buy-in ensures that the norms and values of the organization are accepted and helps minimize resistance to change. If there is a difference in beliefs pertaining to the organization's norms and values, that clash will lead to an ineffective organizational culture, creating a disconnection between productivity and desired outcomes.

A common question shared by many new and senior supervisors is, "How can I change the current culture of the organization?" Overhauling organizational culture may be difficult due to

Managerial Leadership **BRIEFCASE**

Ensuring Your Organization Is Equipped for Business

As an EMS officer, you want to make sure that your section, division, or organization is equipped for business. To do so, you must first review the organization's big picture, at which point you will have an idea how to manage, adjust, and implement organizational spokes and the 5 BPs. The 5 BPs must be clearly defined for all members of the organization to understand them; they must also be continuously monitored to ensure they will serve as a starting point for future organizational spokes. Taking an organizational snapshot and conducting a big picture review should not be one-time tasks, but rather ongoing processes that help you keep a close eye on the overall value-added organizational spokes and business priorities. Making an organization equipped for business is not only about operational components, but must also include leadership behavior and organizational culture. As an EMS leader, you must make sure that you are looking at the entire forest and not just the singular trees in front of you.

the deeply rooted beliefs shared by most of the employees. Some organizational cultures may need an overhaul, whereas others may serve as a benchmark. There is no doubt that an organization-wide culture can exist only if the people directly involved accept the norms and values set by the leadership team. That is, multiple cultures may exist within the organization if the norms and values set by the leadership team are not embraced by the rest of the organization. If you are dealing with a large organization, you will most likely deal with individuals who have different norms and values. It takes a coordinated approach and support from senior staff members to ensure that employees accept the desired norms and values of the organization. A healthy organization, however, will have a single positive working culture that is woven throughout the entire organization.

As a new manager at any level, it may be difficult to break away from a culture that continues to promote complacency and to replace it with a positive, inclusive culture that will benefit the organization, its members, and its customers. EMS officers should attempt to make changes to the organization's culture slowly. This will improve buy-in from the team and will facilitate a transition into a new culture. Although an EMS officer can begin to introduce a positive and productive organizational culture, it will take a majority of team members supporting the new culture to ensure that the organization continues to move in the right direction. It will be your responsibility to align your team's goals with the goals of the organization. By continuing to show a commitment to customer service, quality process outcomes, and doing what is right for the organization, you and your team will set the example for all members of the organization, which will then lead to employee buy-in. Once you have buy-in from the team members, you will start to develop a positive and robust culture. That is the key—the team needs to believe in what you are asking them to do, and they need to be part of the process.

Becoming a Market Leader
Communication and Collaboration
As with many facets of business, communication and collaboration are essential to the success of the organization. Therefore, establishing good communication among all members of your team

Success in the BUSINESS WORLD
Focus on Organizational Culture
In business, organizational culture is often referred to as corporate culture, and it can have a great impact on employee satisfaction and productivity. In recent years, an increasing number of companies have started to focus on creating and maintaining positive corporate culture. Perhaps the most well-known example of this is Google, Inc., which employs a chief culture officer to monitor the company's culture and steer it in the preferred direction.

will help break down barriers and perhaps begin to establish a new culture of inclusiveness within your section. Your team members will be more open to discussing issues and new ideas if there are open lines of communication among all team members and you as the EMS officer. In addition, if team members feel that their opinions matter, they will most likely become highly engaged with your vision for the organization. Most commonly, people resist change simply because they fear the unknown. Healthy dialogue may avoid such resistance and prevent stagnation.

Best Practices

Many organizations become complacent and end up following their competitors rather than working toward becoming a market leader. As a new officer, you should make every attempt to find and implement best practices with every project you are overseeing. Using the 5 BPs, you can begin carving out a plan that will help turn your organization into an industry leader in the field of EMS delivery. For example, the *people* business priority can help achieve successful performance outcomes, strengthen communication, and foster collaboration:

- How does the organization treat its employees?
- Are the employees engaged and passionate about what they are doing?
- Are the right employees in the best roles for organizational success?
- Do the employees have the tools to achieve organizational success?
- Why is treating employees well so important?

As an example, take a look at the airline industry and consider how engaged employees truly made a difference within one specific airline company. During the recession of 2007, several airlines experienced significant challenges. Some airlines had to restructure, others merged with competing airlines, and some simply filed for bankruptcy. During this difficult period in the industry, Southwest Airlines achieved a strong market position when compared to other airlines. It did so by relying on a strong, positive corporate culture, demonstrating that a healthy culture among its leadership, employees, and customers was one of the essential keys to its success.

Another company that has done well by promoting a positive working environment is Google, Inc. Google is known for developing a creative environment where employees are empowered to make decisions and encouraged to follow through on new ideas.

A culture of highly engaged employees is beneficial to every organization, but it is just one piece of the entire plan. What do you think of your organization's culture? Should you find a way to change it? Change may be difficult and can take time, but a positive organizational culture that supports the organization's missions and goals, supports the employees, and benefits the customer is well worth the effort. Although it may be easier for higher-level officers to initiate culture changes than for new officers to do so, one should not sit around waiting for someone else to create a positive organizational culture. It takes just one person to initiate a change that others will follow.

After Promotion

It is completely normal to be nervous on your first day as an EMS officer; nevertheless, if you have established a personal working plan prior to reporting for work, you will be ready for day 1. You passed the promotional exam, you made it past the interview, and you have the necessary experience to be an EMS officer. A group of individuals saw something in you that illustrated qualities of a leader, so do not underestimate your abilities. Now is the time to position yourself for success, and this includes having an organizational plan that will exceed the expectations of your team, your customers, and the organization.

Day 1, Where Do I Begin?

It is Monday morning and you report to work a little earlier than usual in your new role as an EMS officer. In this role, and regardless of the level of responsibility to which you have been promoted, there are some fundamental initiatives that must be considered by all those in a position of managing and leading. You are now responsible for leading team members and ensuring that any systems that fall under your responsibility are managed effectively and efficiently.

First, now that you have been promoted, you will have an opportunity to implement new systems, participate in the hiring process, establish quality initiatives, establish strategic and financial management objectives, and perform other management functions. Therefore, understanding your new role and striving to be constantly well informed about the day-to-day operations will prepare you to adjust, eliminate, or implement organizational spokes that will support the organization's mission. You will most likely have employees reporting to you, so be humble. Just because you have a new title does not mean that you can now begin to ignore the rules. In fact, now more than ever you need to display leadership qualities. You will set the example for others, so be a good listener; be patient; treat others as you would like to be treated; polish your brand; continue to learn; always display leadership behavior; and do what is in the best interest of the team, the customers, and the organization. It is not about you; it is about the organization, especially its people. It is up to you to keep your team engaged and moving in the right direction. If you were not an employee of the organization prior to accepting the new role, make it a point to learn the lay of the land and its people. To whom will you report? Who will report to you? Learn who oversees each section within the organization and have a clear picture of what is expected of you. Your goal as an EMS officer will be to exceed performance expectations, so you need to be clear about what is expected of you.

One of the greatest challenges for a new EMS officer is stepping into a new role surrounded by senior management who expect the newly promoted officer to operate and execute his or her duties just as the officer's predecessor did. You are not your predecessor, and you will make good things happen for your organization. Listen to your supervisor, remain focused, and continue to learn. Do not become frustrated or disrespectful toward a senior officer because you are being asked to step outside your game plan. There is no place for big egos in EMS organizations. Maintaining an open mind to new ideas and new directions is a characteristic of great leaders. This is your time to shine and get your employees, as well as your boss, involved with some of your ideas. It is much easier to embrace an idea or change if team members are well informed, the team (including the boss) has had an opportunity to provide input, and you can clearly demonstrate how this change will benefit the organization. With time, the senior officers and your employees will trust you, but not before they embrace you as a proven leader.

Expecting the Unexpected

You will not be able to plan for everything, of course, because business and organizational behavior is very fluid. However, if you have a plan in place, you will be able to manage the day-to-day operational and administrative demands and be prepared for any unexpected issues that may arise. EMS officers at any level must make every attempt to prepare the organization for its day-to-day demands; however, it is those low-frequency situations that are sometimes overlooked by the leadership team and not planned for appropriately. When an organization operates and conducts its strategic planning without considering the potential for difficult economic times, it will have trouble keeping up. This problem crops up all too often, not only within the EMS community, but within other business organizations. When organizations do not have a plan in place and unexpected challenges arise, they may be unable to adjust appropriately and overcome the challenge. These organizations may end up sacrificing key services or products due to their inability to support those initiatives fiscally, lay off employees, be forced to merge with an other organization or downsize, or, worst of all, go out of business.

This fate befell many EMS organizations that operated during the early 2000s as if they believed that the good times were here to stay. During these years of booming economic growth in the United States, organizations provided employee raises, new services were introduced, new equipment was purchased, and so on. When the bottom fell out of the housing market, however, oil prices went on an upward trajectory, interest rates soared, monetary lending became nearly extinct, and unemployment reached the highest rates seen in years. Many EMS organizations had to make very difficult operational and administrative decisions because they did not prepare for the economic decline. Specifically, these organizations did not have enough monetary reserves to continue operating in the same manner as they had during the days of heady growth.

As the EMS officer, it is now your responsibility to ensure that your division is well positioned for business in good times as well as bad times. One reason certain organizations have been able to survive during difficult economic times is that they have well-developed strategic plans for operating in a very lean environment. There is not a lot of unnecessary spending with these organizations, and they find ways to deliver their products and services in a more effective and efficient manner compared to their competitors. They are able to be successful because they plan and prepare for turbulent times. There should be no reason for an EMS organization not to embrace this kind of business-culture mindset.

Lastly, you or your organization's leadership team must acknowledge that managing an EMS agency or fire department is no different than managing a business and must continuously ask whether the organization can prosper in its current state of production. You are in the services delivery business, so your external and internal customers are at the top of the 5 BPs list.

Promoting a Learning Environment

Upon being promoted to an officer position, you will be expected to be ready at a moment's notice to discuss common business practices, define certain systems and processes, and convey your expectations of the organization. Promoting a learning environment is a must for any organization, but especially for an EMS organization. This is one of the key components of the 5 BPs that will be discussed throughout the text. You should never be afraid to say, "I don't know, but I will get back to you with an answer," or "Can you teach me?" In addition, you need to become as well informed as you can be about the day-to-day operations (systems and processes) of your section or organization. If you are unfamiliar with a system or certain process, take the time to learn about it, because your team members will turn to you for answers. Understanding the systems and processes of the organization will enable you to do a better job as an organizational leader and be ready for questions that come your way.

In addition, you need to stay up-to-date with current business trends. Enroll in classes that will help you succeed in your new position, learn from senior leadership team members, read industry journals, and remain humble. The most junior employee can teach you a thing or two.

WRAP-UP

Concept Review

- It is critical that, once promoted, the EMS officer begin to understand that he or she will need to become familiar with not only the prehospital aspect of EMS, but what is needed to ensure that the organization or division remains viable in offering its services.

- Just as each EMS organization is structured differently, so it is likely that the rank structure and the roles assigned to members will differ among these organizations.

- As an EMS officer, your primary focus must be to ensure that the organization—and not just your division—is moving in the right direction and achieving positive outcomes.

- Five business priorities must be at the core of every organization and must be continuously supported: people, strategic objectives, financial management objectives, learning objectives, and a culture of quality.

- One of the biggest mistakes EMS officers make when initially promoted is getting so involved with the day-to-day processes (micromanaging) that they overlook the people who run the processes.

- As an EMS officer, it is important to implement a vision, mission, goals, performance measures, and objectives to set the organization on the right path for achieving its desired outcomes.

- Although most organizations have a finance section/department, you should not depend on them to solve all your budget questions. Become familiar with some basic financial terminology, and learn basic accounting principles and the financial parameters of your new role.

- A fundamental principle in ensuring that you and your team are successful with the day-to-day operation is to have the right team members doing the right jobs. It is then your responsibility as an EMS officer to encourage your team to learn and grow.

- Implementing a quality improvement program within your organization will be extremely valuable in ensuring that the work being done adds value to the organization.

- Organizational spokes are operational or administrative sections, processes, culture, or anything else within an organization that is responsible for supporting the overall mission of the organization.

- Understanding organizational culture—a set of norms, beliefs, and attitudes that have permeated an organization—is an important step for every organizational leader.

- Establishing good communication among all members of your team will help break down barriers and perhaps begin to establish a new culture of inclusiveness within your section.

- As a new officer, you should make every attempt to find and implement best practices with every project you are overseeing.

- It is normal to be nervous on your first day as an EMS officer, but if you have established a personal working plan prior to reporting for work, you will be ready.

- Regardless of the level of responsibility to which you have been promoted, some fundamental initiatives must be considered by all those in a position of managing and leading.

- You will not be able to plan for everything, but if you have a plan in place, you will be able to manage the day-to-day operational and administrative demands and be prepared for any unexpected issues that may arise.

- Promoting a learning environment is a must for any organization, but especially for an EMS organization.

Managerial Terms

Big picture The overall structure, composition, and direction of an organization.

Equipped for business A concept indicating that an organization has all the necessary plans and resources to function effectively and efficiently.

Five business priorities (5 BPs) The foundation for any organization and a roadmap for all EMS officers. The five business priorities are people, strategic objectives, financial management objectives, learning objectives, and a culture of quality.

Norms Attitudes and behaviors that the organization or individuals within the organization see as normal.

Organizational spokes Components of an organization that support and add value to the organization (the five business priorities) while keeping it moving on the right path.

Values Ideas that reflect what the organization or individuals within the organization believe is right or wrong, good or bad.

Vertical snapshot A look at the basic elements of an organization, from top to bottom.

Case Review: Resistance to Change

Upon assessing the vertical snapshot and big picture of your organization, you determine that you will meet with your team to discuss some strategic initiatives that you will be implementing to improve the EMS division. You explain to your team that you want to make sure your section is equipped for business, and you introduce them to the 5 BPs (people, strategic objectives, financial management objectives, learning objectives, and a culture of quality), which you will be monitoring closely as the initiatives are being implemented. The team's assignment is to work with you to determine (1) whether the 5 BPs are currently part of the EMS division and (2) if so, which organizational spokes are in place to support each of the business priorities. Several weeks go by and you notice that none of the team members has completed the assignment. You gather the team to discuss the issue, and you realize that there is some resistance to the requested assignment. Why is this happening?

Case Discussion

Why do you think the EMS officer experienced resistance from the team about the assignment? Several things may have contributed to the team resisting or rejecting the assignment. Although the issue in this case dealt with the personnel being resistant to change, most commonly it is poor process implementation or the process itself that hinders the achievement of successful outcomes of core initiatives. This chapter addresses why resistance occurs and how to manage it. Later chapters address how to identify poor processes and implement ones that work.

In this case, it appears that the EMS officer was attempting to implement the 5 BPs but did not seek buy-in from the team or sufficiently explain why the 5 BPs were important for the division. Something to consider when implementing a change is to ask for input from your team members. When you ask the team for input, the team will most likely accept the new initiatives with little or no resistance. As the EMS officer, you will have the opportunity to implement new initiatives, but you will find that when an initiative is clearly communicated, feedback is welcomed, and team members are encouraged to participate, change becomes a lot easier for everyone.

Case Review: Logistical Decision

You receive a telephone call from the logistics chief asking about the repair or replacement of a suction device. The logistics chief asks you, as the EMS officer, if you want to do away with the equipment, have it repaired, or purchase a new model suction device. What should you consider before responding?

Case Discussion

At first read, this case appears relatively straightforward: The equipment should be repaired. But is the equipment under warranty? Will it be more expensive to repair the equipment or to purchase a new device? Is that model outdated, making the parts scarce? Should you move toward an initiative that would replace the rest of the suction devices if the current ones are outdated?

In this case you will have to make both an operational and a financial decision. To do so effectively, the EMS officer must have a set of strategic and financial management objectives that parallel the day-to-day operations of the organization or section. These objectives should already be in place, having been created during the strategic planning process. The EMS officer must consider the following issues:

- The life expectancy of the equipment
- How often it is used
- Whether it should be replaced
- How it contributes to patient care
- Whether more advanced equipment is available in the market that would serve the customer better

These are common questions that any EMS officer must be prepared to answer. Do not wait to receive the phone call to begin thinking about these questions. If your organization does not have a capital improvement plan, then begin working on one. Reach out to vendors, other agencies, and your finance section for assistance. Be ready and have a plan.

2

Managerial Leadership

Learning Objectives

After studying this chapter, you should be able to:

- Define the managerial role and its impact on an organization.

- Describe how to succeed as a manager.

- Define the leadership role and its impact on the organization.

- Describe how to make an impact as a managerial leader.

- Explain how to implement managerial leadership in an EMS organization.

- Describe how to ensure ethical behavior.

- Discuss the elements of good time management.

Introduction

As you continue to grow within your organization and become part of the leadership team, you will be asked to manage a section, processes, people, or projects, or possibly all of these simultaneously. The one thing that you can bet on is that people (team members/associates) will be involved with your new assignment. In addition, as you assume your new role, you will hear the terms *manager* and *leader* used interchangeably, even though in reality they represent two different concepts that complement each other. Management is a science, whereas leadership is an art. The ultimate goal for any individual newly promoted to any level of management should be to become an effective and efficient **managerial leader**. In this chapter, we will define managerial leadership as a concept that encompasses the behavior and roles of someone in a key supervisory role—for example, supervising officer, managing officer, or executive officer. Before an officer can become a successful managerial leader, however, he or she must first understand the separate roles of the manager and the leader. Management primarily deals with processes, whereas leadership is all about the people. Although much of the focus in this chapter is directed toward the emergency medical services (EMS) managerial role, the information can be applied by any individual within any EMS, fire, hospital, or business organization.

Understanding the Managerial Role

As a new EMS officer, you will be managing processes, systems, and people. You will need to have effective communication skills and ensure that your team members are willing to work with you as you attempt to accomplish certain tasks—for example, creating standard operating procedures (SOPs), budgeting, developing protocols, conducting quality assurance, training, developing performance improvement initiatives and measures, and purchasing new equipment. As an EMS officer, you will most likely be managing processes and systems that will need to be monitored to ensure there is no variation from the intended outcome. With that said, you must recognize that these processes and systems are always supported by people; because you are leading those people, you must embrace the concept of becoming a managerial leader.

Processes and Systems

The EMS officer will most likely be involved with a variety of assignments that include certain processes and systems critical to completing the assignment. A **process** is a set of steps or actions to achieve an end result, and a **system** is a group of interrelated components working together to ensure a specific outcome. Working and overseeing processes is part of the EMS officer's day-to-day responsibilities. There may be times when processes are followed automatically, without the individual thinking they are processes, but that does not diminish the importance of processes in contributing (through action or steps) to completion of a specific assignment.

Table 2-1 includes examples of EMS officer assignments and the processes required to achieve a successful end result or product. Not only are there processes for almost every assignment required of an EMS officer, but these processes, no matter how small or large, serve as the essential steps in completing an assignment. As the EMS officer, it is your responsibility to ensure that every process adds value to the assignment and the overall organization (and thus adds value to the relevant organizational spokes).

As an EMS officer, you will be expected to know how certain processes contribute to establishing a system. EMS officer tasks include the following:

- Developing SOPs, general orders, bulletins, memos, and other directives: It is essential that all members within an organization work together to achieve the organization's goals and priorities. This can be quite challenging for the employees, however, if the information coming from the leadership team is not clear, is not released in a timely manner, or does not reach all of the employees. Failure to clarify the desired processes and system will lead to an unproductive work environment and employee frustration, ultimately affecting the organization's service delivery outcome. Although an EMS officer may use several methods of communication to deliver critical information to the entire department, certain important directives must remain accessible for future reference. Among these documents are standard

Table 2-1 Sample EMS Officer Assignments and Processes	
Assignment	**Process**
Create a written directive.	1. Gather the appropriate information. 2. Review data outcomes. 3. Write the directive. 4. Be available for questions after the directive has been disseminated.
Create or adjust the EMS division's budget.	1. Gather historical budget data. 2. Determine whether the items requested in the budget are necessary and add value to service delivery. 3. Establish financial management objectives.
Develop medical protocols.	1. Review the latest EMS literature to ensure the protocols are still current. 2. Ensure that all medical protocol adjustments are approved by the medical director. 3. Ensure that the crews have the tools they need to execute the protocols effectively and efficiently.
Develop a quality assurance program.	1. Recruit prehospital EMS professionals to review EMS charts. 2. Implement a system to collect and analyze the charts. 3. Determine what to do when a variation from protocol has been identified.
Develop performance metrics.	1. Determine which key result areas are to be measured. 2. Establish benchmarks. 3. Create performance objectives to achieve the desired outcome.
Purchase equipment.	1. Do research to ensure that the correct equipment is purchased. 2. Determine how the equipment will be purchased (e.g., with budget dollars or a grant). 3. Create a request for proposal (RFP). 4. Establish a vendor selection committee. 5. Select a vendor. 6. Make the final purchase. 7. Distribute the equipment to the field.
Develop an incident action plan (IAP).	1. Identify which equipment will be needed for the event. 2. Identify the incident objectives. 3. Create an incident assignment list. 4. Complete a communication plan.

operating procedures or guidelines (SOPs or SOGs), general orders, bulletins, and memos. Such written communications are instrumental when a specific set of instructions or a directive is being disseminated to the organization and needs to be available for a set amount of time. Having written communication in these cases also helps prevent misinterpretation and confusion. (See the "Communications" chapter for more information on SOPs/SOGs and other written communications.)

■ Creating budgets: As an EMS officer, you will most likely be assigned to oversee a budget that involves EMS support items. You must continuously assess how well your budget is being managed. When items that have been budgeted are being purchased, check the budget and determine whether adjustments need to be made based on the cost of the items. The overall monitoring of the budget must be ongoing, not just addressed during a budget workshop. Taking recurring snapshots of the organization's budget will provide information that will help the EMS officer determine whether the financial management objectives (one of the five business priorities [5 BPs]) have been met. It is also important to become familiar with terms such as *operational budget*, *capital budget*, *zero-based budget*, *baseline budget*, *balance sheet*, *income statement*, *forecasting*, and *balance transfers*. The budget process will be extremely frustrating for any EMS officer who chooses not to set financial management objectives prior to the budget process and does not routinely take the time to assess the assigned budget. (See the "Budgeting" chapter for more information on budget considerations.)

- Creating medical protocols: You may be asked to help revise your department's medical protocols. To do so effectively, you will need to be familiar with the processes of working with other agencies that will be impacted by any protocol changes. Collaboration with other EMS agencies will facilitate the release of the protocols and ensure that the prehospital care providers are clear about expectations, ultimately improving EMS service delivery. As an EMS officer in the department, you will need to take the lead and set the tone for collaboration and inclusiveness among all protocol stakeholders.

- Creating a quality management system: As part of doing business, regardless of which business you are in, quality management is a necessity (and a culture of quality is one of the 5 BPs). A quality management system is the means by which you (and perhaps a team) review specific core processes to ensure that the services delivered are meeting or exceeding the benchmarks set by the organization. For example, you might assign a group of medical professionals to review how well the department's emergency medical technicians (EMTs) and paramedics are delivering patient care. The review may be completed by direct observation or by reviewing patient care reports post incident. No matter which approach is used, a process must be in place to address any variations from the expected EMS delivery service. If a variation from protocol is identified, the case may be forwarded to the department's medical director for further review. Additionally, you and the medical director may establish different levels of severity related to the variations in service delivery and determine how to address each case. The medical director may elect to address the most critical protocol variations, with the rest being addressed by you as the supervising officer. You might also consider establishing a system that encompasses not only a quality assurance process for medical care, but also a quality control and quality improvement component, to complete the continuous quality improvement system. (See the "Creating a Culture of Quality" chapter for more information on quality management programs.)

- Creating performance improvement measures: As an EMS officer, it will be your responsibility to establish performance metrics and to set benchmarks for the EMS division. Analysis of these results will allow you to see how well your division is delivering quality service and where there is a need for improvement. It makes no sense to implement a new system if you have no baseline performance measure of the current system. Reviewing performance metrics and determining whether your division is meeting the targeted benchmarks will provide essential information for making organizational decisions. Every EMS officer responsible for a division or for the organization as a whole must establish, implement, and review performance metrics on a regular basis. Knowing how well the division or organization is performing must be a top priority.

- Purchasing equipment: As an EMS officer, you will almost certainly have the responsibility of purchasing equipment. You will therefore need to become familiar with your organization's purchasing process. You may be asked to obtain purchase quotes from vendors, complete material requisition forms, and perhaps forfeit the purchase of a budgeted item and request the transfer of budgeted dollars to a new line item. If absolutely no budgeted dollars are available, applying for a grant or entering into a partnership with other EMS agencies to offset some of the expenses may be an option. Regardless of the purchasing process in place in your organization, you should not hesitate to seek advice from those who have already done it and to continue to ask questions.

- Creating an incident action plan (IAP): You may be required to create or implement an IAP. In doing so, you will need to ensure that IAPs are completed in accordance with your department's policy, and you may be required to complete a plan for longstanding operations, special events, or even the organization's internal day-to-day operations. Regardless of which type of need prompts development of the IAP, you must gather a variety of information to ensure that the plan is timely, addresses the current issues of an event, and includes the strategic plan that is or will be used in managing the event.

These are just a few examples of the tasks that new EMS officers will face when taking their post. Accomplishing specific tasks such as these requires a firm understanding of both management and leadership and a recognition of how they fit within your new role as an EMS officer.

The EMS officer must be knowledgeable in the processes and systems assigned to him or her. Therefore, it is important for the EMS officer to routinely evaluate these processes and systems to ensure that they are adding value to the organization. To do so, the EMS officer should determine the end goal or desired outcome each process or system is designed to achieve. When attempting to establish or evaluate a set goal, the EMS officer should consider using the SMART mnemonic: specific, measurable, achievable, relevant, and time-bound (discussed further in the "Strategic Planning" chapter).

- Specific: The goal must be specific and not ambiguous. The team members must know what they are attempting to accomplish.

- Measurable: It is nearly impossible to determine how effectively processes or systems are working if they are not being measured. As the EMS officer, you must know if these elements are adding value or underperforming.

- Achievable: The EMS officer must make every attempt to continuously evaluate the goals of processes and systems to determine whether they are achievable, ensuring that processes and systems are continuously improving and ultimately leading to a better end product. The EMS officer must also attempt to stretch the goal in an effort to build stronger processes and systems, but not to the point that it will be impossible to attain.

- Relevant: The EMS officer must ensure that the processes and systems leading to a specific goal are relevant to the core mission of the EMS division or organization. For example, if your response area is entirely urban, it would not make sense to have your team work on an assignment that entailed purchasing gear for wildland firefighting.

- Time-bound: You must set target dates for project completion. The team members must clearly know what is expected of them and how much time they have to complete the project. Many projects never reach a state of completion because there is no preset completion date and the assignment falls off the radar.

People

As an EMS officer, your management duties will center on overseeing the processes and systems that impact the EMS organization or division. In addition, you will manage those team members who are directly involved with the day-to-day operational and administrative duties. Management of the team may include deciding which team member is the best suited for a specific project, answering a team member's question about a specific task, determining whether a team member's performance is adding value to the organization, and so on. When managing the team, the EMS officer is ensuring that the assignments and the core mission of the EMS division are being accomplished. With that said, as an EMS officer, you must focus on not only managing your team, but also on being a great leader and supporting your team. A leader is respected, knowledgeable, and highly engaged with the team. He or she helps each team member achieve that person's full potential and focuses on the greater good for the team and the organization.

A question commonly asked of those in a supervisory position is, "Do you lead or manage your team?" Ultimately, the EMS officer must do both and, therefore, must accept the role of a managerial leader.

As a managerial leader, you will need to develop the ability to prioritize requests for direction. Your team members will seek you out for guidance and, depending how many members directly work for you, it might be a little overwhelming if you are continuously being bombarded with questions and requests. Establishing a "response triage" system will help you address those issues that are time sensitive and operationally critical to the organization. Depending on the time required to address the issues and the level of importance, you can begin to set the least important requests aside for a later time. However, your system needs to include a reminder alarm because you certainly do not want to forget to respond and give the impression to the team

Managerial Leadership **BRIEFCASE**

Good Leadership Traits

Here are a few tools that may help break the ice with your team and set you on your way as you assume your new role.

■ Promise only what you can deliver. If you cannot deliver or you fall short, immediately explain to your team what happened.

■ Be honest with your team. Once they know you are not being honest, regaining their confidence will be virtually impossible.

■ When things go wrong, before placing blame on a team member, remember that you are in charge. The buck starts and ends with you. Rather than asking, "Who did this?", ask, "What happened?" Many times a process—and not a person—is at fault.

■ Give a gift for no reason: Saying "Thank you" goes a long way.

■ Be accessible to your team and be a good listener.

■ Break out of your normal office routine and spend some time with your team. Get to know each team member.

■ Autonomy is critical—and micromanaging kills it.

■ When someone comes to meet with you in your office, do not sit behind your desk. Find a chair and sit next to the visitor.

■ Do not wait for change to happen; you, as the leader, can make it happen.

■ Let your team know that leadership can be executed at any level.

■ You are always on stage, so be an example to others.

■ Be humble.

■ Be loyal to your employees, customers, and organization.

■ Offer positive and constructive feedback.

■ Keep learning and improving your processes.

■ Give clear direction.

■ Develop people.

Poor Leadership Traits

These poor leadership traits are almost a guarantee for leadership failure:

■ Not providing feedback to the team

■ Micromanaging employees

■ Always "shooting the messenger"

■ Never having time for team members

- Not developing, coaching, or mentoring team members
- Not delegating
- Taking all the credit when things are good, but blaming others for mistakes
- Not projecting confidence
- Sabotaging team members' ideas
- Demonstrating poor listening skills

member that his or her question is unimportant. There are several software programs that you can use to track items and even set an alarm to remind you to follow up. Although a question might not seem to be of critical importance to you, it will be for the individual who is seeking an answer. Remember that one of the 5 BPs is people, and your interactions with team members and others will affect the organization.

How to Succeed as a Manager

Once promoted, you may find that the experience of being a manager is not exactly what you expected. Some new managers are comfortable overseeing processes and systems, but have trouble adapting to people reporting to them. Other managers take the post with the intention of making an immediate impact, but that does not always happen. Still other new managers may feel compelled to get the job done without delegating, and soon become overwhelmed. There are many components to a managerial position: people, workflow processes, budget planning, performance metrics, quality methodology, and more. For a new manager to succeed, he or she should prepare in advance for the many challenges that will be presented in the new role.

Success as a manager requires leadership. Although management deals primarily with processes and systems, these organizational resources need oversight by team members, and this is where the "leadership" in managerial leadership is applied. As a managerial leader, you want to ensure that the daily demands placed on the organization are being addressed. If the team members do not believe in you and what you are asking of them, it will be difficult to keep up with the day-to-day business operation. Delivering quality outcomes and ensuring that the day-to-day operations exceed expectations is vital; however, demonstrating good communication skills with members of the organization while establishing a culture of trust and inclusion with your team is just as critical. Management is fulfilling the day-to-day operations; leadership is gaining the needed support from your team to ensure that operational demands are addressed effectively.

One challenge of management occurs when a project develops **scope creep**, in which the participants move away from the intended goal of the project and into other areas that add no value to the project. As the manager, it will be your responsibility to keep the project moving forward within the set parameters. For example, you can be a great manager by planning, organizing, directing, controlling, and coordinating a process. There is a good probability, however, that this project will not be your only priority. In asking your team members for assistance in completing this project, you will have to find a way for them to work cohesively and accept you as a leader. At this point, you will begin to see where the leadership component of managerial leadership plays a critical role. Poor leadership skills will seriously affect the organization's effectiveness in delivering high-quality goods and services, regardless of how well you manage the organization's processes or the systems currently in place.

Understanding the Leadership Role

Leadership is influence, and it's all about your team. Providing your employees with a roadmap of what is expected of them and inspiring them to get to a place where they are successful within the organization should be your goal. This effort will benefit you, your employees, and the organization as a whole. Leaders must be passionate about their role in working with people while keeping the vision, mission, and values of the organization in mind.

Many examples of good leadership can be found outside the world of emergency services. For instance, the Walt Disney Company, the U.S. military, Zappo's, Copa Airlines, and Southwest Airlines are all known for their good managerial leadership culture. These organizations are all very successful at what they do and are very much in tune with their employees and customers. As mentioned earlier in the text, the first of the 5 BPs is always people. To be successful in a leadership role, you need to put your people first within your organization.

One of the first things to consider when accepting the role of EMS officer is the organizational behavior within the organization. **Organizational behavior** is how people behave within an organization, which in turn is a direct reflection of the **organizational culture**. The culture of the organization is what makes the organization function the way it does. It is up to the members of an organization to embrace the expected organizational norms, values, and beliefs set by the leadership team. Therefore, it is critical for your team to believe in you and support your direction as the leader. If they do not, the culture will be severely affected and the organization will not perform as well as it could. As a leader, you must understand that the organizational culture can make or break the organization, and you will need to strive to develop a culture that delivers positive results. This is why people are truly the primary ingredient to any successful organization.

Leadership Styles

Once you understand the organization's culture, you will have a better understanding of the type of leadership style that would be most beneficial for your team. Several leadership styles are commonly referenced in business texts; however, what works best for you and your organization might not fit neatly into one of these styles. Consider whether it would be appropriate to develop your own style, perhaps using elements of the leadership styles discussed here. Keep in mind, too, that different situations may call for different leadership styles; for example, your leadership style in an emergency situation will likely be different from your approach during a budget meeting. It is important to adjust your leadership style according to what will engage your team.

Common leadership styles include the following:

- Directive leader: Creates a dependent relationship with subordinates, who obediently carry out the leader's orders. The directive leader provides clear directions and objectives as to how a task must be completed. This approach will work well with team members who are not sure how to complete the task or who need continuous guidance. This type of leader, however, may be looked upon as a micromanager, and the directive leadership style does not work well with those who know their job expectations.
  - Example: An EMS officer has been assigned to complete a large EMS project and will be supervising temporary employees who are unfamiliar with the tasks needed to complete the project. The EMS officer will need to provide clear instructions as to how complete each task.
- Coaching leader: Focuses on guiding the team, challenging the team, and taking them to the next level. This leadership style works well when team members want to learn and face the organizational challenges head-on. The coaching leader focuses on motivation, trust, and learning. This leadership style is not appropriate, however, if the team members are not willing to accept the coach (personally) or what the coach is trying to accomplish. Such a leader may come across as a micromanager.
  - Example: The EMS officer is responsible for overseeing the day-to-day operational and administrative duties for a large EMS department and uses a coaching leadership approach to ensure that the team remains focused and executes the processes as expected to get the job done. In addition, this coaching leader challenges the team not only to deliver a quality product, but also to achieve the performance goals set at the beginning of the year. The EMS officer will need to provide support to the team by creating an environment of collaboration and trust, but making sure not to get in team members' way.

Managerial Leadership BRIEFCASE

Establishing a Brand

As a leader, you will need to be conscientious in maintaining your personal brand. Just as a corporate brand is important, so is establishing and maintaining a positive personal brand. If you display a sense of being upset or unapproachable, that is how the employees will see you. Regardless of your intentions as a leader, how you carry yourself is how others will perceive you.

■ Consensus leader: Seeks agreement without hurting subordinates' feelings. This leader relies on group consensus when making decisions, making sure that all team members have an opportunity to be part of the decision-making process. Such a leader may appear to be indecisive in always seeking the group's input before making a decision and may create some discontent among team members if a decision is made without their input.

  - Example: The EMS officer is interested in purchasing a piece of equipment that will benefit patient care. Before the EMS officer makes the purchase, he or she seeks input from the employees to determine whether the purchase will be worthwhile.

■ Affiliative leader: Has an empathetic relationship with employees. The affiliative leader works to establish cohesion and harmony among team members. This leader places employees first and often praises them. Such a leadership style may cause the leader to overlook troubling situations affecting an employee or the entire group.

  - Example: The EMS officer routinely praises staff for doing a great job. In addition, the EMS officer frequently meets with the staff individually and as a group to ensure that there is a harmonious culture and to address issues before they get out of control.

■ Expert leader: Believes that knowledge is power and that being right and efficient is more important than establishing a relationship with team members. This leader is knowledgeable, perhaps an expert, in the responsibilities assigned to him or her. Such a style can, however, lead to lost opportunities for team member input and to team member frustration.

  - Example: The EMS officer assumes the role of leader with most assignments and believes that his or her own input is most accurate.

■ Charismatic leader: Gathers followers by having a charming personality. The charismatic leader has the talent to highly engage the audience and is very effective in conveying a message. This leader may, however, focus more on himself or herself than on the overall good of the organization. For the charismatic leader, most commonly the focus is all about the leader's presence, personal goals, and perception by the audience.

  - Example: The EMS officer is extremely friendly and outgoing with the team members, leading to a sense of community following the leader.

■ Situational leader: Puts himself or herself in a leadership role during challenging situations. This leader is able to adjust and lead the team in different business environments, but may experience difficulty in adjusting leadership styles to meet the needs of the organization.

  - Example: The EMS officer is faced with day-to-day operational and administrative challenges. Therefore, he or she must be ready to address patient care issues, protocol violations, patient complaints, billing questions, and other challenges. Situational leadership is the most important leadership style because it emphasizes the leader's ability to lead during changing circumstances.

■ Servant leader: Is available for the team members and puts the needs of the members first. The servant leader's priority is helping the team members succeed. This leader works to ensure the team keeps moving in the right direction, supports each team member in achieving his or her goal, and promotes a good working culture. This form of leadership style is more of a support role for the team members; therefore, it is not recommended in situations where quick decisions are needed.

- Example: The EMS officer plays a supportive role and does what it takes to ensure the team is well positioned to succeed as a group and individually in the tasks assigned to them.

■ Autocratic leader: Does not seek input from team members. This authoritarian leader always has the last word. Under certain circumstances—for example, when quick decisions need to be made and the leader is a subject-matter expert—this form of leadership may be beneficial; however, it can be extremely demoralizing to team members and will ultimately lead to team member frustration and underperformance.

- Example: The EMS officer assumes the leadership role in purchasing new ambulance units for the department without seeking input from the paramedics or fleet technicians.

■ Participative leader: Works cooperatively with employees to get the task completed. The goal with this form of leadership is to get everyone involved and working together. This leadership style seeks the participation of all team members, but the leader is still in charge and has the final say. Participative leadership promotes a good working culture and, by seeking out employee input, engages employees and improves morale. This leadership style will not work well if the members of the organization are not interested in the work being done and do not believe that their ideas will be considered.

- Example: The EMS officer assumes the leadership role in reviewing the department's medical protocols. As a participative (democratic) leader, he or she involves the team members in the decision-making process about which protocol needs to be updated or eliminated before addressing the topic with the department's medical director.

■ Transformational leader: This leadership style goes to the very core of the organization's culture and the employees. Transformational leadership plays a critical role when the organization needs to "reboot" the way it is doing business by establishing a new vision for the organization and getting everyone on board. This form of leadership is most useful when the organization is seeking a new direction, as long as the leader's vision is one that is well suited for the organization.

- Example: An EMS division is unproductive and experiencing numerous problems related to quality of care. A new EMS officer is brought into the organization with the goal of transforming the service delivery into one characterized by high performance and positive, high-quality outcomes.

■ Laissez-faire leader: This leadership style is non-authoritarian and offers minimal guidance to the team. The laissez-faire leader allows the team members to work independently and at their own pace. Team members feel that they are provided the opportunity to get the job done without being micromanaged, providing a stress-free environment and productive working environment for the team. However, poor outcomes may result due to the lack of supervision.

- Example: The EMS officer is responsible for several projects, which he or she assigns to team members. The EMS officer then allows the team members to complete the assignments at their own pace and with little direction.

A good leader knows and understands the team members' full potential. This is vital in ensuring the team members are assigned tasks that match their strengths. A good leader will be able to detect when a team member is underperforming and will assist that individual in getting back on track. A good leader also knows when to step out of the way and let the team members maximize their potential. As a leader, you have the opportunity to create an environment of learning and motivation, promote a positive work environment, and support a culture of inclusion among organizational communities.

Making an Impact as a Managerial Leader

If you are promoted from within your own organization, you may have an advantage over someone coming in from another organization who is promoted to the same role—but there are positives and negatives to both situations. The primary advantage to being promoted from within is that you are already familiar with the processes and systems, culture, and people of the organization, as well as the internal and external factors that promote or threaten the organization's mission. However, prior familiarity with the organization does not mean you can become complacent and just stick to the status quo. Your job is to help the organization achieve its full potential and exceed service delivery expectations.

The primary advantage of joining a different organization as a manager is that you can provide the members of the organization with a new perspective on how to do things and perhaps look at processes and current systems from a different point of view. However, as a new member of the organization, you will not be familiar with its culture, people, processes, and systems, and will have to focus on learning these details as a first step in managerial leadership.

Regardless of whether you are hired from outside or from within the organization, there are certain guidelines you should consider (**Table 2-2**).

Implementing Managerial Leadership

As an EMS officer, it is important that both your management skills and your leadership skills are constantly being refined. The EMS officer will continuously work with processes and systems that will require management expertise. The EMS officer also will need to set an example as a leader and understand the true role of a leader within an organization. When these two roles are combined, it is no longer simply a manager or a leader, but rather a managerial leader, who must be driving the organization or division.

Table 2-2 Guidelines for New Managers	
Do	**Don't**
■ Spend time learning the organization. ■ Be patient in making changes and listen to your team members. ■ Ask questions and seek feedback. ■ Meet with not only members of your organization and your team members, but also with members of the community. ■ Manage your time wisely: You will be busy getting adjusted to the new role and your employees will want your attention. ■ Spend some time with your team members individually. ■ Speak with other managerial leaders within the organization and get to know them. ■ Make a point to celebrate accomplishments. ■ Promote your team members and help them grow. ■ Deliver on your word.	■ Don't make immediate changes unless they are absolutely necessary. ■ Don't spend large amounts of time away from your team, especially early in your managerial leadership role. ■ Don't have a know-it-all attitude. ■ Don't exclude your team from the decision-making processes that affect them. ■ Don't keep secrets from the team to make yourself look good. ■ Don't micromanage. ■ Don't embarrass, belittle, or be condescending to anyone. ■ Don't ask your team members to do something you would not do. ■ Don't take the credit for the team. ■ Don't assign a project if you are not familiar with it. ■ Don't make promises you cannot deliver.

Success in the BUSINESS WORLD

Working Together

Certain organizations have demonstrated a great deal of talent at managerial leadership. One of those organizations is the Walt Disney Company. The leaders within this organization emphasize that it's not the magic that makes things work; it's the work that makes it magic. This statement illustrates how important people are to the organization and the importance of coming together to achieve the magic. As a managerial leader, you need to make sure that the processes, systems, and people are aligned to achieve the most successful performance outcomes.

Similarly, Southwest Airlines has been one of the most successful organizations within the air travel industry, and it attributes much of its success to the company's employees. The Southwest leadership team infuses the organization with a high-performing culture that has led to high employee satisfaction and a low turnover rate. One factor that Southwest Airlines attributes to the success of its organization is the relationship between team members and managers. The leadership team encourages employees to be themselves and to be creative. In turn, the airline has been widely lauded for its superior performance, having the fewest delays, fewest complaints, and fewest mishandled bags.

How can you start yourself on the road to becoming an effective managerial leader? First, you must be honest with your employees. Do not pretend you have all the answers and are fluent with all organizational processes and systems when that is not the case. Doing so will cause you to lose credibility with the staff.

This is one of the many reasons why every managerial leader must consider using the 5 BPs within his or her organization. The 5 BPs will not only help the organization move in the right direction, but will also provide the EMS officer (managerial leader) with a plan of action to ensure that he or she addresses the necessary management and leadership responsibilities.

Establishing the 5 BPs as a Managerial Leader
People

First, meet with your team and get to know them. Your team is watching your every move, so you will need to establish the tone for the culture you are striving to achieve. Listen to what team members have to say. When you meet with them, do not rush into making promises or immediate changes (unless clearly warranted); just listen. There will be plenty of time for changes and to assign the work you want to see done. Let your team know that you are here for them and that together, as a team, you will do many great things for the organization.

You may encounter some team members who are eager to get their message to you and others who are on the shy side. Let them know that you are also eager to get to know them and will be meeting with them as a team and individually. Understand that they, your team members, are stakeholders within the organization and have a lot invested in its success. This is the time to assess your employees' competencies, commitment, focus, and other characteristics. Try to find out who is engaged and who is not. For those who are not engaged, try to determine why.

In addition, if you have not done so already, take a snapshot of the organization by meeting with other department heads and getting to know them. Schedule a business appointment, but not to discuss an issue; rather, take the time to introduce yourself, listen to what they have to say about the organization, understand their role within the organization, and get to know them as colleagues.

Avoid these common mistakes made by managerial leaders when working with people:

- Feeling that you are better than other members of the organization
- Implementing change immediately without understanding the organization and its people
- Not understanding key business priorities and not having a strategic plan
- When an issue arises, being quick to blame someone without listening or investigating the entire event
- Complaining to your team members about other leadership personnel
- Not listening to team members and ignoring customer feedback
- Not promoting a learning environment
- Micromanaging

- Not being open to input from team members
- Showing no interest in team members' accomplishments

Strategic Objectives

As a new managerial leader, you will have to set the direction for your division, section, or even the organization. It is important that you have a strategic plan that will serve as a compass for where you want the organization to go and keep it on a steady course. The plan should center on the organization's strengths, weaknesses, opportunities, and threats (SWOT analysis). The strengths and weaknesses are obtained from within the organization itself, while the opportunities and threats focus on the external challenges. After conducting a SWOT analysis, you can begin to develop goals, objectives, strategy, and tactics for the organization (discussed in the "Strategic Planning" chapter). You can also find guidance in the organization's vision statement, mission statement, values, and goals.

The **vision statement** identifies where you want the section, division, or organization to be in the future. It serves as the compass of the organization. For example, the organization's vision may be to become the industry leader when caring for patients in the prehospital setting, promoting healthy living, and being customer-centric.

The **mission statement** identifies what you are doing now as an organization. An example of a mission statement is, "The XYZ EMS Division is a quality-driven service delivery organization that provides prehospital emergency medical care to the citizens and guests of our community."

Values consist of the core beliefs living within the organization. If you cannot support or believe in a value, then it is not a value you should consider for the organization. Organizational values include traits such as honesty, integrity, professionalism, respect, and collaboration. As the EMS officer, it is important to gather your team and determine which values are important to the members. These values may either echo or add to the values of the organization. Commonly, the organization will have a vision, mission, values, and goals clearly identified for the organization as a whole. Once the EMS officer and the team members have established the values for the division, then the group can begin to build and support the values as you move forward.

Goals are set targets (short or long term) that organizational members attempt to achieve. Clearly defined goals and objectives are critical to keeping all the organizational team members focused. They provide direction and a clear picture of what the organization and/or the functional

Managerial Leadership BRIEFCASE

Listen to the Team

One of the most important things you can do as a managerial leader is to listen to your team members. You should gather as much information as necessary to make an informed decision. If you take action without being properly informed, you will ultimately regret it.

group is attempting to accomplish. For example, a goal set for an EMS department might take into account revenue from EMS transport collection, cardiopulmonary resuscitation outcomes, response times, and customer surveys collected.

If you have ever felt lost or confused and had no idea where to start a project, you most likely did not have a plan. A critical mistake that managerial leaders make when newly promoted is to continue the same inefficient routine that has been in place prior to their assumption of the EMS officer role. EMS supervisors must ask the tough questions: How are we performing as an organization or division? How can we get on track and become more competitive if we are underperforming? Where do I want this organization, section, process, or team to be 1, 3, and 5 years from today? Unless you have a plan, you may feel as if you are stuck inside a mirrored house at an amusement park. You need to set the organization on a path that will be beneficial for years to come, know which services and goods the organization is committed to providing, establish and evaluate the service delivery metrics, and determine the core values you want to instill within your organization. Unless you create a plan and execute it appropriately, the organization, your employees, and you will never find your way out of the mirrored house.

Financial Management Objectives

Although many organizations have a budget office, accounting department, finance section, or similar department to provide assistance with financial matters, ultimately it is your responsibility as an EMS officer to manage your section's budget. Establishing financial management objectives allows you to see the big picture from a budget perspective and to remain fully informed regarding your financial resources. It is extremely difficult, if not impossible, to operate any business entity without the appropriate allocation of funds. As a managerial leader, you will need to know the following details:

- Where the money is coming from to support day-to-day operations
- Which expenses the organization incurs on a day-to-day basis
- Which operating and capital expenses will be incurred for the year
- Whether there is any money left in reserves from last year
- How to forecast for future purchases as you move forward

Reviewing strategic objectives will help you decide where to allocate some funds as you plan the section's financial management objectives. Although you will not need a finance or an accounting degree to work with budgets, you should become familiar with the terms associated with budgeting and some of the most common budgetary processes used within your organization. Being unfamiliar with what is being discussed and perhaps not understanding what is assigned to you as part of the process will simply lead to underperformance and frustration.

Without financial management objectives and familiarity with your assigned financial responsibilities, it will be difficult for you to make appropriate budgetary decisions.

Forecasting expenses and revenues is critical, but also difficult to accomplish. Take the time necessary to review your strategic plan and align the plan with the financial management objectives. Unplanned events are also likely to occur, so be sure to prepare as best as you can and do not drop your guard.

Learning Objectives

Now that you have been promoted, it is more important than ever to continue the learning process. You will not be able to make difficult decisions quickly if you are not well informed or if you become complacent about learning. In addition, within the 5 BPs' learning objectives, your team members must be included in the process of continued learning. It is now your responsibility to ensure that your team members have the greatest opportunities possible to learn and grow.

Learning objectives may consist of formal education, specialty classes related to the work environment, certificate courses, seminars, and conferences. The goal when establishing learning objectives must be to ensure that the team members are prepared to function in their current roles and prepared to handle the organizational challenges ahead. Consider working with your organization's leadership team to develop a formal managerial leadership training program for the employees who are currently or may someday be in a managerial role. Regardless of which title someone has within an organization, each person has the power to initiate change. Accepting this concept and encouraging others in the organization to embrace this approach allows ideas and positive change to permeate throughout the organization. If employees feel empowered and believe they have a say within the organization, they will support the organizational mission.

If you do not encourage your team members to grow and learn, you are not performing all of your responsibilities as a managerial leader. One reason that many managerial leaders fail is because they are afraid that an employee will know more than they do. Your role as managerial leader is to create a positive learning environment, promote learning, and surround yourself with the most talented group of team members possible. This will benefit the organization, the employees, and you. You can learn from your employees, and having a high-performing team under your leadership will benefit the organization. It is a good idea to seek ways of promoting formal education; however, you can also develop an educational program within the organization that will benefit the employees.

For example, you might speak with the organization's finance manager to see if he or she would be willing to review some simple budgetary processes with your team and other members of the organization. In addition, you might ask the human resources director to address some departmental policies and their importance. You should also consider asking an information systems (IS) representative to provide a brief introduction to the software currently used by your organization, discuss the appropriate steps for troubleshooting, and include tips for maximizing efficiency using the current department software. Lastly, you might ask the fire chief or other members of the department's senior staff to address key points pertaining to managerial leadership. A learning program does not have to be an expensive, complicated, or tedious experience. The key is never to stop learning, and it is up to you to keep this objective moving forward. Surround yourself with talented, enthusiastic individuals, and you will grow as a leader.

Culture of Quality

It is not enough to have a good product or service; you need to have a system in place that will consistently ensure that your product or service is continuously measured and evaluated. For this reason, performance metrics and benchmarking must be part of every organization. If you are not measuring the organization's performance, it will be practically impossible to know how well the organization is performing. A variety of quality management programs are available; however, you will need to obtain buy-in from the organization's senior leadership team to ensure that the quality initiative will be successful. (See the "Creating a Culture of Quality" chapter for more information on quality management programs.)

The Walt Disney Company and Southwest Airlines, for example, emphasize the importance of delivering nothing less than a high-quality service. There is no doubt that this emphasis on delivering such high-quality service has made these organizations the successes they are today. Likewise, if you plan to excel as a managerial leader, then you need to deliver quality at all levels of service and product delivery. You and your team need to buy into this philosophy and not settle for anything less, as the level of dedication to quality will be noticeable in the long run. The implementation of a quality methodology initiative will help the organization become more efficient and effective, save the organization money, keep customers happy, streamline processes, improve systems, and create a high-performing culture among team members.

Organizations that have opted not to incorporate a quality initiative into their daily operations commonly encounter a drop in productivity from their employees, a decrease in customer satisfaction, less profitability, and more variation (waste) in the goods or services being provided to customers. Imagine if your organization did not have a quality program as part of its day-to-day operations. For example, if you were the EMS officer overseeing an EMS division, how would you know if your paramedics were performing according to the standards required by the medical director? How would you know if the paramedics were following the

Managerial Leadership **BRIEFCASE**

The 80/20 Rule

The 80/20 rule, also known as the Pareto Principle and the Law of the Vital Few, is a rule that all managerial leaders must keep in mind. It states that 20 percent of something results in 80 percent of the outcome. For example, 80 percent of EMS delivery complaints involve 20 percent of EMS responses. When analyzing your operations, look for that 20 percent that is creating 80 percent of the poor outcomes and do not get bogged down with every issue brought to your attention.

appropriate protocols? How would you handle a patient complaint? How would you determine how productive the organization is if you have not established organizational performance benchmarks? Would you be able to save the organization money by streamlining processes? How or when would you know that the processes the organization is using are outdated? It would be extremely difficult to operate in today's competitive market without a quality initiative within your organization.

Ethics

Ethical behavior is the expected rule of conduct within a culture. To ensure high ethical standards, organizational leaders must clearly determine what is considered ethical behavior within the organization and then share that information with internal and external stakeholders.

Ethical behavior must start at the top, and organizational leaders must both demonstrate such behavior themselves and promote it in others. An organizational code of ethics underlines for all employees the expectations of the organization in terms of ethical behavior, how ethical practices reflect the organization's culture, and the ramifications of unethical behavior. The code of ethics should also include examples of unethical situations and common ethical questions and answers. An ethics compliance officer, if in place, can respond to employees' ethics-based questions and enforce the organization's ethics policies. Ethics training also plays a critical role in ensuring employees are informed about policies and procedures pertaining to ethical behavior.

Key strategies when facing an ethical dilemma include the following:

- Gather all the information and get to the root of the problem before making a decision.
- Consult the code of ethics and relate the situation to socially accepted options.
- Seek advice from the leadership team, your immediate supervisor, human resources, or an ethics compliance officer.
- Consider the dilemma as it would appear on the news and be perceived by the public.
- Research similar situations and how they were resolved.

The organization's leaders must promote an environment of honesty, integrity, professionalism, and trust. Although policies and training will not eliminate unethical behavior, organizational leaders must have a clear plan in place that has employee buy-in and becomes part of the organization's culture.

Time Management

When you assume the role of an EMS officer and managerial leader you will need to organize your time wisely. You will be expected to attend meetings, meet deadlines, and answer team questions while performing other operational and administrative duties like reviewing patient care charts for quality assurance, implementing protocols, determining key performance indicators and performance measures, addressing customer complaints, and conducting EMS service delivery presentations for external customers. The goal is to be as effective and efficient as you can be and to take care of issues immediately. When you spend time addressing the same issue over and over, you are wasting time and not adding value to the organization. The following tips can help you stay on course:

- Determine the order of priorities. If your boss is expecting an assignment from you, the issue is time sensitive, or it is a pivotal issue for the organization, it's a priority.

- Use a notebook or a note application to keep track of your ideas, assignments, and to-do lists. Be sure to set reminders and deadlines. Once the tasks have been completed, remove them from the list.

- Keep a specific notebook for your important and high-priority business documents. The notebook may also contain meeting minutes, memos, contracts, and similar documents. The goal is to have the high-priority documents organized and readily available if you should need them immediately.

- When you receive an email to which the sender expects a reply, if an immediate response is not possible, then flag the email and respond as time permits or at the end of the day. You could also save the email to the draft folder so that at the end of the day you can review all the emails in the draft folder and respond accordingly. You have created a system that includes the emails you need to respond to in an organized and timely fashion. This saves you having to scan through all the emails in your inbox to find which emails you need to respond to at the end of the day. This organizational method will be extremely helpful, especially if you receive a lot of emails and don't have time to respond immediately.

- Give yourself a minimum of 1–2 hours a day for yourself. Block it off in your calendar and make sure the time is spent completing your assigned projects and planning. This time is not for meetings or interruptions. This is your time to get work done.

- Block off time to address concerns, answer questions, and visit team members at their work station(s).

- Make every attempt to avoid meetings on Monday mornings or on Fridays. Mondays are usually the busiest time in the office. Take Monday mornings to address any issues that occurred during the weekend and/or to prepare for the week ahead. Use Fridays to tie up any loose ends that might be lingering from the week and to get ready for Monday.

- Spend time with your family and always let them know how much you care and appreciate their patience when it comes to you working long hours. They need to know how much you care about them.

- Take a break during the day and don't forget to take some time for you. Even if it's for 5 minutes, clear your mind of any pressing issue, stretch and move around, and think about what you have accomplished and what makes you happy. Managerial work can be very stressful, and relaxing and taking a few moments away from the stress can keep you from getting overwhelmed.

WRAP-UP

Concept Review

- As you assume a supervisory role, you might hear the terms *manager* and *leader* used interchangeably, but in reality they represent two different concepts that complement each other.

- As an EMS officer, you will most likely be managing processes and systems that will need to be monitored to ensure there are no variations from the intended outcomes.

- Sometimes processes are followed automatically, without the individual thinking they are processes, but that does not diminish the importance of processes in contributing (through action or steps) to completion of a specific assignment.

- Management of the team may include deciding which team member is the best suited for a specific project, answering a team member's question about a specific task, determining whether a team member's performance is adding value to the EMS division, and ensuring that the assignments and the core mission of the EMS division are being accomplished.

- If a new manager is to succeed, he or she should prepare in advance for the many challenges that will be presented by the new role.

- Leaders must be passionate about their role in working with people while keeping the vision, mission, and values of the organization in mind.

- Once the EMS officer understands the organization's culture, he or she will have a better understanding of the type of leadership style that would be most beneficial for the team. Different situations may call for different leadership styles, however, so it is important to adjust the leadership style according to what will engage the team.

- The primary advantage to being promoted from within is familiarity with the processes and systems, culture, and people of the organization, as well as the internal and external factors that promote or threaten the organization's mission.

- The primary advantage of joining an organization as a new manager is the ability to provide the members of the organization with a new perspective on how to do things and perhaps look at processes and current systems from a different point of view.

- For an EMS officer, it is important that both management and leadership skills are constantly being refined. The EMS officer will continuously work with processes and systems that will require management expertise. The EMS officer also will need to set an example as a leader and understand the true role of a leader within an organization.

Managerial Terms

Goals Set targets (short or long term) that organizational members attempt to achieve.

Managerial leader An individual who combines both the manager's and the leader's skills.

Mission statement A statement that identifies what you are doing now as an organization, the purpose of the organization.

Organizational behavior The way people behave within an organization.

Organizational culture The behavior of the organization's members as a result of the organization's norms, values, and beliefs.

Process A set of steps or actions to achieve an end result.

Scope creep A phenomenon that occurs when the project objectives are not met because the project has grown beyond the desired outcome. It commonly results from a lack of clearly defined objectives, poor communication among the project manager and the team members, and absence of a check system that alerts the team that they have deviated from the initial intent of the project.

System A group of interrelated components working together to ensure a specific outcome.

Vision statement A statement that identifies where the organization should be in the future. It serves as the compass of the organization.

Case Review: What Does Linen Have to Do with Saving Lives?

An EMS officer receives a call from a hospital administrator informing her that her crews are taking too much linen, towels, and pillow cases from the hospital to stock their ambulance units. The administrator tells the EMS officer that this practice is costing the hospital too much money and the hospital administration has opted to discontinue it. It will be the EMS officer's responsibility to find a way to purchase (nonbudgeted) linen or to come up with a plan to convince the administrator that the crews will discontinue taking excess linen and keep the current practice.

When the EMS officer addresses this issue with her crews, they tell her, "We take only what we need—and besides, after we use the linen, we return it back to the hospitals, so they cannot be losing money." The EMS officer asks herself, "Am I managing an EMS system or a laundry service?" However, this is part of the EMS operations and it is the EMS officer's responsibility to find a way to remedy the issue, resulting a win-win outcome for all.

Case Discussion

What would you do in this scenario? The EMS officer in this scenario needed to make some difficult decisions. Should the EMS officer purchase the linen and include it as part of the department's inventory, or should she attempt to work with the hospital administration to work out some sort of agreement? One thing the EMS officer knew for sure was that the department did not budget for the purchase of linen, towels, or pillowcases because the local area hospitals had provided these items for more than 15 years. Therefore, the EMS officer had to find a way to convince the hospital administration that the crews would be cognizant of the expense and would work on not taking additional linen.

In this case, the EMS officer played the role of mediator between the crews and hospital administration. The hospital administrators agreed to continue providing the crews with the linen, as long as they took what they had dropped off at the hospital in a one-for-one exchange. The EMS officer was successful in averting a potential budgetary disaster simply through communication and collaboration. The EMS officer met with the hospital administrators and explained how the process worked from the prehospital perspective. Subsequently, the EMS officer met with the crews and explained the hospital administration's concerns. Lastly, the crews were invited to meet with hospital administration and worked on achieving a compromise. This win-win outcome for all was made possible by the EMS officer's clear understanding of the process and the officer's own role in achieving a successful resolution.

Case Review: No Recognition

A division chief of training notices that an employee appears to be disengaged and not giving his usual 100 percent. The division chief makes it a point to meet with the team member and find out why his work performance has diminished. During the conversation, the team member states that for several years he has been assigned to multiple roles and not one "thank you" has ever come his way. The only time he is noticed is when he is sick or out of town and his roles are delegated to someone else for that short period. The division chief informs the team member that it is because he does such a great job that no one really addresses his performance on a regular basis. The division chief apologizes and acknowledges that he needs to do a better job of letting all members of the team know how much the organization appreciates their contributions. Furthermore, the division chief makes it a priority to meet with the members of the team to address any concerns they may have and to review their accomplishments on a weekly basis. The employee conveys that he does not need any special treatment; however, it would be nice to know that the organization appreciates his work.

Case Discussion

Do not wait to thank your employees until their annual performance evaluation. If team members feel that their supervisor is proud of the team members' work and know it because the supervisor voices his or her appreciation, then the team members will take ownership for their work and most likely continue to perform above expectations. The division chief deserves a lot of credit for admitting that he was wrong and for being willing to correct his mistake.

3

Building the Team

Learning Objectives

After studying this chapter, you should be able to:

- Discuss the process for hiring the right team member.

- Discuss the process for leading the team.

- Identify and describe management components in building a team.

- Discuss the EMS officer's role in conflict resolution and negotiations.

- Explore the use of personality assessment tools in understanding team members.

- Discuss the EMS officer's relationship with the human resources department.

- Describe how to deal with disengaged team members.

Introduction

Each member of an organization plays an integral role in the success of the organization. Building a productive and competent team will help the organization be successful. The managerial leader must embrace the fact that the team will often look for direction, necessitating that clear goals, expectations, and communications be established with the team members so they know what is expected of them. As mentioned earlier in this text, the organizational spoke necessary to all organizations is a positive working culture based in communication and collaboration. This is an important consideration when building a team.

We have all been part of a team. Teams go beyond sports; family, coworkers, and classmates are team members in your day-to-day activities. But what does it take to build a winning team?

Hiring the Right Team Member

There is no doubt that as a supervising, managing, or executive officer you will have to hire team members, or at least be part of the hiring process. The hiring process is extremely important, and a lot of time and money are spent on hiring the right person for the job. When selecting a team member, try to select someone who will complement the team's existing talents and bring value to the team.

Posting a Position

One of the most important things you will do as an EMS officer and managerial leader is to ensure that your employees understand what is expected of them at work; therefore, the EMS officer must ensure that all the positions assigned have clearly defined job descriptions. A job description is not a set-in-stone list of the duties that will be performed by the employee who accepts the position, but rather provides a foundation for the employee as to what is expected from him or her. The content that is included in a job description varies among organizations. You should always check with the human resources (HR) department for guidance. Although the HR team will provide excellent information on organizational requirements, the specific job functions and skill requirements may have to be included within the job description by the EMS officer before the job is posted. Consider the sample in **Figure 3-1** when creating a job description.

Characteristics of the Class

The EMS Quality Assurance Technician reports directly to the Division Chief of EMS. This position will carry a variety of responsibilities in support of the administrative mission of the EMS Division. Although the Quality Assurance Technician may be assigned any task per the Division Chief of EMS, the primary responsibilities are as follows:

Examples of Duties

(Note: The listed duties are illustrative only and are not intended to describe each and every function that may be performed in the job class. The omission of specific statements does not preclude management from assigning specific duties not listed herein if such duties are a logical assignment to the position.)

EMS Division

- Oversee all EMS quality assurance, quality control, and performance improvement programs.
- Assume the duties of the office manager when needed.
- Research and develop new equipment.
- Coordinate medical legal issues.

Figure 3-1 Sample job description. *(Continues)*

- Coordinate EMS coverage for special events.
- Serve as project manager for new EMS initiatives.
- Serve as the department's Infection Control Officer and be responsible for the management of organizational exposures, vaccinations, and post-exposure prophylaxis (PEP).

Requirements

Education and Experience

- High school diploma or GED
- Associate's degree
- Bachelor's degree (Preferred)
- Quality methodology program certified (Preferred)
- Paramedic with 3 years' minimum field experience as a paramedic
- Minimum 3 years' EMS system quality assurance experience
- Strong skills in using computers, Windows operating system, and most common office software applications
- Excellent interpersonal skills inclusive of the ability to work with diverse groups
- Demonstrated presentation creation and delivery skills
- Proven ability to provide and deliver excellent customer service
- Clean recent driving record

Special Requirements

- Must obtain a valid chauffeur's or noncommercial class "D" driver's license prior to employment
- Must successfully complete a physical ability test
- Must be in good physical condition, as determined by a medical examination given by a licensed physician as prescribed
- Must be able to work irregular schedules
- Certificates from the following list are required based on the area of assignment:
  - Certification in Advanced Life Support and Prehospital Life Support
  - Certification in Emergency Pediatric Care

Figure 3-1 Sample job description *(continued).*

Once the job description has been completed and thoroughly reviewed by the HR department and the EMS officer, then the open position can be posted for advertisement. Such postings may be found on most HR department websites, within the HR department, and in other departments within the organization.

Evaluating Applications

A job advertisement will be posted for a set date—typically for 1 or 2 weeks. It may be posted either for internal candidates (organizational members) only or for internal and external candidates. Once the job advertisement has closed, the EMS officer will need to evaluate the potential candidates.

If numerous applicants responded to the posting, you will need to establish a plan of how to prioritize them. The first thing to do is to determine which candidates are qualified for the position. Just because someone applies for a job posting does not mean that that person is qualified. Second, you may want to consider creating two batches of applications: one batch containing the applicants who meet the job qualifications and a second batch containing the applicants who exceed the job qualifications.

Evaluating the applications, references, and resumes will not only provide insight into the candidates' professional history, but will better prepare you when interviewing the candidates and asking pertinent questions. If there is enough time to interview all the applicants, you should make every attempt to do so. This will eliminate any controversy pertaining to preferential hiring and will show you were fair and diligent with your assignment. If there is limited time and the position must be filled immediately, then you may need to narrow the applicant pool by selecting only a few of the most qualified candidates to be interviewed. You will need to make sure that you document why those individuals were selected versus the rest of the applicant pool. There is no doubt that there will be times where you may have to hire someone fairly quickly; however, making every attempt to take your time when deciding who to hire will be worthwhile in the long run.

Interviewing Candidates

Before interviewing candidates, check with the HR department to see whether you should use a pre-set template for scoring each candidate after his or her interview. Many organizations will have the interviewers score the candidate based on how the candidate answered questions and how prepared he or she was for the interview. Each question may have a numerical value, or perhaps a checkmark will be made under a plus or minus column, with these marks later being tallied to achieve a final candidate score. Depending on the final interview score, each applicant is ranked compared to the other applicants.

When conducting an interview, you should make every attempt to have at least two interviewers besides yourself present. This will allow for one interviewer to ask the questions while the other members of the panel are listening and documenting key answers that will help you in making a final decision about which candidate to hire. It is critical that the members on the interview panel know exactly which skills and talent you are looking for in a candidate before the interviews begin.

During the interview, the questions asked may be job specific, scenario based, or both. They may even already be assigned by the HR department for you to use during the interview. As an EMS officer who is assigned to do the hiring, however, you will most likely be required to create the questions yourself. The HR department will typically leave the technical, job-specific questions to the division leaders to create—but be sure you check on this point before you begin scheduling candidates for the interview process.

If you are interviewing many candidates, make sure that you allow enough time to meet with each candidate and to answer any questions the applicant may have. It is difficult to make a decision during a 30-minute interview, so you may want to consider implementing an internship period in which the top three or five candidates participate in a one-day hands-on evaluation.

The following tips may help during the interview process:

- Set the date for the interview and let the candidate know that he or she has been chosen for an interview.
- The interview panel should consist of the section head and selected senior team members. Having a diverse interview panel is critical; therefore, every attempt must be made to satisfy this objective.
- Make sure that credit for their special assets is given to those who are eligible—for example, military service, bilingual, specific education and/or training.
- Prior to beginning the interview, introduce the panel to the candidate, offer a little history about the organization, explain what the position entails, and discuss expected performance outcomes.
- Ask questions that will place the candidate in different scenarios pertaining to the current organizational processes and systems.
- Find out what the candidate knows about the organization. You may be surprised by how many candidates do their homework and research the organization before attending the interview. This will give you insight into how motivated the candidate is to join the organization.
- Upon completing the interview process, ask the candidate if he or she has any questions and convey a time frame as to when a decision is expected to be made.
- Be professional at all times and be prepared to answer the candidate's questions. It is normal for a candidate to spend some time asking questions about the organization's vision, mission, values, and goals; job expectations; salary; work hours; work flexibility; professional development; and so on. A candidate should have every opportunity to get to know your organization, just as you are attempting to get to know the candidate.

Choosing the Best Candidate

When hiring a new employee, it makes sense to hire the candidate with the most talent. To help with this decision, consider the following:

- Does the candidate have the skills to add value to the organization's processes and systems? A candidate can be extremely skilled, but those skills may not align with or add value to the organization.
- Does the candidate have the potential—and is he or she motivated—to grow within the organization? Ask the candidate to provide some examples of how his or her contributions in previous employment positions made a significant impact to the organization.
- Does the candidate have the personality to fit with the organization's culture?
- What stresses the candidate and how would he or she handle these pressures? Be sure to ask for real-life examples of when the candidate had to deal with a stressful work situation.

Spend the time and money upfront conducting a thorough interview and selecting the right candidate. Do not be too quick to hire someone just to fill a position; doing so may create significant team and underperformance issues in the future. Make it a point during the interview to ask specific questions that directly focus not only on the expected work assignments, but also on whether the new hire would be a good fit within the current working culture. It will be more expensive and time consuming in the long run to hire the wrong person. Go beyond the resume, the job description, and the interview. Get to know the candidates and make a serious commitment to hiring the right person from the start, even if takes a bit longer to do so.

Leading the Team

Establish a Plan

The newly promoted EMS officer must first establish a clear direction, expectations, and distinct plan for the team. In doing so, the EMS officer must ensure that all team members understand the vision and mission of the organization and division (if applicable). In addition, all team members need to know that they have an important role within the organization and they are valued. If the team members do not understand what is expected of them or what the mission of the organization is, then you have not clearly stated the vision and it will be difficult for the employees to embrace a team approach. As the EMS officer, you must promote a positive working culture that fits your organization and division. In addition, every team member must know how important it is to support the positive working culture, especially during the many challenges they may face together.

Understand Your Team Members

The EMS officer must also make every attempt to learn the strengths and weaknesses of his or her employees. Once the officer has a good understanding as to where team members can make significant contributions using their strengths, the organization will begin to see positive outcomes. Because weaknesses can hold back employees from performing at their very best, the EMS officer must work to remedy any weaknesses in team members to help them, and by extension the entire team, succeed. If the team member demonstrates continuous underperformance in one area, however, adjusting the team member's responsibilities may help that individual achieve the desired outcomes. It is not enough to ensure that the team members have talent; placing them in the right environment is essential to capitalize on their maximum potential.

Get Buy-in from the Team

As the EMS officer, you must seek buy-in from the team members and listen to what they have to say. Team members need to know that what they say matters and need to understand where they fit into the big picture. If the team members do not feel that they are part of the team, their participation and enthusiasm will wane.

Research Other Organizations' Methods

It is paramount that as an EMS officer you look at how other EMS and non-EMS organizations build winning teams. Seek out organizations that are considered benchmark, gold standard, or industry-leading organizations; the lessons learned from this research can yield valuable insights about building winning teams.

Management Components

As an EMS officer, there is no doubt that you will be responsible for the oversight of your team at work. One of the biggest mistakes new EMS officers make is believing that their team does not need nurturing and support from the managerial leader. There are five components to managing teams:

1. Coach and mentor the team.
2. Empower the team (avoid micromanagement at all costs).
3. Have confidence in the team.
4. Collaborate and communicate with the team.
5. Be available for the team (be a managerial leader).

As an EMS officer, your goal must be to achieve high-quality outcomes and exceed every expectation set by the organization's leadership team and your customers. The key question, then, is how do you go about accomplishing this task? First, you continue to ensure that the five business priorities (5 BPs) are being addressed as they pertain to the organization or your area of responsibility. The first business priority is "people." No matter where you are on the leadership ladder, the same rule applies: You and your organization will not be successful without excellent support from the people who perform the day-to-day operational and administrative duties. Therefore, you as the EMS officer must create a plan that conveys a message to your team about the organization's culture, vision, and mission, and about your own commitment to helping the team members all succeed. All members of the team must understand the importance of what you are trying to accomplish and appreciate how every member's role is important to the success of the team. When formulating this plan, take time to do your homework; learn what it takes to build a winning team and what you need to do to get there.

Seek out organizations that have proven track records and learn what they are doing to build and keep a winning team performing at a high level. For example, how do companies such as the Walt Disney Company, Google, Southwest Airlines, and Zappo's achieve a positive working culture that leads to a winning team environment?

If there is one thing these organizations have in common, it is the high value they assign to their employees and their commitment to promoting a culture of support and inclusiveness across the organization. To build a winning team, the EMS officer must demonstrate commitment to the success of the team and highlight the importance of each member's contribution to the overall goal of the division. As you begin to create a plan to build a winning team, it is paramount that you keep the following considerations at the top of your list.

Coach and Mentor the Team

As an EMS officer, you will certainly be a coach as you direct your team in day-to-day operational and administrative assignments. When **coaching**, the EMS officer is primarily focusing on tasks, usually for short periods of time, and is performance driven. **Mentoring**, in comparison, goes beyond coaching and deals with a broader scope of influence. A mentor works with a mentee (someone who is seeking guidance) and establishes a relationship to improve the mentee's personal growth, professional development, and related needs. As a mentor, the EMS officer will be more closely involved with the team member's personal, long-term growth. The mentor's relationship with the team member consists primarily of being a personal advisor and goes beyond the work environment.

As an EMS officer, you must always be ready to serve as a coach and understand the privilege of being a mentor. A managerial leader should make every attempt to serve as a mentor and/or a coach for those around the leader, but especially for the members of his or her own team (**Figure 3-2**). Being a coach and mentor is essential in building winning teams, in that the EMS officer has an opportunity to promote the division's culture and vision with the team members. In addition, by serving as a coach and a mentor, the EMS officer will be able to convey a clear message for all team members to follow, and may also serve as an advisor for the team members. If the team members understand the message that is being conveyed by the EMS officer, understand why they are doing what is asked of them and what the end product is, and know that the EMS officer (coach-mentor) will be there to support each member along the way, their actions will begin to lay the foundation for a winning team.

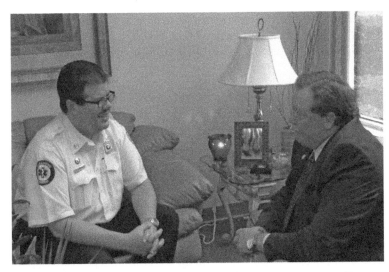

Figure 3-2 An EMS officer should make every attempt to serve as a mentor and/or a coach for his or her team members.

Your team is a clear reflection of your expectations as an EMS officer, so be open to coaching and/or mentoring as you begin laying the framework for your division to become a high-performing team. As a coach and a mentor, you must take the time to know your team members and understand who they really are. Often, we work with people and yet have no idea what they do or do not like, which personal goals they have, where they want to be in 5 years, and whether they are married or have children. The time you spend becoming familiar with the members of your team on a personal level will pay huge dividends in the future. Every managerial leader must support and cultivate each team member's professional talent so all members may continue to learn and grow personally and professionally.

Coaching a team in an office environment is very similar to a football coach's work during a football game. The quarterback calls the plays in the huddle; however, the actual play calling is most likely performed by a coach on the sideline who has a broader picture of the game. This is where you, as a managerial leader and coach, need to use a wide-angle lens versus a narrow lens. To coach a team is a great honor and comes with a lot of responsibility.

As a coach, it is your responsibility to get your employees to a level where they can succeed. Your goal as a coach is to get your players playing at the positions where they do best and to provide them with every opportunity to succeed. Many team members are let go or demoted for underperforming, yet when placed in another role they may very well blossom. Get each employee in the right position. It is your job as a managerial leader to ensure that all the links of the team are strong enough to support the organization's mission. It does not matter if you are surrounded by strong links; if just one link is weak, it will be nearly impossible to complete your objective. Identifying your team's strengths and weaknesses offers an opportunity for you to shape the team, begin to mold team members for future leadership roles, and reinforce the notion that you care about their future. It is also an opportunity to provide candid feedback and seek input from the team members.

When a managerial leader has been asked to serve as a mentor by a team member, this opportunity is not only a great honor and extremely rewarding, but also comes with an enormous amount of responsibility. When serving as a mentor, you should make every effort to learn from the mentee, just as that individual will be learning from you. The first step for the mentor and the mentee is to develop a relationship where both mentor and mentee acknowledge that being candid with each other is a top priority and feedback is encouraged. The mentor must make every effort to help the mentee succeed professionally and personally. Second, develop a plan that will establish a foundation for the guidance the mentee hopes to receive from the mentor—for example, guidance with professional growth, managing co-workers, or resolving conflicts. Third, when agreeing to be a mentor, make sure that you are truly committed to helping the mentee as long as he or she needs it. Fourth, being a mentor means that you must be a role model; therefore, be sure to act accordingly. Fifth, remember that the relationship is all about the mentee.

Open communication and candidness must always be encouraged. Your team members are the ones in the trenches doing the work, so if you listen to what they have to say, you will likely be rewarded with successful outcomes. This does not mean that you have to accept every plan or suggestion they provide, of course. Nevertheless, you should recognize that the input you choose to ignore might be the piece of information that could have saved your project in the long run. It will be difficult to establish a working relationship if the EMS officer and team members are not candid with each other. To grow professionally and get to the root of any issue, both parties must be honest with each other or the relationship will ultimately fail.

As a coach or mentor, you will need to keep things interesting and fun to keep the team members engaged, especially for those personnel who have been with the organization for a while. If the team members have been doing the same tasks for several years, they may lose interest in their current work assignment. Ask team members if they would be interested in doing some different types of projects or assignments. For example, if a team member is routinely assigned to review medical charts, he or she could be reassigned to EMS research and development. If a team member is routinely assigned to a medical response unit, he or she could be reassigned to help with EMS training. The key is to change things up and keep the team engaged. If the team members are happy with their current roles, great; if not, make it a priority to engage them and tap into some hidden talent. Perhaps you might implement a social fun lunch Friday or stress-free break day; that is, you could invite the team members from other sections to spend some time with your team, and ensure that everyone has an opportunity to get to know each other during lunch or during breaks. It is important that you get everyone involved and provide options for the team members, either professionally or personally, so they can decide what works best for them and to help them achieve their full potential.

Empower the Team

Avoid micromanagement at all costs. As the coach and mentor for your team, you must make sure that you provide the necessary tools and information that will allow each team member to perform at his or her very best. Empowering the team members to do what it takes to perform at their very best and allowing them to make decisions that will exceed the expected outcomes will not only add value to the customer service delivery, but also build a sense of confidence among the team members. The team members need to feel that they are part of the organization and not just collecting a paycheck. If they believe their contributions to the organization are making a difference, they will have ownership of their performed duties.

As the coach and mentor, you must be available for the team members to assist them and answer their questions. At the same time, you should not get in their way. A number of things may demoralize the team members and lead to frustration and underperformance, and one of them is being a micromanager. Micromanaging your team must be avoided at all costs because it will serve as a roadblock to becoming a successful team. Let the team members know what is expected of them, provide them with the tools to get the job done, be available in case they need you, then turn them loose and let them soar.

New leaders may have a difficult time taking a step back and allowing their teams to execute the tasks that have been assigned to them. This not only creates frustration among the employees, but will also tie up the leader with specific tasks versus focusing on the bigger

Managerial Leadership **BRIEFCASE**

Promoting a Learning Environment

Once you are promoted, team members will look to you for answers. You must remain knowledgeable in your area of responsibility or you will begin to lose credibility. Even so, the emphasis of promoting a learning environment does not apply only to you, but also to your team members and all members of the organization. The moment you and your team stop learning and keeping up with industry developments, you, your team, and your organization will stop moving forward. Learning can be formal or informal; the key is to continue to grow and learn within the organization. Perhaps you and your employees might work toward achieving a formal college degree or a certificate in continuing education, or both. It is also important to embrace any continuing education course that is being offered by your own department or the organization's HR department.

organizational picture. Having the freedom to work autonomously is great—but you must make sure that individuals are doing what they feel passionate about and that they are knowledgeable about the work assigned to them. Having a team member who is not skilled for a position work autonomously is a recipe for disaster. Imagine a quarterback playing fullback or wide receiver. Each member of the team must have an assigned role, do it well, and be trusted enough by the manager to get the job done. Promoting a culture of inclusiveness and letting team members know that their contributions are vital to the success of the organization provides some owner-ship to the team members and serves as a great motivator. The team members will maintain a sense of purpose toward the organization if they feel as if they are part of the team and not just a drone collecting a paycheck. Sharing outcomes and results—that is, showing the team members something tangible that they help put together—creates ownership.

You as the managerial leader will assume many roles, and one of those is coach and mentor. Your team will look to you for guidance. In turn, you should get to know your team members and their aspirations. Find out what their dream jobs would be both within the current organiza-tion and outside the organization. You might be surprised by the answers, but these answers could lead to improvements in the organization and the division of duties.

The feeling of being empowered to do a job is a tremendous boost to an employee's confidence and serves as a great motivator. If team members feel that they cannot make any decisions with-out your approval, suggest new processes, or resolve customer issues without you being present, this will not only diminish the morale of the team, but also affect your role as a managerial leader, potentially ruining your relationship with your customers due to poor performance. As a managerial leader, you always want to avoid micromanaging your team. Ask yourself the following:

- Are any internal or external forces keeping the employee from performing at his or her best?
- Does the employee have the appropriate training for the position?
- Is the employee given every opportunity to succeed?
- Do the team members have the tools to succeed?
- Are you, as the EMS officer, available to provide feedback and guidance?

Provide your team with the tools they need to complete the project asked of them, give them sup-port, and let your team take charge of their success.

To empower your employees, you must first establish a rapport with your team and listen to what they have to say about the business and its processes. Listen to their concerns. Find out what gets them fired up and piques their interest. It is your job as a managerial leader to find ways to energize your team; therefore, you need to make every attempt to identify what motivates them. Unless you ask, you will never know. While understanding that every team member is dif-ferent, there are still some basic steps that the EMS officer can take to empower a team to carry out the day-to-day operations of the organization:

1. Keep the team informed of the operation so they can make the appropriate decisions when dealing with customers.
2. Promote constant communication among all team members, including yourself. If your team believes that you are not being honest and open with them, they will retreat.
3. Once your team understands what is expected of them, leave them alone to do their job. As the coach, your job is to assist the team members in achieving their full potential.
4. Treat your employees with respect. You are empowering your employees to do the job you hired them to do, so give them the respect they deserve and let them perform their duties. You will crush the employees and the likelihood of them ever doing something on their own if you embarrass, belittle, or micromanage them.
5. Give recognition when earned. Employees often hear from management only during their annual evaluation, if they get one, or when they have done something wrong. Make it a point to let the team members know that they are doing a great job. Further, it may be appropriate to acknowledge the top performers during team meetings or to visit the employees at their workstation and let them know how proud you are of them. Recognize a team member or members for a job well done and make it personal. Send a handwritten letter to the employees letting them know how much you appreciate their hard work and what a great job they are doing.
6. If your team is meeting its full potential, see what you can do to take them to the next level. Always support your team and provide learning opportunities to help them reach their goals.

Instill Confidence in the Team

Instilling confidence in your team is one of the greatest things that you can do as a managerial leader. Displaying a sense of confidence in yourself, too, will help convey a message to the team that you are in control and can handle whatever issues arise. If team members believe in

Managerial Leadership **BRIEFCASE**

Realistic Expectations

You might have observed someone in a management or leadership role funnel projects or tasks to subordinates who were not prepared or equipped to complete the requests being assigned to them. Asking your team members to complete a project is acceptable if the project falls within the employee's job expectations, and if the employee has the appropriate training to complete the project, enough assistance to complete the project, and clear direction from his or her manager as to what is expected of the project. Never set up your team members for failure; make sure that you give them every opportunity to succeed.

themselves, and they know that you believe in them as well, you may be surprised at what they can accomplish. It is your responsibility to create a positive environment by providing your team with the tools they need to be successful and then by letting them do their job.

There is no doubt that your team will face difficult decisions; part of your role is to prepare them for times like these. If a team member makes a mistake, take the time to support the individual and not tear him or her down. The team member will most likely feel terrible about the mistake, and reminding the person what a poor job he or she did helps no one. Instead, take that opportunity to let the individual know how he or she can improve, but point out the positive aspects of the situation and build from there.

Confidence is gained through action; therefore, the sooner you set the stage for your team to succeed, the more quickly their confidence will begin to grow. The team members will become more confident as they begin to tackle issues together and start to see the positive results. Celebrate your team's winning accomplishments and acknowledge their losses, but do not let the losses set the team back. Encourage the team to regroup and continue to move forward toward your goal. By doing this, you as the managerial leader will demonstrate your confidence in the team and motivate the team to perform at a higher level. Team confidence will grow, boosted by the EMS officer's positive and encouraging actions toward the team.

Promote Collaboration and Communication

Promoting collaboration and ongoing communication among all team members is one of the key ingredients in building a winning team. As the EMS officer, you must encourage maximization of work performance from all team members. This can certainly be achieved through collaboration. When promoting collaboration, you are bringing a diverse group of team members together to achieve a desired outcome. This allows for additional sources of input into projects and process workflow, but also demonstrates the power of working together by achieving the desired outcomes.

Managerial Leadership **BRIEFCASE**

Communication

If you are wondering why certain processes and systems are not working or are performing at levels less than expected, before looking at the process itself or the team's lack of productivity, ask yourself if your directions and expectations have been clearly explained to the team. Many times leaders are quick to blame the team when the culprit is, in fact, poor communication between the leadership and the team members. Once you address the communication factor, then you can take a look at the processes.

In addition, maintaining open lines of communication throughout all phases of an assignment and on an ongoing basis for day-to-day operational and administrative duties will foster cohesiveness among the members of the team. Keeping your team informed about projects, competitive business forces, performance measures, and any issues pertaining to the day-to-day operational or administrative duties is as critical as encouraging team members to offer input.

It can be very difficult to reach a consensus when team members are trying to make a decision. This is where the power of collaboration and communication plays such a critical role. As a managerial leader, you must make every attempt to become an effective communicator, support the concept of collaboration, and promote a state of being in control. If you appear indecisive or walk away from difficult situations, your team will have a difficult time accepting you as their leader.

If a team member does not know his or her role, it will be difficult for that person to work efficiently and contribute in a way that moves the team or the organization in the desired direction. If a team member knows his or her role and chooses not to follow it, you must make every effort to determine why the team member is choosing to underperform. If you have made every effort to assist the team member in becoming engaged with his or her daily duties and the individual still chooses to underperform, then it will be time to dismiss the member from the team.

If you have a winning team, celebrate your accomplishments and let your team know that they are the reason for the success. If your team falls prey to a losing streak, it is your responsibility to get them back on track. Avoid the attitudes described in **Table 3-1**.

Be Available for the Team

You will not be a successful managerial leader if you are not available to your team. If you think that you can be successful at leading your team by sending e-mails, conducting conference calls, sending text messages, and not being present to meet with them face to face when issues are present, you are mistaken. The team needs to know that you are always there for them. If you will be out of the office for an extended time (e.g., project, travel assignment, vacation), make sure you set aside some time to meet with your team and let them know you will be out of the office. In addition, let them know if someone will be covering for you and/or how they can reach you in case of an emergency.

If you are assigning a project to your team, you need to be available to answer questions, work through problems that are holding back the team, and demonstrate to the team that you are there with them every step of the way. If you are not available, your absence will simply create tension and frustration among the team members. Moreover, being available demonstrates that this project is important to you and that you trust the team with getting it done.

Do not wait until it is time to complete your team's annual performance evaluation to spend time with the team members. At that point, the attention will come too late. In addition to being in the office and speaking with your team on a daily basis, make it a point to meet with your

Table 3-1	Avoiding Negative Attitudes
Attitude	**How to Avoid It**
Point the finger	Don't jump to say, "It's not my fault we are doing so poorly." Promote the philosophy that you win as a team and lose as a team. There is no time for pointing fingers, and doing so will simply create a divide among team members. The team needs to learn from its losses and move on. It is your responsibility to get the team on the right path and to keep moving forward. Don't forget: You are the leader, so it all starts and ends with you.
That's not my job.	If you are a member of the organization, then regardless of your role it is your responsibility to help move the team and the organization forward to the set goal. It is not uncommon for someone in a managerial leadership role to acquire a sense of entitlement—that is, the attitude that as the "Boss," the individual is not required to assist with any of the day-to-day operational or administrative duties. This approach is completely opposite of how and what a managerial leader should be doing within the organization. Certainly, EMS officers will have many assigned responsibilities; however, they need to set a good example when they are asked for help and take the time to assist a co-worker. They must make every attempt either personally to assist or to find another way to get the work done. Neglecting to assist will send a message across the organization that the EMS officer is not a team player. This, in turn, will create discontent among the team members and they will be hesitant to support any future initiatives.
I don't have time.	Make time. When you are at work, nothing else matters except helping your team and making sure the organization is successful.
I'm a great leader and that's why we succeed.	If you can do it better, great. Don't advertise that fact, but show the team how to get the job done. Promote collaboration, confidence, and a winning environment. Although you may be a great leader and very well informed on how to get things done, nothing will happen without your team. They will make it happen for you.
I don't want to do this job anymore.	No one says you have to do the same job for a lifetime, but don't quit in the middle of a project. This kind of behavior is not good for you, the team, or the organization. How you carry yourself as a managerial leader and set the tone for the team will go a long way toward getting things done. As with any position, there is a high probability that at some point the EMS officer will want to be promoted and move up the chain of command. This process is important for the organization because it allows for a fresh perspective and ideas to fill the position, while also enabling the former EMS officer to learn new skills and expand his or her role within the organization. These opportunities must be encouraged and supported by the senior leadership staff. If the EMS officer is seeking to be promoted within the organization into another role, he or she must also make sure not to abandon the team in the midst of a project or other large commitment. If the EMS officer must assume the other position in a short amount of time, then that individual must appoint a project coordinator who is well informed about the current project and the desired outcome. The exiting EMS officer must also make every attempt to inform the new EMS officer of which projects are in process and be available if any questions should arise. The former EMS officer must also inform his or her new boss of the current projects he or she is leaving behind and ask for some flexibility in assisting the new EMS officer if the need arises.

team members individually as often as you can. This will allow for candid conversations and will build a stronger relationship between you and your team members. During this time, you should turn off your cell phone and ask not to be disturbed. This is the team member's time with you, so make it worthwhile and show the individual that you truly care.

Commitment to the Team

Understanding that your team is the most important asset is paramount in achieving organizational business success. As a new managerial leader, establishing a healthy relationship with your team members should be one of your first priorities. Demonstrating your loyalty, trust, commitment to their growth, and a culture of inclusiveness between you and your team members is critical. If you study successful organizations, you will notice the following characteristics:

- The members in leadership roles coach and mentor junior employees.
- There is collaboration between senior and junior employees.
- There is confidence and trust among the team members.
- The managerial leaders are available for their team members.

As a managerial leader, you must also create an environment where your team members believe in you and begin to gain confidence in your decision-making ability. This will set the stage for guiding the organization and/or division in the right direction. Every EMS officer should cultivate effective communication and key managerial leadership characteristics as part of his or her managerial leadership ethos (belief or distinguishing character trait). If a managerial leader has clearly demonstrated high moral values and ethical standards, has integrity, is honest and knowledgeable, and encourages open dialogue among all team members, the receivers of the message will most likely embrace the leader's message.

Managerial Leadership **BRIEFCASE**

Leadership Training

If you create a climate of winning, your team will aspire to be winners. If you choose to promote a nonwinning climate, then that is what your team will aspire to achieve. The choice is up to you. Many organizations implement leadership programs that groom future organizational leaders. If the organization invests time and energy in preparing these future leaders, this is not only a great investment for the organization, but will also help instill the organization's vision among all members. Although some organizations have established formal leadership training initiatives, as a manager you can implement formal or informal leadership training with your team members. This allows you to establish your goals, vision, and mission for your section, and your team is part of the entire process.

If your team has never worked with you, they may be reluctant to follow you as an EMS officer/managerial leader immediately. They will likely do what you say because you are their new boss, but you do not want robots working for you. Instead, you want team members who remain engaged and believe in what you tell them. Once you have demonstrated to your team that you are a managerial leader of high standards and are knowledgeable with the current business operations, then you need to move toward setting a plan for a culture of communication. There is no doubt that confidence and implementing a new culture will require some time; therefore, you need to work on it every day. You can get started with this endeavor by showing respect, listening and providing feedback, eliminating noise, knowing your team, and rolling up your sleeves.

Showing Respect

Always be respectful to those with whom you speak. Get to know your employees and show them that you care about both their personal and their professional lives. Ask them for input pertaining to the business operations and input on what you can be doing better as an EMS officer/ managerial leader. You must always make time to listen to your employees. Mutual respect is critical when communicating, especially during candid discussion.

Listening and Providing Feedback

Listen to what the other person is telling you and provide feedback. Don't answer a telephone call, write an e-mail, engage in conversation with another person walking by, or become preoccupied when a team member is speaking with you. This is the team member's time, so make it worthwhile for the person and take the time to listen and pay attention. If a team member feels that he or she is not important to you, then why should you be important to the team member?

When providing feedback, offer it in a positive tone, be specific, and make sure that the individual understands what you expect. (See the "Communications" chapter for more discussion on

Success in the BUSINESS WORLD

Gold Standard

Southwest Airlines is considered a gold standard organization: The ticket agents are courteous and eager to assist the customers, the flight attendants interact with the passengers during the flight, and the captain routinely makes it a point to welcome the passengers on board and to keep them informed about the flight. The airline offers perks that other major airlines do not, and it has a good record for being on time for departures and arrivals. Of course, it is the employees who make all of this success happen. Southwest Airlines has won the "Triple Crown" of the airline business—given to airline companies for outstanding service—more often than any other airline organization. Like any successful organization, however, Southwest Airlines must continually improve to keep its market share.

listening and providing feedback.) If you are providing negative feedback, it will be your responsibility to work with the team member and to give him or her every possible opportunity to get back on track. Each team member deserves a chance to grow within the organization. Although you see the individual at work, you may not know about particular issues affecting the individual outside work that may be causing the employee's underperformance. Here is an opportunity for you to step up and truly be a leader by attempting to get to the root of the problem and helping the employee through a difficult time in his or her life and/or professional career.

Eliminating Noise

Eliminate noise from the background. When distracting events are going on around you—for example, construction, crowds of people, conversations taking place, a constantly ringing telephone, other team members coming into your office to ask questions, or customers waiting for service—it will be extremely difficult to communicate effectively. You must try to avoid getting involved in lengthy, important conversations when in a noisy environment. Unless the discussion relates to an operational issue that must be resolved immediately, wait until the noise around you quiets down or move the conversation to an area that is not noisy.

Noise is not limited to loud chatter or interruptions, however. Noise can also come in the form of the participants' emotions or biases. It may be difficult to speak with a team member when that person (or you) is upset or distracted. This is where you must apply your skills to diffuse the situation or bring the focus back to the situation at hand. During these situations, it is critical to let the speaker know that what he or she has to say is important to you. Gaining the person's confidence is a key part of communication during these times. Wait until the individual is done speaking before offering your input. If the team member does not trust you, he or she will not open up to you. (Noise is also discussed in the "Communications" chapter.)

Promoting Open Communication

A team member may listen to what you are saying, yet may not understand how to accomplish the task being asked. Make sure that everyone understands what you are saying and always encourage the team members to ask questions, especially when they do not understand what is being asked of them. Promote an atmosphere of open communication. You want your team members to be open and not to keep things to themselves because they are afraid to ask. This is especially important if team members know of potential conflicts ahead if the team follows a certain path. Encourage team members to participate and engage with one another. Such actions will foster great relations and solid communication among the team members.

Rolling up Your Sleeves

If you roll up your sleeves and demonstrate to your team that you are not afraid to get your hands dirty, they will be more likely to accept you as one of them. Again, this will foster good relations with the team members, which will lead to healthy communication among all members.

Furthermore, being in the trenches with your team members allows you to observe their work—together and as individuals—and provide feedback about their performance. This will make any feedback you may have, good or bad, easier to accept on their part, as long as you avoid micro-management. Many managerial leaders lose respect from their team members because they become disconnected from the team and are unsure which role each team member is responsible for fulfilling. As the managerial leader, you must understand which tasks your team members are responsible for and be able to offer support if the need arises. You do not have to be proficient at every job the organization executes, but understanding what it takes to complete the tasks will prepare you to make more effective and efficient decisions, help you understand which tools your team needs to perform effectively, and help you develop better plans during strategic and business planning sessions.

Meetings

If you ask most employees to name the one thing that sets them back in their workday, their answer is usually "a waste of time." High on the list of sources of wasted time are unnecessary and over-long meetings. It is not unusual for someone who either does not know how to run meetings or just loves to hear himself or herself talk to sequester the team in a small conference room for several hours, repeating the same topics from previous meetings. In these situations, nothing gets accomplished. Unnecessary or poorly run meetings can kill morale and dampen passion for the job.

Although regular meetings with your team are important and provide a great opportunity to ensure that everyone is on the same page, these meetings must be productive and efficient. When planning a meeting, you must be prepared with all the materials and information necessary so that the meeting runs smoothly and on schedule:

- Make sure there is a reason to have the meeting.
- Create an agenda and share it with the team prior to the meeting.
- Make sure you announce speaking time limits to ensure that there is enough time to cover each topic in the agenda and to give all the participants ample time to speak. As the host of the meeting, you must make sure that only a certain amount of time is allotted for each topic or you will run the risk of not covering the material and not allowing all the participants the opportunity to speak. If you need more time on a particular topic, ask the participants if, considering the time constraints, they would rather continue discussing the topic or schedule another time to continue this discussion and move on to the next topic on the agenda. Assign a team member to keep you on track with the agenda and timing.
- Attempt to keep the meeting short, or at least no longer than it has to be.
- Make sure everyone at the meeting has had an opportunity to speak and knows what is expected of them at the conclusion of the meeting.
- If the meeting will go beyond the scheduled time, make sure you take breaks.

When holding a meeting, try to involve everyone at the table. If you are the only one doing the talking, team members will become bored and you will most likely miss the opportunity to capture some good ideas from the participants. There is a high probability that after the first 15 minutes you spend speaking at your team, they will stop listening and start thinking about what they are going to do on the weekend, what they will have for dinner, who is picking up the kids from school, or whether someone will call them so they can be excused from the meeting. Say what you are going to say, listen to what your team has to say, make sure that the topics discussed are clear before concluding, and encourage the team members to take action.

At the end of the meeting, be sure to go around the table and ask those attending the meeting if they have any questions or if they would like to discuss any particular issues prior to the conclusion of the meeting, such as a project timeline question, clarification on a topic discussed during the meeting, scheduling a topic for the next meeting, or perhaps requesting some time to present a topic at the next meeting. The goal is to make sure that before the meeting breaks up, every participant has had an opportunity to speak and, as the host of the meeting, the EMS officer has made every effort to make the meeting productive for everyone.

As an EMS officer, you will most likely be attending meetings with organizational staff members, customers, hospital personnel, vendors, and so on. It is not uncommon for two different meetings to be scheduled on the same day and time. If they conflict, it may be necessary for someone to attend one of the meetings on your behalf. If you plan to send a substitute to a meeting, be cognizant that this person may have a full plate and that adding more duties will not be fair or productive for the team members. Always be considerate of others when asking for assistance.

Success in the BUSINESS WORLD

Industry Leaders in EMS

Although we have discussed some of the approaches taken by non-public safety organizations, there is no doubt that many EMS, fire, police, and other public safety organizations promote the importance of building winning teams to ensure the delivery of quality service. For example, the Phoenix Fire Department; New York City Fire Department; Miami–Dade County Fire Department; King County Medic One in Seattle, Washington; Wake County EMS System in North Carolina; Medstar EMS in Texas; and Sunstar EMS in Pinellas County, Florida, are all organizations that have gone beyond the status quo and are committed to being industry leaders by having the right people in the right place and creating winning teams.

Conflict Resolution and Negotiations

As much as we attempt to avoid conflict, as a manager you will undoubtedly have to deal with such a challenge. When thinking about the root cause of a conflict, the matter really boils down to a disagreement between at least two parties. Perhaps you, the manager, are one of the parties in a conflict. Regardless of who is involved, you must demonstrate the exceptional qualities of a managerial leader and make every attempt to negotiate a win-win solution for both parties. The following guidelines will help resolve conflicts:

- Get to the root of the disagreement by conducting a thorough interview of everyone involved. Interviews of key personnel should be done separately (initially) with another neutral member present besides the EMS officer. Once you have obtained enough information about the root cause of the conflict from all individuals involved, then you can meet with both individuals at the same time in an attempt to seek an amicable resolution.

- Listen to both parties.

- Encourage both sides to be open and candid.

- Find a positive point in each party's position.

- Ask what it would take to find a common ground.

- Seek the parties' input on how to resolve the conflict.

- Understanding that this conflict is important to both parties, be sensitive when supporting one side.

- Always remain professional. Resolving conflicts is one of the most difficult responsibilities you have as a manager.

- If mediation by an EMS officer is proving ineffective, the organization's HR department may have an employee relations officer assigned to assist in resolving conflicts between personnel.

Resolving conflicts between team members becomes significantly easier if you have already taken the time to know your team members on an individual basis, both personally and professionally. It may take a while to get to know team members if the EMS officer is new to the team or when working with a new team member.

Personality Assessment Tools

A personality assessment tool can provide important behavior information to the EMS officer about the team members. Such an assessment will provide information about an individual's behavior pattern or key personal and professional strengths, depending on the tool used; this information can then be used to support team members in achieving their full potential, and to improve communication. Such tools also help when dealing with conflict resolution, as the EMS officer will now have a good understanding of each individual's behavior pattern. After the team member or members complete the assessment tool, the EMS officer can review the outcome profile from the assessment and gain better insight into how the employee perceives key elements of behavior or what the employee's personalized strengths are, depending on the assessment tool used. This will help the EMS officer be better prepared when dealing with team members during different situations and will ensure that the EMS officer has a thorough understanding of how best to help each team member succeed.

Some behavior assessment tools provide specific behavioral style or personal strength information about the individual taking the assessment. For the managerial leader, these results can offer insight valuable for understanding team members, colleagues, and those around you better.

When deciding to implement an assessment tool, contact the organization's HR representative and ask for guidance as to which behavioral assessment tool to use. It is not uncommon for HR to have an assessment tool already in place and ready to use for those who choose to participate in its application. Some organizations may mandate the assessment tool, whereas others may leave the choice of tool up to the managers and employees. Regardless of which assessment tool is used, it is highly recommended that the EMS officer make every effort to learn what makes individual employees perform at their very best and to manage conflict effectively by understanding the team members' behavioral styles.

DISC Profile Assessment Tool

The DISC profile assessment tool uses four dimensions—dominance, influence, steadiness, and conscientiousness—to describe the employee's behavioral pattern. This tool can prove invaluable to the managerial leader, especially during conflict resolution and when working with new teams. The information gathered in the DISC profile assessment can help you address each individual in the manner to which he or she will respond most effectively.

How It Works

After a participant completes the DISC assessment, which should take no more than an hour, the participant is provided with a report that shows his or her DISC dimensions and explains how they represent the participant's behavioral patterns according to that person's responses during the online assessment. In addition, the report will include the participant's strengths, weaknesses, tendencies, needs, and preferred environment. The report not only shows the participant's highest-rated dimensions, but also provides information regarding how the participant uses each of the dimensions (dominance, influence, steadiness, conscientiousness).

Interpreting Results

Evaluating only the highest-rated dimensions will provide only a partial picture of the team member. The EMS officer, when evaluating employees' DISC dimensions, must look at all four behavior styles and consider how they relate to the employee. Although there are no guarantees, the following are a few examples of certain roles accompanied by their most likely highest-rated dimension:

- It is not uncommon for those individuals in authoritative roles to have a high "D" (dominance) dimension. The "D" dimension reflects someone who takes action, desires an environment of power and authority, accepts challenges, and tends to make quick decisions.
- Someone who strives to be a leader may score a high "I" (influence). The high "I" focuses on influencing and persuading others, as well as coaching and counseling.
- An employee with years of seniority may be a high "S" (steadiness). The high "S" prefers the status quo and a predictable routine, is a good listener, and enjoys helping others.
- A person involved with quality measurements and outcomes may score a high "C" (conscientiousness) dimension. The high "C" tends to focus on key details, check for accuracy, and desire opportunities to ask "why" questions.

In addition to identifying the participant's behavioral patterns, the DISC assessment provides other reports that offer the participant a greater understanding of his or her leading dimensions and also provides information about how the person is likely to use the nonprominent dimensions. This information is extremely valuable. As an EMS officer, you will have several employees reporting to you and understanding their dimensions will allow you not only to lead more effectively, but also to maximize the employees' potential and to address conflict more effectively if needed.

Other Profile Assessment Tools

Other assessment tools that can prove helpful when determining employee behavior traits, the means by which individuals come to certain conclusions, and personal behavior strengths include Myers-Briggs Type Indicator (MBTI), the Emotional Intelligence Appraisal, and the Clifton Strength Finder. While all of these assessment tools can be helpful to the manager in learning about the employees, they may also be helpful to the employees in learning about themselves.

Once the employee has completed taking the assessment, the managerial leader should review the outcome with him or her individually and establish a path that will build on the strengths identified in the assessment screening. This will allow the leader not only to understand the employee's strengths, weaknesses, and behaviors on a professional level, but also to demonstrate to the employee that the leader is genuinely involved with that individual's personal growth within the organization. Some organizations are now including an assessment tool as part of the hiring process and then sharing the results with the candidate's prospective manager. Having a better understanding of how each member of your team and/or the organization perceives and responds to certain situations will prove beneficial when attempting to resolve conflict and negotiate a win-win outcome for everyone.

When the Manager is Part of the Conflict

Conflict resolution is something that, as a managerial leader, you should expect to address regularly. Conflict, in which two parties hold different views on a specific topic, may arise between subordinates or between external customers and members of the organization. Conflict resolution can become much more difficult, however, when you are one of the parties involved in the conflict. As a managerial leader, you should make every attempt to resolve the conflict as you would with any other conflict—by seeking a win-win outcome for both you and the other individual. You must make every effort to understand the other individual's point of view and to place yourself in his or her position. Depending on the situation, however, you as the EMS officer may need to resolve the conflict by issuing a direct order. The goal is to consider what the other individual's position is and how you can best resolve the conflict.

If the conflict cannot be resolved between you and the individual, it will then be time to step back and allow someone else to assist with the conflict resolution. This scenario poses a significant challenge not only because it involves you, but also because it will be difficult for you to remain neutral. Therefore, it is important to ask for assistance in resolving the conflict immediately.

You can take several steps to ensure that a conflict between you and someone else is addressed appropriately and resolved quickly with the goal of a win-win outcome for both individuals:

1. When an EMS officer is engaged in a conflict with someone and there are no signs of the dispute being resolved, it is important to seek a neutral party (mediator) to help resolve the conflict. This needs to be done immediately, because ignoring the conflict will simply create frustration and make matters worse.

2. The mediator must be someone who does not have ties to either party. Seeking assistance from the HR team is important to ensure that both parties are appropriately represented and have an opportunity to express their position.

3. If the conflict is between you and a direct report, after the conflict is resolved you will need to continue working with this employee. Regardless of the outcome, the managerial leader must look at the long-term picture. It is important for you to make every effort to get past the conflict and begin the healing process. You are both on the same team and as the managerial leader you must set the example and lead the way.

Working with the Human Resources Department

The HR department is a common organizational spoke in EMS and other organizations. It consists of a variety of trained professionals whose primary goal is to be fair advocates for the members of the organization, to provide employment resources, and to ensure no discrimination occurs in the workplace. In addition to addressing employee issues, managerial leaders should use the resources provided by the HR department to assist in the development and growth of their employees.

Every organization is different; however, the HR functional working team will most certainly work closely with the organization's leadership team to ensure that all employment advertisements and job descriptions have been thoroughly reviewed before posting them for the public to see. When there is an internal open position, a posting and an application for the position can usually be found online or within the HR office. The job postings remain in place for a set period of time, with this span being determined by the HR department or the functional working group's leader who is seeking to hire. Once the posting period has closed, all applications are forwarded to the functional working team's leader for evaluation, interview, and selection. Once a selection is made, the new employee will meet with an HR representative prior to coming on board to collect and complete the following items:

- Compensation and benefits
- Tax information
- Retirement information
- Professional certifications
- Background check

The HR department can also assist in employee development by offering courses and resources geared toward both managers and employees. Although each HR department will have specific resources for its employees, most offer the following standard resources:

- Diversity training
- Americans with Disabilities Act (ADA) information
- Training to prevent sexual harassment
- Recruitment of potential employees to fill vacant positions throughout the organization
- Risk management guidance
- Workers' compensation
- Family Medical Leave Act information
- Performance evaluation resources
- Health insurance information
- Employee assistance programs
- Workplace safety information
- Employee training and development programs
- Employee privacy information
- Training to prevent discrimination

Union and Contract Relationships

If the organization has a union, the HR team will also work with the organization's management and the collective bargaining team. There will be a labor contract that managers must consider when making decisions that impact the members of the organization. The collective bargaining team and the management team negotiate to create a labor agreement contract. During this process, the following items are commonly negotiated:

- Wages
- Staffing profile (the number of personnel needed to meet the organization's service delivery outcomes and the required certification to meet the job requirements)
- Drug testing
- Certification requirements
- Holidays
- Overtime
- Discipline
- Grievances
- Jury duty
- Management rights
- ADA issues
- Probation

According to the concept of *management's right*, management has the right to make management decisions outside of the negotiated union contract to meet the needs of the organization, but only in extreme operational circumstances. Going outside the negotiated labor agreement can happen only if there is an immediate need or potential negative impact to the organization or its employees. For example, the union contract might state that once an employee wins a bid into a station, management cannot reassign that employee to report to another station during that shift. However, if management needs to staff a position at a certain station and that employee is the only one qualified to fill that role, then management may need to reassign that employee for that one shift. In this example, management needed to ensure that a specially trained provider is available at a specific station. The reassignment could be the result of certified employees calling out sick or the lack of specially trained employees to fill that position. This practice could generate a grievance on behalf of the employee if an article in the labor contract specifies that once an employee wins a bid at a station, he or she will not be reassigned to another station.

As another example, the union contract may include language that precludes lower-ranking officers from filling certain positions, such as a district chief's position. The language may state that only promoted district chiefs can fill the district chief open slots. However, if there are no districts chiefs immediately available to fill an open district chief position, management might consider staffing the position with a lower-ranking officer to cover for the day or until a district chief agrees to work the shift. This action, no matter how justified, could easily trigger a grievance from the district chiefs if a lower-ranking officer were assigned to cover a district chief assignment in violation of the labor agreement.

Similarly, management may opt to relocate an EMS transport unit regardless of whether the crew bid into a specific station and expected to work within the area into which they bid. For example, suppose a department currently has two EMS transport units responding out of one station. A noticeable increase in requests for service occurs in another part of the department's service delivery area that has only one EMS transport unit available. Management might then decide to move one of the two EMS transport units from its current location to the area experiencing a higher call load.

These are just a few of many examples of union–management issues that you may encounter as an EMS officer. Management must have a clear justification as to why the actions were taken and understand what is considered management rights versus what has been agreed upon within the labor management agreement contract. If a specific article has been agreed upon and included in the contract, then management has every right to follow through with that action. In contrast, if there is no article clearly identifying what management wants to do, the actions must be clearly justified or they will be considered a violation of the labor agreement.

Grievances

Filing of a grievance is the next step once a violation of the contract has occurred. Regardless of the infraction that occurred before a grievance is generated by an employee, there must be clear evidence that the labor contract had been violated to warrant such a claim. The grievance process is commonly included in the labor agreement. When a grievance has been issued by a union member, the goal is to have both parties—that is, a union representative and members of the leadership team—address the issue and come to a resolution without having it escalate to the next step. If the management and union team cannot agree on a solution, then the matter will go to mediation, in which a third party attempts to resolve the dispute between the parties. If the matter remains unresolved, then it goes to arbitration, where both parties agree to have a third party rule on the matter.

If an employee believes that a disciplinary action has been wrongfully meted out to him or her according to the labor agreement, that individual will likely initiate the grievance process. Therefore, if the EMS officer is authorized to discipline employees, the officer should take several steps to ensure resolution of a grievance is handled correctly and does not violate any article of the labor agreement. Although each organization will handle grievances differently, the following steps may provide some guidance on how to address a potential disciplinary issue while ensuring **due process**:

- After an employee allegedly commits a serious workplace infraction, the department's internal affairs department or a senior leadership member assigned to the case completes a formal investigation to ensure that all the facts have been gathered. Depending on the level of the infraction (commonly outlined in the organization's policies and/or labor agreement), discipline can range from verbal counseling, to written counseling, to suspension without pay, to termination.

- Once all the facts have been collected and reviewed by the organization's assigned internal affairs investigator, the investigator determines whether, in fact, the employee has committed a workplace infraction. If there is not enough evidence or the employee is clearly not guilty, then the case is dismissed.

- If there is enough evidence to find the employee guilty of the charges, then a hearing panel is assembled to review the case. A hearing panel commonly comprises leadership members from the employee's organization and a union representative. If the hearing panel determines that the employee is guilty, the panel may provide a written statement to the internal affairs officer as to why the hearing panel believes the employee is guilty. The internal affairs officer will then submit the hearing panel's decision to the person assigned to issue the discipline (e.g., chief, deputy chief, or other high-ranking member of the team).

- If the employee does not agree with the discipline, he or she may choose to issue a grievance against the disciplinary motion. At that point, the organization's leadership (every department is different) may elect to review the disciplinary action or keep it as is. The employee will then have an opportunity to request a mediator to review the case.

Discipline is just one component over which an employee may initiate a grievance if the disciplinary action has violated the labor agreement. As the EMS officer, before initiating any discipline to an employee, you are responsible for investigating the allegations thoroughly and determining whether the employee has violated the labor agreement. If so, you are most likely well within the scope of your authority to issue discipline without the employee grieving it at a later time. The goal is to be fair and diligent with the issues presented to you as the EMS officer.

Every organization has its own policies pertaining to discipline and how it is included in the labor agreement. Therefore, it is important that you are aware of the grievance and disciplinary process within your organization.

When a disciplinary hearing is called for, it is critical that the process be fair to the employee(s) and that all parties are addressed with respect. The goal is to obtain all the facts and to provide enough time for the employee to gather all the information needed to address the hearing panel. The goal, on behalf of both parties (management and the employee), is to find a resolution to the issue and, regardless of the outcome, to maintain the employee's dignity.

Disengaged Team Members

As an EMS officer, your role will be to encourage your team members to perform at their very best, work collaboratively to achieve the organization's performance goals, and promote a culture of inclusiveness. However, the EMS officer must always be alert for those individuals who are disengaged or who choose to work in unproductive silos.

The disengaged employee will try to do as little as possible and is minimally committed to the organization and to completing his or her assigned work duties. In addition, the disengaged employee will not go out of his or her way to exceed organizational goals or expectations. The EMS officer must make every effort to identify these individuals before they become actively disengaged.

Actively disengaged employees will resist change, often find a reason not to agree with the leadership team, and make an effort to make things difficult for the organization. They may consider themselves to be informal leaders because they disagree with the organization's culture and its perception of how the employees are being treated. This form of behavior can be extremely distracting to other employees. The EMS officer must find a way to detect this form of behavior early and prevent it from spreading throughout the organization. Disengaged—and especially actively disengaged—employees can be detrimental not only to the team, but also to the organization as a whole by undermining the organization's mission.

When faced with a disengaged or actively disengaged team member, it is important to consider how that individual became disengaged. As an EMS officer, you must attempt to get to the root of the issue if you plan to help the team member and prevent his or her attitude from impacting other employees. If the team member is considered actively disengaged, there is a possibility that you may not be able to reverse the situation; the team member is likely ready to move on from the organization. The following interventions, however, may prevent an engaged employee from becoming disengaged or actively disengaged:

- Say "thank you."
- Provide clear direction and maintain open lines of communication.
- Ensure that team members know what is expected of them.
- Ensure that team members have the necessary tools to get their job done.
- Seek input from the team and let the members know that what they say matters.
- Do not lie to the team.
- Celebrate achievements.
- If there is an issue, roll up your sleeves and help.
- Discuss the organization's culture with team members and find out what it means to them. This will ensure that everyone is on the same page.
- Do not wait until an employee evaluation is due to address performance concerns. Your input on employee performance must be ongoing.

- When a team member appears to be disengaged, address the issue immediately and let the team member know that you are there to support him or her.

The goal must always be to find ways of ensuring that the team members remain focused and engaged. As the EMS officer, however, you must also make the difficult decision of when to terminate an actively disengaged employee; when doing so, you must think about the other employees and the greater good of the organization.

Organizational Silos

As the managerial leader, one of your many responsibilities must be to promote a culture of inclusiveness where input is welcomed and encouraged. It must be known across the organization that every team member is valuable to the organization and plays a critical role in its success. If, as the managerial leader, you give the impression that you do not believe in promoting this type of culture, your employees will want to stay away from you, and you run the risk of creating organizational unproductive silos. Although **organizational silos** (functional working teams) are at the very core of most organizations, the EMS officer must make every effort to detect productive versus unproductive silos.

Organizational silos are groups of individuals within an organization who are assigned to work in a specific division or department—for example, logistics division, EMS division, finance division. These silos are typically benign if the team members embrace the culture of the organization. Most organizations are designed to work in silos because each division will have different responsibilities throughout the organization.

When assessing the effectiveness of a silo within the organization, the managerial leader must determine whether the silo is productive or unproductive (**Figure 3-3**). Productive silos communicate, work alongside other functional working teams, understand the goal of the organization, and support its culture. Unproductive silos commonly do not communicate with other functional working teams throughout the organization, tend to work independently, and do not support a culture of collaboration. The unproductive silo creates a disconnect between the team and other functional working teams within the organization. This, in turn, creates an underperforming environment. The underperforming environment arises because not all functional working teams of the organization are communicating with each other, making it difficult to determine a central goal for the organization. In addition, the members in each unproductive silo may develop adversarial tendencies toward other members of the organization who are not in their silo.

As an EMS officer, there are several things you can do to prevent unproductive silos from forming within your organization. First, promote a culture of inclusiveness and set a clear goal that every team member understands. The managerial leader must emphasize to all members of the organization that their input is vital to the organization and their role is important. As the EMS officer, make it your responsibility to set up meetings with other functional working teams and begin to share ideas and projects. Take the first step in breaking down barriers and

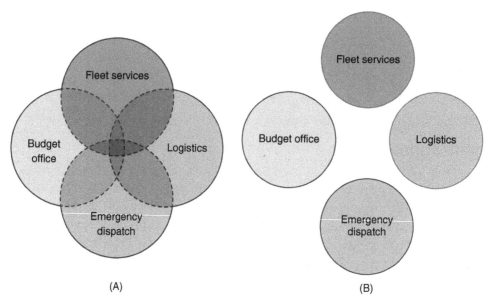

(A)   (B)

Figure 3-3 A. Productive organizational silos work well independently but also with the rest of the organization. **B.** Unproductive organizational silos work independently and do not collaborate or communicate well with other facets of the organization.

promoting collaboration. Demonstrate how functional working teams are more efficient when they work and communicate effectively with each other. If the employees are working in silos because they fear or are resistant to change, explain why change is taking place, compare the current situation with the proposed change, and explain the role they will be playing once the change is implemented. Silos are expected to be part of most organizations; as the EMS officer, you must promote a culture where silos remain highly productive and add value to the organization's service delivery outcomes.

Managerial Leadership BRIEFCASE

Working with Disengaged Employees

If you have a disengaged employee or employees on your team who refuse to accept change, you must attempt to find why they have become so disengaged or why they are so resistant to change. As a managerial leader, you will need to show not just the disengaged employees, but all of your employees, why you are pursuing change. They need to see the facts and appreciate what this change will bring to the organization and to them. Be prepared to answer any questions they may have to alleviate their concerns, include them in the decision-making process, and stay the course. Ultimately, if they remain disengaged or resistant to change, then perhaps their services and talents will be better suited to another organization.

WRAP-UP

Concept Review

- Each member of an organization plays an integral role in the success of the organization. Building a productive and competent team will help the organization be successful.

- When selecting a team member, try to select someone who will complement the team's existing talents and bring value to the team.

- To lead a team, you must take the following steps:

  - Establish a plan.

  - Understand the team members.

  - Get buy-in from the team.

  - Research other organizations' methods.

- One of the biggest mistakes new EMS officers often make is believing that their team does not need nurturing and support from the managerial leader. There are five components to consider when managing teams:

  - Coach and mentor the team.

  - Empower the team.

  - Have confidence in the team.

  - Collaborate and communicate with the team.

  - Be available for the team.

- Demonstrating your loyalty, trust, commitment to their growth, and a culture of inclusiveness between you and your team members is critical.

- Resolving conflicts between team members becomes significantly easier if you have already taken the time to get to know your team members on an individual basis, both personally and professionally.

- Using a personality assessment tool can provide important behavior information to the EMS officer about the team member(s).

- The human resources department consists of a variety of trained professionals whose primary goal is to be fair advocates for the members of the organization, to provide employment resources, and to ensure no discrimination occurs in the workplace.

- When faced with a disengaged team member, consider how that individual became disengaged. Attempt to get to the root of the issue to help the team member and to prevent his or her attitude from impacting other employees.

Managerial Terms

Coaching A method of directing, instructing, and training a person or group of people with the aim to achieve some goal or develop specific skills.

Due process The opportunity for an individual to know the charges and have evidence considered prior to disciplinary action.

Mentoring A developmental relationship between a more experienced person (a mentor) and a less experienced person (a mentee).

Organizational silos Groups of individuals within an organization assigned to work in a specific division or department—for example, logistics division, EMS division, finance division.

Case Review: Absent Leader

Julie, a manager overseeing logistics, is called to the chief's office, where she is told to report to human resources in the morning. When Julie arrives at the HR office on the following morning, she meets with one of the HR representatives, who informs her that her team has filed a complaint against her. The complaint is centered on Julie not doing her fair share of the work, demanding too much of her employees, treating them unfairly, not addressing team personality issues, and never being around when they need her. Julie is taken aback and denies all of the allegations. She even points out examples of when she helped a certain team member with projects and states that she is always available for her team by cell phone or e-mail when not in the office. Julie is not dismissed from the organization; however, she is required to take leadership, team building, and communication training.

Case Discussion

After the meeting with the HR representative, Julie meets with her team and is able to repair the disconnection and serious concerns of the team members. Still, this is a situation that must be avoided at all costs by every managerial leader. After a total team breakdown, it is very difficult to regain the trust of the team, and the manager will most likely feel some resentment owing to the team's betrayal. Of course, the goal is to ensure that the team is working together, to promote and use open lines of communication among all members, and to be present to support the team.

Even if a managerial leader has the best plan and intention to promote a healthy work environment, there will still be times when some team members will not be content. Therefore, as a new managerial leader, you will need to continuously work on cultivating, building, engaging, and maintaining healthy communications with all team members on a regular basis. Being available by e-mail and cell phone is helpful, but it is not a substitute for face-to-face time with your team. They need to know that you are there for them.

It is common to become defensive when told that you are not doing a good job, but as a managerial leader you need to remember that the team's effectiveness and environment starts with you. To prevent a case similar to Julie's, make it a habit to conduct a self-evaluation of your managerial leadership skills on a regular basis, ask your team for input on how you are doing as a managerial leader, and have another individual in a leadership role evaluate your performance.

This was a tough case because Julie believed she was doing everything correctly as a managerial leader and supporting her team; however, she was completely off-base as far as her team was concerned. Rest assured that if you have done everything possible to promote a positive work environment and some team members are still unhappy, the issue could very well be with them. You cannot necessarily please all members all the time. This fact of life is why being present and understanding each team member's contribution to the organization will help you determine which employees are contributing to and promoting a positive organizational culture and which ones are trying to break the team apart.

Case Review: Weekly Meetings

During his weekly senior staff meeting, Chief Hill discussed the importance of gathering information for a SWOT analysis. In addition, he wanted the members to look into gathering the information and to bring the information back to the weekly senior staff meeting for review and discussion. When the senior staff team reported for the following weekly meeting, the chief requested the assigned work from the members. Unfortunately, some of the team members had not completed the assignment, and several of the members ended up working on the same topic. The outcome resulted in frustration, embarrassment, and the appearance that the chief and the senior staff members were a bit disorganized.

Case Discussion

Chief Hill could have taken several steps to avoid this severe miscommunication:

- Provide a clear message of the goal he was attempting to achieve
- Make sure that all the senior staff members knew what he expected from them before ending the meeting
- Clearly identify which team member should complete each task
- Set a deadline for project completion
- At the end of the meeting, recap the expectations and ask if there were any questions

These are just a few actions to consider when assigning a team project. In any case, the message must be clear. Everyone on the team must know what is expected of him or her, and the roles must be clearly identified. The chief should have considered using a planning worksheet, which could have been completed by the chief or an assistant and then distributed after the first meeting to the team. At that point, the team would have a document showing what was expected of the team for certain tasks, thereby avoiding the confusion that occurred in this case. Included here are two worksheets that might be helpful for any manager when assigning tasks or addressing specific organizational issues (**Figure 3-4** and **Figure 3-5**).

Action Item Planning Worksheet			
Action Item	**Action Item Goal**	**Responsibility**	**Due Date**
Strength	Determine the organization's strengths.	Jennifer	Monday, June 25
Weakness	Determine the organization's weaknesses.	Steve	Monday, June 25
Opportunity	Determine the organization's opportunities.	Stephanie	Monday, June 25
Threats	Determine the organization's threats.	Jack	Monday, June 25

Figure 3-4 Sample action item planning worksheet.

Action Register Worksheet			
Meeting Group: Weekly Senior Staff Meeting			Date: May 22, 2015
Problem	Action Taken	Target Date of Completion	Responsibility
Excess station inventory	Set supply ordering levels	July 1, 2015	Logistics Chief Smith
EMS units responding emergency to nonemergency requests for service	Memo to EMS crews and dispatch team clarifying appropriate response assignments	May 25, 2015	Communication Center Chief Jackson

Figure 3-5 Sample action register worksheet.

CHAPTER

4

Communications

Learning Objectives

After studying this chapter, you should be able to:

- Identify and describe the basic components of the communication process.

- Describe how to communicate effectively with employees, customers, and colleagues.

- Describe how to communicate effectively verbally.

- Describe how to communicate effectively in writing.

- Identify barriers to effective communication and explain how to overcome them.

- Describe the EMS officer's role in media relations.

Introduction

A managerial leader can expect to spend the majority of his or her time at work being engaged in conversation—with colleagues, with team members, with senior leadership members, and with customers, among others. During these exchanges, it is not enough just to convey a message. That is, the information must be clear and concise, and the sender of the message needs to make sure that the receiver understands it.

Your success in the art of communicating effectively will make or break the success of many of the actions you initiate as an emergency medical services (EMS) officer. You do not have to be in a high-level position to understand that communicating effectively is essential in all aspects of life. Most day-to-day communication is second nature to many of us—the question is whether you communicate *effectively*. Communicating effectively can determine your team's acceptance of you as a leader, the success of a project, your marketability for promotion, and specific outcomes during a crisis situation. Effective communication, therefore, is a skill that must be mastered.

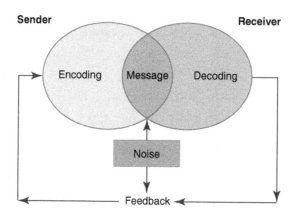

Figure 4-1 The communication process flow (Shannon-Weaver communication model).

Communication Basics

The basic elements of the communication process are as follows (**Figure 4-1**):

- The **sender**: The person who is trying to communicate.
- The **receiver**: The person with whom the sender is trying to communicate.
- The **message**: What the sender is trying to communicate.
- The **medium**: The format through which the sender is trying to communicate.
- **Encoding**: How the sender formats the message.
- **Decoding**: How the receiver interprets the message.
- **Feedback**: The response from the receiver to the sender based on the message received. Feedback can be verbal, nonverbal, written, or a combination of these.
- **Noise**: Any internal or external element that affects the message being received as the sender intended. Noise may include sounds such as sirens, traffic, or a phone ringing, or it may consist of visual distractions such as emergency lights or body language. Noise can also include the receiver's bias toward the sender, the message, or the situation. In fact, any of the communication barriers discussed in this chapter can be considered noise.

As an example, suppose an EMS officer is speaking with a team member about an upcoming project. The EMS officer (sender) approaches the team member (receiver) and informs her that she is being assigned to help with a new customer service initiative for the organization (message). The officer speaks (medium) clearly and uses professional language (encoding), but the team member misses part of what he is saying because someone nearby has just slammed a door (noise). She knows the officer wants her help with a project, but she does not know what the project is about (decoding). The officer notices that the team member looks confused (feedback), and the team member asks the officer to repeat the details (feedback). The officer, who had also heard the door slam, repeats the assignment (message), and the team member confirms that she now understands it and would be happy to participate (feedback).

Communicating effectively is paramount both at work and in daily activities outside of work. To achieve this goal, we must focus on communicating with clarity. The sender of a message must ensure that when communicating, verbally, nonverbally, or in written form, the message (encoding) is clear, an appropriate medium is used to deliver the message, and the message is simple for the receiver to understand (decode). If the message is not clear, the receiver will have difficulty understanding it.

The clarity of a message can be impacted by poor grammar, use of an ineffective medium to deliver the message (e.g., sending a time-sensitive message via e-mail when the receiver is nearby and not at a computer), an attempt to cover multiple topics in the same message without making clear transitions, use of a monotone without any inflection to provide guidance as to where a verbal conversation is heading, absence of a clearly defined topic, use of technical or uncommon words, noise that disrupts the communication process, or inclusion of only brief information when discussing a complex subject matter. Good communication requires practice and considering the message from the receiver's perspective.

Good communicators make it a habit to say what they are going to say clearly, confirm that the message was received, and use transitions when they shift to another topic. Using transitions helps prevent confusion, clearly defines the new topic, and keeps the receiver engaged. The following is an example of a transition being used during a conversation:

> We have determined that it is too expensive to purchase an ambulance unit due to the amount of equipment and size of this acquisition. Now let's talk about purchasing a quick-response non-transport unit instead.

The second sentence makes it clear to the receiver that the sender has moved from discussing the ambulance unit to considering the quick-response non-transport unit. With such a transition, the possibility for confusion is reduced.

After sending a message, it is important that the sender ask for feedback and/or that the receiver provide some feedback to the sender. Feedback ensures that the correct message has been received; if it has not, any confusion can be addressed at this point, before the misunderstanding is compounded further. The process of communicating effectively encompasses not only sending a clear message, but also being a good listener and verifying that the message has been received.

Communicating Effectively

Effective communication is essential for your success as an EMS officer. Many individuals who experience difficulty when they assume a new position as an EMS officer do so because they fail to appreciate the importance of communicating effectively. Expecting team members to understand what you are telling them without providing them with clear direction and without asking for feedback to ensure that they understand the directive will most likely result in a poor performance outcome. Not only is this method of communication ineffective, but it also creates frustration and leads to underperformance from the team members. As a supervisor, you need to make sure that your message has been fully understood before moving on.

When you have been promoted and are meeting with your team for the first time in your new capacity, consider your communication strategy to ensure that you clearly communicate your message to all members of that team and, later, to the larger organization. When you begin to communicate with your team, you will most likely use a variety of communication methods—for example, one-on-one conversations, written memos and e-mail, meetings or briefings, or perhaps question-and-answer sessions during presentations.

Face-to-face communication should be considered the first choice for most messages. Considering the challenges presented by busy work environments and the prevalence of multiple office locations, however, face-to-face communication may pose a bit of a challenge and may not always be possible. The best communication method often depends on the message to be communicated, along with any logistical, financial, or time constraints. When you are facing these types of constraints, you can choose from several communication platforms to overcome the potential barriers. You will need to become familiar with the communication platforms that not only work best for you, but also are most likely to get your message across in a clear and concise manner.

Verbal Communication

When attempting to communicate, you need to make sure that the message was received and understood by the receiver. Face-to-face communication is typically preferred because it reduces the possibility of miscommunication and adds value to the encounter. The sender can see whether the receiver understands the message by observing the receiver's body language. The sender can ask questions to ensure the receiver understands the message, and the receiver can provide immediate feedback to the sender.

When using verbal communication, your message must be clear, concise, and to the point, especially if you will not have a lot of time to discuss the message. Introducing a message and leaving it for someone to interpret with no opportunity for immediate discussion can

Managerial Leadership BRIEFCASE
The Medium of Communication
Communication may take place through either a physical or a mechanical medium. In a physical medium, the speaker can be seen—for example, during a meeting, an interview, or a presentation, or while speaking at the scene of an emergency. With a mechanical medium, the communication is written. This type of medium can comprise a letter, an e-mail, a Tweet (i.e., Twitter message), and even the documentation of a patient care report.

create confusion. If you do not have enough time to discuss your message, make a point to follow up with the person or team later to address any questions they may have.

Verbal communications, particularly face-to-face conversations, can be greatly impacted by nonverbal communications, such as your mannerisms and your attire. With this type of communication, it is imperative that both the sender and the receiver focus on the message being delivered. However, even when the sender and the receiver appear to be engaged with the message that is the subject of the dialogue, an unintended message may be sent. Regardless of how engaged each individual is with the current discussion, if either the sender or the receiver appears to be looking away, has shoulders down and arms crossed, is reading e-mail, is looking at his or her phone, or is speaking to other team members as they walk by, that behavior will imply that the message is not being well received.

When engaging in verbal communication, both the sender and the receiver should actively participate in sharing the message, while their body language simultaneously shows engagement. For example, eyes must be focused on each other, with shoulders back and both hands interlocking fingers. The participants must ignore the noise around the discussion and not take phone calls or speak to other individuals not involved with the discussion. Facial expressions are extremely important and convey a message of their own. If the sender is conveying a positive message but presents with a serious facial expression, the disconnect between the message and the body language may create a distraction and confusion about the true message. Similarly, if the receiver appears to have an angry facial expression when receiving good news, it may appear that the receiver is not happy about the news. As these examples demonstrate, when communicating, it is important for both parties to be aware of the message being delivered, to ensure that the message has been received and understood, and to make every effort to display appropriate body language during the conversation.

The following sections outline typical situations in which an EMS officer uses verbal communication and identify additional considerations for communicating effectively in those situations.

Informal Conversations

Most of an individual's verbal communications are informal conversations. Informal conversations do have a role in the workplace, even at an EMS organization. As with any workplace interaction, however, certain guidelines must be followed to ensure that you conduct yourself professionally.

The decision to use formal versus informal communication will depend on the audience, the setting, and the message you are attempting to deliver. Informal conversations are more relaxed and conversational. It is not uncommon for an EMS supervisor to visit an EMS crew at their station and have an informal conversation about local politics, sports, or recent or future organizational events. It is also common to receive phone calls from crew members asking for advice about a non-work-related matter.

Knowing when it is appropriate to use informal versus formal communication is extremely important for the EMS officer. Although informal conversations may be appropriate in certain settings, the EMS officer must still conduct himself or herself as a professional. A colleague may share a joke that others may find offensive or share rumors about another colleague. It would not be appropriate to engage in such conversations, and you may even consider warning the colleague against such conversations in the workplace. For a team to work together well, the members must share trust and respect, and this cohesiveness can be lost when unprofessional comments and behaviors make members of the team uncomfortable. As the EMS officer, you must set an example of what is acceptable at the workplace.

Meetings

Meetings are a necessary component in every organization. In EMS, meetings can range from one-on-one updates on a task or a disciplinary issue to formal interdepartmental conferences. How you participate in these gatherings will impact the effectiveness of your communication and the productivity of the meeting.

In your capacity as an EMS officer, you are likely to lead meetings and serve as the chairperson of a committee many times. It is critical to be well prepared for these roles and to identify the specific topics you want to address before meeting with others. Prepare a written agenda well in advance and share it with your team. This forewarning will allow team members an opportunity not only to see what will be discussed during the meeting, but also to prepare for the meeting. During the meeting itself, how you present yourself will influence what is accomplished through the meeting and how you are perceived by the attendees. Consider your volume and tone of voice when you are speaking at such gatherings. Do you present yourself as someone who knows it all and is talking down to the attendees? Do you speak with appropriate inflection or in a monotone? When attendees ask questions, do you roll your eyes? Are you preoccupied with doodling or texting? Are your arms crossed, giving the impression that you are upset or closed off?

When you are leading a meeting, you must set a positive tone, encourage participation, and demonstrate that you are highly engaged with the topics being discussed. Make sure to use vocal inflection when you are speaking, as it will indicate how you want to convey the message. If you speak too loudly, it might appear that you are upset; conversely, if you speak too softly, attendees will have to strain to hear you and your message will be lost.

When attendees are speaking, make sure that they are not interrupted and follow up with feedback on their comments or questions. This kind of response will signal to the attendee that you are acknowledging his or her participation and input. Avoid distractions such as doodling, clicking a pen over and over, texting, and taking phone calls. If you need to answer the phone or respond to a text, excuse yourself. If you are waiting for a text or a phone call prior to the start of the meeting, let everyone know that you may need to step away for a few minutes. When you are chairing a meeting, all eyes will be on you—so preparing ahead of time will be essential.

Meeting with your team is important and is a great opportunity to ensure that everyone is on the same page regarding administrative and operational duties. Keep meetings focused, listen to attendee feedback, and follow up with attendees after the meeting if necessary. You want to be sure your messages and the other messages conveyed at the meeting were received correctly by the attendees.

Video Conferencing

In-person meetings are ideal in that they limit the opportunities for miscommunication, but they may be difficult to accomplish if you are meeting with different business partners across the state or country, must deal with multiple functional unit locations, or face time constraints that prevent all attendees from gathering at one location. In such cases, video conferencing may be a valid alternative to an in-person meeting. Video conferencing permits individuals to be in different locations, yet see (face-to-face) and speak with each other. This type of meeting can be inexpensive and can take place anywhere there is an Internet connection, as long as the participants have hardware and software capable of connecting to each location.

Video conferencing offers many advantages: It is an opportunity to engage in face-to-face exchanges; multiple individuals can share in the conversation; it saves money on travel; and the technology can be set up quickly. Because the image is being transmitted by a camera, however, it may be difficult to capture the other person's body language. Furthermore, the picture can be grainy, can freeze, or could be put on pause, preventing the viewer from capturing the entire scene. Also, if the connection is poor, not only will the image not be available, but the sound may be interrupted as well. This will cause the message to be distorted between parties and may cause miscommunication.

Phone Conferencing

Phone conferencing is similar to video conferencing, but without the visual images. Phone conferencing allows multiple individuals to attend a conversation using the same telephone line. This technology is beneficial when multiple individuals need to meet but, due to travel expenses or time constraints, cannot meet in person, and not all attendees have access to video conferencing.

When the phone conference date is set, the participants are given a phone number to call and a specific code that allows them entry into the phone conference. The phone conference will have a host who is responsible for selecting the topics for discussion and ensuring that the items on the meeting agenda are addressed.

Phone conferencing is quick to set up and inexpensive, but does have the disadvantage that the host and other participants are unable to see one another. When using either video or phone conferencing, you will be engaged in verbal communication; therefore, you must have a plan that will ensure your message is clear and is properly received.

Presentations

Delivering a presentation is an often-feared task, but success can be achieved by preparing thoroughly, relaxing during the event, and keeping the presentation simple. Opportunities for presentations include department EMS/medical in-service educational programs; orientation for new hires; town hall meetings to discuss the EMS system; and when requesting the purchase of equipment during budget workshops in front of a city, county, or town board.

Be sure to get a good night's sleep the night before any presentation. Also, it is very important to dress appropriately for the occasion. There is no doubt that being knowledgeable about the material being delivered supersedes every other aspect of the presentation, but your attire, a clear message, your personality, and the ability to keep the audience engaged are also essential components of an effective presentation.

Know the Material

Be sure you thoroughly know the material that you will be presenting. Your audience will see you as the subject-matter expert during the presentation, so do your homework well before the day of the presentation. It is your responsibility to deliver an organized, clear, and concise message. The goal is to capture the audience's attention within one to three minutes after beginning your presentation. The following tips will help you develop and give an effective presentation:

- When creating the presentation, make it easy for the participants to follow along and be sure to provide materials that will illustrate your point.
- Avoid busy slides—for example, those with multiple charts and photos, excessive text, and too many bullet points. Select an appropriate background color, background image, and font size.
  - When selecting a background for a slide, make sure that the color and graphics do not distract the viewer from focusing on the main point: your message.
  - If you will combine images with text, try not to exceed three images per slide, and keep the text to short statements.
  - Keep the font size to no less than 30 points, and make it larger if the presentation is being given to a large group.
- Capitalizing every letter in any written medium gives the impression of aggression or yelling at the receiver, a situation you want to avoid.

Keep your presentation simple and easy to follow. If its complexity overwhelms the audience, they will disengage from the presentation and the message will not be received.

Anticipate the Unexpected

As much as you might plan for the ideal presentation, you must also make contingency plans in case a component of your presentation does not fall into place. The day before the presentation, make sure that all the equipment is in working order, your handouts are ready for distribution, and you have a backup plan for every aspect of the presentation (e.g., extra handout materials, light bulbs for projectors, audio-visual equipment).

Know Your Audience

If you will be presenting a topic that is familiar to the audience, then you may use terminology that is related to the topic at hand. In contrast, if your audience is new to the topic, be sure to lay out the information in a way that is easy for newcomers to understand and follow during the presentation.

Become Familiar with Your Surroundings

You may be asked to give a presentation somewhere besides the environment in which you work—for example, at a local library, college conference hall, church hall, home owner's association community room, or restaurant. Regardless of where the presentation will be held, you must prepare well in advance not only by developing the material to be presented, but also by familiarizing yourself with the presentation location. Will the presentation organizers have the audio-visual equipment necessary to support the presentation, or will you need to provide all such equipment? How many attendees are expected to be present? How much time will be allotted for the presentation, and will it be followed by a question-and-answer session? Is the room conducive to a presentation? It is critical that you establish a list of what is needed to ensure that no surprises interfere with your ability to deliver a successful presentation on the scheduled date.

Plan Your Time

Before presenting, determine how much time you have to get your message across. Try your best to stay within the time frame given to you. Depending on the content and your presentation style, you will need at least 30 to 60 seconds per slide and at least 15 minutes for questions and answers after the presentation. Going over the allotted time will make you appear unprepared, and if another speaker will follow you, you will be taking that person's time. Practice your presentation several times to ensure you can finish it in the allotted time and you are well versed with the material.

Emergency Response

Once promoted to the rank of EMS officer, depending on the organization's rank structure, you may work in a front-line unit, serve as an area supervisor, or oversee an entire functional workgroup (division). As the EMS officer is promoted through the ranks, his or her involvement with patient care will diminish. It is important, regardless of your rank, to understand that as an EMS officer you will be dealing with internal and external customers and must know when and how to adjust your communication to ensure your message is received. (See the "Customer Service" chapter for more discussion of internal and external customers.)

When communicating with a patient (external customer), that conversation may occur during an EMS transport, during an interfacility transport, or after the patient has been released from the hospital. The EMS officer may also have to communicate with the patient's family, friends, and even bystanders. Therefore, the EMS officer must be able to communicate effectively with the patient and other external customers in these situations. If the EMS officer is rendering care to a patient during a medical emergency, then the communication must be directed toward the patient, explaining which interventions are being provided, as well as toward the officer's partner.

When treating a patient, the EMS officer will need to convey a sense of calm and demonstrate that the situation is under control—not just for the patient, but for everyone else on scene as well. If the EMS officer is barking out orders or running around the scene in a state of panic, he or she will most likely lose control of the scene, thereby creating undue stress for the patient, who is already experiencing a taxing medical emergency. Similarly, if the EMS crew appears confused about the situation or treatment, or if the crew's attention is focused on something besides the patient, the impression will be that the crew is disengaged. The way EMS personnel communicate with patients, family members, friends, bystanders, and other prehospital providers while on scene will set the tone throughout the emergency situation.

Verbal communication, body language, and the actions taken toward patients/customers not only set the tone for scene management, but also establish a positive relationship between the providers and those who are sick or injured. When dealing with a patient and other personnel at the scene, it is important to speak clearly, without raising your voice. Body language must reflect a calm control of the scene, and the crew's action must center on improving the patient's state of well-being.

Every EMS officer must assess the environment in which he or she will be communicating and then make the appropriate adjustments to be most effective. Depending on the incident and the EMS officer's rank, it is not uncommon for the EMS officer to assume command of the scene. The EMS officer will need to take a macro view of the scene because his or her responsibility extends beyond patient care and into the operational components of the scene. For example, the officer's tasks may include addressing questions about patient care, coordinating the activation for aeromedical transport, determining the hospital to which the patient will be transported, requesting the appropriate equipment needed for patient extrication, and addressing the family's and friends' concerns.

The EMS officer, regardless of rank, will also need to communicate effectively with the other EMS personnel or organizational team members (internal customers). Communicating with an employee or colleague during a prehospital emergency differs from communication in an office environment. At an emergency scene, the pace of getting the job done is much quicker and minimal supervisor–employee guidance occurs because the crew members are trained to handle the situation. When communicating with an office staff member, especially one without EMS experience, a different communication approach should be employed. Using a management and leadership style appropriate for an emergency scene in an office setting is likely to create frustration among team members. Likewise, communication styles appropriate in an office setting would create confusion and frustration among responders and patients at an emergency scene, where an authoritative and decisive approach is expected and appreciated. Adjusting communication styles is critical to ensure that the message is well received.

Crew Resource Management

To improve communications during stressful situations, many organizations have implemented **crew resource management (CRM)**. The CRM concept was introduced during a NASA air safety workshop, and spread from there to the airline industry, where it had a markedly positive effect in improving safety. At the time, the airline industry was facing an increased rate of airplane crashes with catastrophic outcomes. Investigators noted that the majority of the airplane incidents were the result of human error. After the implementation of CRM, the airline industry began to notice a decrease in airplane crashes, and organizational leaders from other industries took note of the power of CRM. During the past 30 years, improved technology and better built planes have certainly played a critical role in preventing crashes; however, CRM has been an important part of reducing cockpit errors as well.

CRM is a multidisciplinary management system with the primary goal of improving safety and efficiency by focusing on leadership, communication, situational awareness, teamwork, decision making, and use of all resources available to meet the goal. Every person must be empowered to question a plan of action he or she feels is unsafe. Therefore, implementing a CRM system must be a top priority in those organizations where team members work under stressful conditions, time is critical, and the smallest error can mean the difference between life and death. The CRM system provides a foundation for the organization to reduce the likelihood of catastrophic incidents as well as a safety mechanism to stop a crisis from growing.

As the EMS officer on scene during a prehospital emergency, you must listen to those around you, just as you expect for those around you to listen to your directives. The focus is not just on having a checklist, protocols, policies, and procedures, but also on engaging in teamwork and being able to process information quickly to solve problems. During an emergency or other stressful situation, effective communication among team members is essential, regardless of rank. If the lowest-ranked team member notices a critical problem being overlooked, he or she should feel comfortable bringing that issue to the team's attention. CRM entails a culture change in which all team members embrace an ongoing commitment to the team's effective functioning, supported by the senior leadership team. It is up to each organization to develop the CRM system that works best for its members and helps ensure safety and efficiency throughout the organization.

Written Communication

Although written communication is a standard mode of communication within most business environments, it may be the most challenging means of getting the intended message to the receiver. With this type of communication, you cannot see the receiver's body language, the receiver may interpret the tone of the message as being offensive, and you are not readily available to answer any immediate question the receiver has. If the written communication is handwritten rather than typed, the writing must be neat and legible to avoid confusion. Regardless of the format of the written communication, correct grammar, punctuation, and syntax are necessary not only to reduce misunderstanding, but also to maintain professionalism and authority.

When written communication is used, you should be systematic in organizing the topics covered by that communication. If your message topics are organized inefficiently, the reader will be distracted by the chore of processing the information appropriately. Keep the message short, introduce your topic statement, include examples that support your message, and conclude the message.

When using any form of written communication (e.g., e-mail, report, memo, letter), make every effort to include a statement within the body of the message that questions are welcomed. If several days pass without a response to your message (especially if a reply was requested), consider following up with an e-mail or telephone call to ensure that the message was received and that the receiver has no questions. This will help address any concerns or confusion on the part of the receiver.

Memo or Bulletin

A memo is used when a specific message is being sent to members of the organization or between functional working units. A bulletin is used to post a specific message for all members of the organization. Both memos and bulletins are used for internal communication between organizational members and are less formal than letters. Each organization will have a certain way of crafting its organizational memos and bulletins; therefore, it is important that you become familiar with your organization's template for writing memos and bulletins.

Letter

A letter is used when sending a message from a person or on behalf of the organization to another party outside the organization. It is more formal than a memo or bulletin and can be either short or long in content.

The EMS officer will be called upon to respond to patient care complaints, inquiries from other healthcare organizations and state EMS regulatory organizations, and other administrative and operational agencies. A letter may be an appropriate form of communication when the EMS officer needs to provide a formal response to an internal or external customer, request information, or convey a formal message of gratitude. For example, a customer may request a letter clarifying his or her transport bill, a family member may request an explanation as to why the patient was not transported to the closest emergency department, or the EMS officer may want to commend a crew for its outstanding service.

Letters must be written on the appropriate department stationery. It is also important that the letter be formatted appropriately, including the date, the recipient's and sender's addresses, the name of the recipient's business if applicable, the recipient's name and title, and the sender's signature. Lastly, if the letter needs to be viewed by other individuals besides the recipient, be sure to include a courtesy copy (cc:) notation at the bottom of the letter and send a copy to the other individuals designated as recipients.

Letters are a formal way of communicating. They are sent not only to convey a message, but also to document in writing that a formal message has been sent and the date on which it was sent. This type of communication provides documentation if a reference should be required in the future.

Standard Operating Guidelines or Procedures

Standard operating guidelines (SOGs) and standard operating procedures (SOPs) are documents containing a set of instructions to assist employees with the management of operational and administrative conditions. No one can predict every scenario an employee will face, but SOGs/SOPs serve as a reference point for employees when dealing with different operational or administrative conditions and provide a standard of operation across the organization.

Depending on the organization's SOG/SOP implementation policy, the document may be created by a group of individuals who make up an SOG/SOP committee, the organization's leadership team, or subject-matter experts within the organization. It is important to become familiar with your organization's preferred format before attempting to create an SOG/SOP on your own.

Essentially, SOGs provide guidance on how to address certain business activities and SOPs include the steps required to accomplish the activity. The SOG can be in text format and will commonly consist of the following:

- Purpose: The reason for the SOG
- Guidelines: The guidelines for performing specific activities addressed within the SOG

Like an SOG, an SOP document is typically in text format, but it is more detailed than an SOG and includes the steps required to achieve a certain activity. SOPs may include the following sections:

- Purpose: The reason for the SOP
- Policy: The organizational policy that is the reason for establishing the procedure
- Responsibility: Who is responsible for following the procedure
- Procedure: A step-by-step approach on how to meet a specific organizational activity

Once created, the SOG/SOP must be approved by the organization's chief executive officer or the chief of the department prior to dissemination. It is then assigned a file number, a title (indicating whether it is a guideline or a procedure), and a functional level unit that is responsible for maintaining the document. The SOG/SOP must be evaluated at least once every 12 to 18 months.

SOGs and SOPs are business processes that serve as references when team members are faced with certain organizational activities, especially those that occur frequently. Use of SOGs/SOPs ensures consistency across the organization. It is not uncommon for SOGs and SOPs to be used interchangeably, but as an EMS officer you should become familiar with all of the documents that your organization uses.

E-mail

E-mail is one of the most widely used communications media today and can be very effective. It allows the sender and the receiver to have immediate access to a written message and can be used for communicating with internal or external customers. Although e-mail is typically not accepted as a formal medium of communication, it can still be very effective in getting messages across to single or multiple recipients very quickly.

The EMS officer will use a variety of communication tools on a daily basis and should always consider which tool will be most effective for the message and recipient. Benefits to using e-mail include the following:

- It is an easy way to reach individuals or groups quickly with the same message.
- It facilitates sending multiple document attachments to another party.
- It can be sent from anywhere that has Internet access.
- The process is quick, allowing the recipient(s) to get the information quickly.
- It creates an electronic record that facilitates keeping track of communications.

Although this medium is considered an informal avenue of communication, it is still necessary to demonstrate professionalism when sending e-mail messages. Spelling, grammar, and punctuation are just as important with e-mail as they are in other forms of written communication. The immediacy of e-mail can also impact its professionalism if you write the e-mail while you are rushed, angry, or frustrated. It is all too easy to write an e-mail quickly and click the send button; once it is sent, however, you cannot get the e-mail back. Take the time to proofread your e-mails before sending them. If there is a chance your attitude while writing the e-mail could negatively affect the message you really want to send (and how you want it to be received), step back from the e-mail and come back to it when you are calm and collected and can reply with less emotion.

When you receive an e-mail, it is important to respond to the sender to let him or her know the message was received, even if you cannot immediately make a full reply to the content of the message. This response notifies the sender that the e-mail reached you and that there were no technical issues (e.g., hardware/software problems, incorrect e-mail address) that kept the message from its destination. Because e-mail is so ubiquitous and individuals are used to receiving quick replies, you must consider how a sender will react if you do not send a timely reply. If you will be away from e-mail for longer than usual (e.g., when on vacation or traveling), it is best to set an automatic reply to inform senders (1) that you do not currently have access to your e-mail, (2) when you will be able to respond to their message, and (3) how they can get in touch with you if the need is urgent (or who to contact in your stead).

When e-mail serves as the preferred means of communication in the workplace, every employee must understand the organization's e-mail policy. Using e-mail for non-work-related activities could potentially be considered a dismissible offense depending on the organization's internal policies. When using any business-owned computers, smartphones, or other electronic devices for communicating, the EMS officer must ensure that the e-mail pertains to organizational business. The EMS officer, at a minimum and as part of the job, should have access to a computer and smartphone, but must always remember that this equipment does not belong to the EMS officer, but rather to the organization. Therefore, any communication using such devices must be related to business. When assigned to a department-owned workstation computer or other electronics that have e-mail capability, the user must avoid the following activities:

- E-mailing Health Insurance Portability and Accountability Act (HIPAA)–protected patient information
- E-mailing an employee's or coworker's confidential information (e.g., home address, personal telephone number, background history, Social Security number, driver's license number, financial information)
- E-mailing non-work-related information
- E-mailing non-business-related documents
- Sending threatening e-mails
- E-mailing passwords
- E-mailing complex and lengthy information

Many organizations require disclaimers to be included in all organizational e-mails. If you receive e-mails, then most likely you have noticed disclaimers or confidentiality notes at the bottom of the messages sent from a particular business or organization. Such disclaimers are used to protect the organization or the individual sending the e-mail. For example, the disclaimer may state that the information included in the e-mail is confidential and not for sharing, or that all employees have been trained in proper e-mail etiquette and that improper use of e-mail is not condoned by the organization. A disclaimer could also include specific organizational policies to prevent legal issues among internal team members (e.g., sending threatening or harassing e-mail, distributing employee photos, or releasing confidential information). It is important to keep disclaimers short, place them where the recipient can easily see them, and use font characteristics that can distinguish the disclaimer from the actual message (e.g., italics).

When communicating through this medium, the EMS officer must ensure that whatever is being e-mailed pertains to organizational business and is not of a sensitive nature. As the EMS officer, you will be looked upon as a leader and must set a professional tone when communicating, regardless of the format used. Therefore, when using e-mail, you should keep the tone upbeat, open and close the message with positive remarks, stay within the business parameters, avoid e-mailing protected/confidential information, suggest a time to discuss the matter in person if warranted, and not respond to an e-mail when you are upset. Remember also that e-mail recipients cannot see you; they can only read the e-mail. For this reason, you should pay special attention to how you construct the e-mail because it will be a direct reflection on you and the organization.

Text Message

Text messages allow for quick, informal, to-the-point messaging between two or several individuals. The advantages of this communication medium are that it is informal, the process is easy to master, the sender can attach images and recordings, and messages can be sent from anywhere using any electronic device with text messaging capabilities. For example, if you will be late to a meeting, you can text your assistant or the meeting organizer to let him or her know about your delayed arrival. If you are not sure where you are supposed to meet or at what time, you can text a colleague and ask him or her to text you the time of the meeting and directions to the location. Text messaging is not used as a means of formally communicating a message or conducting official business, but it may be used to assist with day-to-day work activities.

Texting language often includes abbreviations such as TTYL (talk to you later), BTW (by the way), IMO (in my opinion), and PWT (point well taken). This shorthand is convenient, as long as the receiver is aware of the meaning of the abbreviations. It cannot be stressed enough that text

Managerial Leadership **BRIEFCASE**

E-mail and Public Records

Communicating via e-mail has become part of day-to-day business operations. While we use this medium on a routine basis, we should not forget that e-mails created and exchanged for official governmental agency business can be subject to inspection under a public records request. This requirement pertains not just to e-mails, but to all written documents, recordings, photography, and data used for official government business. Check with your organization's legal counsel to see what is considered a public record in your state.

messaging must be used only in an informal business environment with the intent of obtaining or sending a brief message and should never include any confidential information. Additionally, if you are sending a text message while on duty, using a device provided to you by the organization, then you must ensure that the text message is work related. Personal text messaging while on duty, especially using a device belonging to the organization, may be considered a violation of the organization's social media policy and may be subject to investigation. Become familiar with your organization's texting policy before you start messaging.

Organization's Website

The use of a website to promote an organization and its services and to keep customers informed of current or future events is essential, especially for public safety organizations. The creation of a website is typically handled by an organization's information technology division; however, as an officer within the organization, you may be called upon to provide some input. Websites are an outstanding form of communication that may be the first place customers go when seeking information about the organization or when they have questions about its service. A website may provide the customer's first impression of the organization; therefore, it must create a positive image of the EMS system.

Although graphics, photos, sounds of sirens, flashing lights across the screen, and animations are attention grabbing and relevant to the organization, such "bells and whistles" may distract the customer and distort the message the organization is attempting to provide its customers through the website. Therefore, when creating a website, the golden rule should be to make it customer friendly and keep it simple. When deciding which color to use for the background, think about the psychology associated with different colors. For example, blue reflects peacefulness and tranquility, red suggests an intense emotion and power, black represents authority, yellow is cheerful, and white represents innocence and trust. The background colors will certainly be a deciding factor in attracting or deflecting your customer's attention.

Avoid clutter or placement of too much information on a single page. The main page should display the organization's name, logo, vision and mission statements, telephone number, address, and a brief summary of the organization's core services. If the page becomes too busy, it will be difficult to navigate, causing your customers to become frustrated. Be sure to add navigational buttons where they will be seen easily to assist customers in working their way through the site and finding answers to their questions. Including photos on the website is certainly advisable; however, they should be limited in size and quantity. If you would like to display multiple photos, consider including them as a slide show on the main page.

Important legal/rights considerations arise when including photos, however. You should avoid posting photos that are confidential or clearly identify a patient. Posting a photo of someone without his or her written consent can create legal problems if that individual feels his or her privacy has been violated. Also, copyrighted material should be used only if the author or rights holder gives permission or if the organization has a license to use the material. It is not sufficient to include a copyright line for the original source; you must have express permission from the owner to include the material on your organization's website.

Public safety organizations should consider setting aside a page for current or potential public safety events. During natural or human-made disasters, community members will need public safety-related information, and websites are a frequently visited resource during these times. (See the "Customer Service" chapter for more information on the use of an organizational website.)

Social Media

Social media encompass any form of written communication, photographs, videos, or audio that can be shared through multiple mass media and electronic sites. Examples include blogs, podcasts, texting, Twitter, Facebook, Instagram, Flickr, and YouTube. Social media serve as a good platform through which to promote services provided by the organization, department–community events, and employee recognition. This platform is also beneficial when certain public safety concerns arise—for example, severe weather, wildfires, evacuations, and other events during which the public will need to be informed. In today's world, where so many people have cell phones or other devices that can readily access social media sites, public safety organizations must do everything possible to take advantage of this platform. Keeping the public informed of public safety issues and drawing attention to the services provided by the organization are extremely important. As an organizational leader, you need to promote both the organization's brand and the services it provides. Social media represent a great venue to do so because of the low cost and easy accessibility of such media.

Although social media can certainly add value to public safety organizations, the individuals responsible for posting content must be well informed of their organization's social media policy. If no such a policy is in place, the organizational leaders must seek advice from the organization's city, township, or county attorney. In particular, none of the content posted to social media can include confidential or protected information. The organization's social media policy should specify what is considered confidential and protected information; examples include photographs of patients, any copyrighted material, protected health information, and personal data (e.g., name, home address, Social Security number, driver's license number). In addition, photos taken by

Managerial Leadership **BRIEFCASE**
Caution with E-mail and Social Media
A good rule is not to write an e-mail or social media post when you are upset or do not have all the facts. Also, do not list a recipient until you are sure that an e-mail is ready to be sent. E-mails and social media posts have a way of finding their way around the organization and your community.

departmental personnel while at an emergency scene must not be posted on any social media site unless the organization's leadership team has authorized its use in that capacity.

There should be only one source for releasing and posting departmental information. It is imperative that members of the organization avoid using their personal social media accounts to post any departmental information, as this practice could lead to publication of conflicting information and create confusion among community members. Moreover, when posting any departmental information on a personal site, the individual posting the information will be responsible for the information being released, and there is a high probability that posting department information without approval will lead to discipline or even dismissal.

Employee Reviews

The EMS officer is required to conduct employee performance evaluations on a regular basis. Written evaluations of employees are most commonly done on an annual basis. Those in a managerial leadership role, however, should not wait to compliment or advise an employee about his or her performance until the annual employee evaluation rolls around. Verbally acknowledging an employee's good performance is essential and should be done more often than once a year.

Similarly, if the employee is underperforming, the EMS officer should not wait until the annual written evaluation to address the employee's performance issues. When working with a new hire, the EMS officer should consider meeting with the new employee at 30 days, at 90 days, and then as needed to monitor the new employee's progress. The EMS officer must be candid about the new employee's performance; if not, the evaluation process will be unfair to the new employee. The EMS officer must not expect an employee to know how well he or she is performing if the individual does not receive timely feedback.

If the evaluation will include discipline, performance improvement benchmarks, or situations that may potentially result in conflict, the evaluation must be documented and signed by both parties. In addition, if the employee has a history of not understanding what is expected of him or her, having a human resources representative attend the meeting as an observer must be considered. Once an evaluation is completed, the EMS officer must not wait another year to meet with the team member. Regardless of whether performance benchmarks have been established, meeting with each of your team members at least once each quarter will promote ongoing communication about performance. Such feedback demonstrates that you care about the employees, and the meeting creates an opportunity for you to share the employee's progress or offer assistance if the individual needs it.

Positive or negative evaluations must be viewed as an opportunity to show the employee you want to help him or her succeed within the organization. If the evaluation is negative, you must convey to the employee what he or she needs to do to get back on track for success. If the evaluation is positive, your communication style must be one of support and celebration. The underlying purpose of the performance evaluation is to ensure that, as the EMS officer, you are doing everything possible to help the employee succeed. Remember that people are at the top of the five business priorities (5 BPs). Conveying encouragement and support to employees to help them do their very best must be the organization's top priority.

Evaluations of senior employees may be more challenging for a new manager, but the EMS officer must address such a performance evaluation in the same way as with junior employees—by being candid, pointing out positive work performance outcomes, and discussing where improvement is required. When providing a written evaluation or verbal feedback to an employee, the EMS officer must be fair, honest, and respectful; address the concerns; promote the positive aspects of performance; and ensure the employee understands the performance expectations.

Before setting up a performance review meeting, be sure to give the employee a few days' notice and provide the individual with a pre-evaluation form **(Figure 4-2)**. These forms are designed to give employees a chance to identify concerns, goals, project accomplishments, and any other topics they would like to discuss during the meeting. When conducting an employee written evaluation or verbally addressing an employee's performance, the EMS officer must commit to sending a clear and concise message—one that avoids the possibility of any misunderstanding.

Media Relations

As an EMS officer, you or your designee may be called upon to deal with the media. During a significant crisis, the media (TV, print, and/or online) will want to speak to the organization's leader to obtain information about the incident. Many organizations have appointed media relations specialists or public information officers (PIOs) to deal directly with the media. These representatives most commonly have an established relationship with the media representatives within their local jurisdiction.

When establishing a professional relationship with the media, the PIO must routinely reach out to the media outlets by calling or visiting the studio to meet the assignment editors (television) or news director (radio). By establishing these contacts before a crisis occurs, the crisis management team will know who to reach out to during a crisis. This will be a win-win situation for the media agencies and the organization: The media agencies will have a contact within the department in the event they need to get department information for a story, and the department will have a contact within the media agencies for when they need to get a message to the public.

If your organization is dealing with a small or large event that has the potential to affect lives, you can expect not only local media attention but also national and international media coverage. To ensure all media agencies receive accurate information about the event, the assigned spokesperson must have the information approved for release by the organization's leader or the incident commander. During a crisis, a set of command structures must be established to ensure that everyone knows their role, including who will be addressing the media. Especially during a large event, the organization may activate a Joint Information Center (JIC) to keep all PIOs in a central location and thereby ensure that all agencies working the incident release the same information.

EMPLOYEE SELF-EVALUATION FORM

Name:	Dept./Ofc:
Title:	Date:

<table>
<tr><td colspan="2" align="center">Performance Review
(form does not become part of employee personnel file)</td></tr>
<tr><td colspan="2">1. Goals and Objectives/Performance Expectations</td></tr>
<tr><td colspan="2">Please list and discuss major objectives and projects covered by this review. Briefly discuss the status of each. (Add additional pages as necessary).

</td></tr>
<tr><td colspan="2">2. Accomplishments/Achievements</td></tr>
<tr><td colspan="2">Please list and briefly describe your most important accomplishments during the past appraisal period.

</td></tr>
<tr><td colspan="2">3. Unusual Circumstances</td></tr>
<tr><td colspan="2">List and briefly describe unusual circumstances, changed priorities or special problems that have occurred during the appraisal period.

</td></tr>
<tr><td colspan="2">4. Performance Appraisal</td></tr>
<tr><td colspan="2">Briefly describe your assessment of your overall performance for the last evaluation period.

</td></tr>
</table>

Figure 4-2 Sample pre-evaluation form for employee performance.
Courtesy of Brevard County Fire Rescue

Technology has provided a conduit through which to convey information to the media in real time. Most commonly such information will be disseminated as a media release via e-mail, posted on a social media site, or faxed to all the media assignment editors and/or on-scene reporters.

Anyone assigned to disseminate information must be mindful of the Health Insurance Portability and Accountability Act. No HIPAA-protected health information can be released to any public or media agency. This includes patients' medical history, current medical condition, address, or any other patient identifiers.

Although press releases are the most common medium for releasing information to the public, other methods may serve as information outlets and may prove beneficial for a specific event. The spokesperson or the organization's leadership team may opt to use the following methods for disseminating information:

- Social media
- Department or organization website
- Press conferences
- Direct one-on-one interview on camera or phone

Regardless of the media platform used, the spokesperson must always remain calm, display a professional appearance, be confident, and know the subject matter (**Figure 4-3**). The individual assigned to work with the media representatives must be well informed on the topic and must feel comfortable discussing the release in front of a large gathering. He or she will be considered the subject-matter expert and will field all the questions from media representatives. When filling this role, credibility is key, so do not lie or guess at information. If you do not have an answer, it is okay to say, "I don't know; I will get back to you." You could also reply, "I can't address that issue right now because I don't have all the information" or "We are currently looking into that matter and will let you know when we find out." Stay away from "No comment"; this response gives the impression that you or the members of the organization are hiding something.

Managerial Leadership BRIEFCASE

Additional Responsibilities of a Public Information Officer

In addition to being the department's spokesperson, the PIO may be assigned other duties (e.g., as a community public safety liaison) in which he or she continues to promote the organization's brand and establish a professional working relationship with local and national media agencies. When the EMS officer is asked to address the public during an educational event or during a crisis, he or she must coordinate with the department's spokesperson and/or the department's leadership team to ensure that a consistent message is being disseminated.

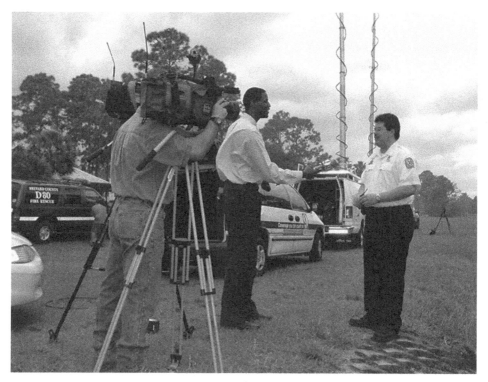

Figure 4-3 The EMS spokesperson must always remain calm and professional when interacting with media representatives.

Courtesy of Melanie Silvestry

Media Releases

When creating a media release, keep it simple. The media will want to know the five Ws: who, what, why, when, and where. Always be sure to include the following information in a press release **(Figure 4-4)**:

- Date and time of the incident
- Topic or name of the incident (if assigned)
- Press release number if you plan to send out multiple press releases
- Body of the message, including the five Ws
- Coding (###) at the bottom of the release to indicate the end

News Interviews and Press Conferences

When conducting a media interview, either on the radio or on camera, you will need to prepare what you will say before you take the microphone. When engaging in this form of verbal

Release of Information
Jones & Bartlett Fire District

Public Information Release

Contact Name: Lt. James Smith
Contact Title: Public Information Officer
Office Telephone: 978-443-5000

FOR IMMEDIATE RELEASE
Jones & Bartlett Fire District Recruit Graduating Ceremony

Date: June 10, 2015

(Viera, Fl.)- June 20, 2015- Jones & Bartlett Fire District will be hosting a graduation ceremony for 30 fire fighter recruits. The fire fighter recruits have endured 8 weeks of rigorous firefighting, brush fire, hazardous materials operation, driver apparatus, and medical training. Upon graduation, the recruits will receive their new station assignments. The ceremony will take place at 6:00 pm in the Jones & Bartlett County Commission Chamber. We ask that media representative arrive 15 minutes prior to the beginning of the ceremony.

(###)

Figure 4-4 Sample press release.

communication, as with other forms of communication, the goal is not to confuse the listeners and to deliver a clear message. Therefore, keep it brief, stick to the subject matter, do not overwhelm the listeners, use transitions, and keep it simple.

The spokesperson must also consider, depending on the crisis, conducting a set of press conferences throughout the event period. This practice will ensure that the media are organized at a central point for gathering information and that they hear the message from an organizational member, such as chief officers, elected officials, and law enforcement officers.

When conducting any form of interview, but especially on-camera interviews, spokespersons must not only be well prepared as to what they will be saying, but also ensure that their body language is professional and that the situation is under control. Appearing to be disheveled, disengaged from the questions being asked, messaging someone during the interview, or displaying distracting facial expressions during critical events will give the wrong impression and create uncertainty among the viewers of such interviews. When facing the camera or conducting a briefing in front of reporters, the spokesperson will be the source of information and will be representing the organization. The community will be listening to the message being delivered and, depending on the presentation, will determine how the situation is perceived by everyone.

If the interview is being recorded rather than being broadcast live, you may have the opportunity to start over and re-record your segment. Speak in clear, concise statements that can be used as sound bites whenever possible because the news media will likely abbreviate your interview and you want to ensure that your message is represented accurately. However, do not just tell the reporter what he or she wants to hear. Speak honestly and professionally on behalf of your organization for the benefit of the public.

Scene Access

It is the media representatives' job to gather the information, so they will want to get as close to the scene as possible. If the scene is unsafe, members of the media will most likely understand that at the current time they will not be allowed to get close to the incident. However, this is not a rule and every effort must be made to inform the media that the scene is unsafe (to ensure their own safety and to maintain scene control), identify a location where they can receive the information until they can be taken to the site, and continue to provide information. In the absence of such EMS actions, media representatives will undoubtedly seek information elsewhere, but the information they find may not be accurate.

If the incident scene is safe, your organization should have a plan that allows media access to the scene when escorted by a designated member of the organization. Furthermore, the PIO should establish a media staging area where he or she will be available to answer questions. It is the PIO's responsibility to get to know the media representatives in the jurisdiction before a crisis occurs.

Many departments use social media, such as Twitter and Facebook, to keep the media informed of unfolding incidents in real time. The media representatives will give you every opportunity to keep them informed; take advantage of this opportunity. If you do not provide the information, they will find it elsewhere.

Barriers to Effective Communication

As a managerial leader, you need to know your employees, your customers, and the best means to communicate effectively with all of them. No matter which form of communication you use, the key is to keep communication a two-way street. Just as you expect your team members and customers to listen to what you are saying, so they also need to know that you are listening and paying attention to what they are communicating. When engaged in a conversation, it is good practice to offer feedback. This practice will not only ensure that you understand the message correctly, but will also tell the speaker that you are actively listening to what he or she is saying. This type of culture, in turn, leads to inclusiveness and candor.

Effective communication requires elimination of barriers. Communication barriers are not specific to external noise, such as construction, telephones ringing in the background, notification of e-mails, emergency vehicles with lights and sirens driving by, or coworkers talking outside your office. Rather, they also include internal factors. For example, you may notice that what you are asking of your group is not getting done, or perhaps it is getting done too slowly. Although your first inclination may be to blame the team, the underlying issue may be ineffective communication. For example, your assignment, or message, may not have been clear enough, or there may be communication issues among the team members. If team members are divided into groups and not all team members are in the same building where the project is being managed, this decentralization can certainly pose a problem because the team members may be experiencing difficulty communicating between locations. Communications can also suffer when a computer server is inoperable and team members cannot send any project documents, plans, or illustrations electronically to the other team members.

Barriers to effective communication can be divided into four categories:

- Personal barriers
- Physical barriers
- Process barriers
- Semantic and language barriers

Personal Barriers

Personal barriers originate with the person who is either attempting to convey a message or receiving the message; they occur when the sender or receiver is not committed to communicating effectively. This kind of barrier can arise when the sender is not prepared to convey the message and the message is not clearly defined. This will make it difficult for the receiver to thoroughly understand the message being delivered. Personal barriers can also become an issue when the receiver is not listening to or focusing on the message being sent, or when the receiver does not absorb the entire message because he or she is distracted during the conversation. Such a break-down in communication keeps the message from being delivered. Personal barriers may also present a problem if the sender or the receiver has a preconceived notion about the individual delivering or receiving the message. Such an assumption may take the form of not having confidence or believing the other party lacks the knowledge to understand or deliver the message accurately.

Performing certain tasks while a subordinate is attempting to speak with you or ignoring a message because you believe the individual is not well informed about EMS delivery are examples of personal barriers that will impede communication.

When sending a message, make sure that the topics are clearly defined, include appropriate transitions to avoid confusing the listener, and ask for feedback from the receiver to ensure the message has been received and understood. If you are the listener, ask questions, take notes, and provide feedback to ensure that you have received the correct message. Remain engaged when someone is speaking with you and do not let personal bias interfere with the communication. Taking the time to listen to or deliver a message, without preconceived assumptions, will demonstrate that communicating effectively is important to you.

Physical Barriers

Physical barriers to communication fall into two categories: noise and distortion. Noise barriers can be environmental in nature—for example, construction taking place outside your office, telephones continuously ringing within the work space, employees congregating outside your office to discuss their weekend plans, employees coming into your office to ask questions, or a colleague who speaks very loudly and whose workstation is close to yours.

Distortion barriers are any disruption in effectively sending a message or decoding the message being sent. For example, there may be too much distance between the sender and the receiver (such as being in different locations), the chosen method of communication may not be effective, the climate in a room may be too hot or too cold and cause the receiver not to be fully engaged, or even road signs may not be clear with their intended message. Physical barriers caused by noise or distortion will cause a message not to be delivered effectively and must be addressed immediately.

Regardless of the type of physical barrier that is preventing or interfering with communication, the goal must be to identify the barrier and then either adjust to it or move away from the barrier.

Process Barriers

Process barriers occur whenever there is a breakdown with any of the processes that make up the communication system. The communication system begins with the sender crafting a clear message and selecting an effective medium to deliver the message. The message is then broken down and processed by the receiver, who provides feedback to the sender. A process barrier is any interruption to this communication process:

- Sender barrier: The sender fails to send the message.
- Encoding barrier: The sender is unable to state the message clearly.
- Medium barrier: The sender uses the wrong platform to convey the message.
- Decoding barrier: The receiver is unable to break down and understand the message being sent.
- Receiver barrier: The receiver does not pay attention to the message being sent.
- Feedback barrier: The receiver does not provide feedback, which leaves the sender wondering whether the message was understood.

Addressing process barriers can be quite challenging because these barriers encompass all of the processes that make up effective communication. Therefore, as the sender of a message, you must focus not only on being able to send the message effectively, but also on ensuring that the message is clearly presented and easy to understand. Furthermore, the sender has to ensure that the medium by which the message is sent is effective and can be accessed by the receiver. Next, the sender must follow up with the receiver to ensure that the message was delivered and understood correctly. This step, which is intended to ensure that the receiver has decoded and understood the message, provides an opportunity to clarify questions or feedback between the sender and the receiver. The sender must take the initiative to overcome process barriers when communicating by having a clear message, using the appropriate method for message delivery, and then following up to ensure that the message has been received and understood by the recipient. This will ensure that all steps within the communication process have been addressed and that no process barriers are present.

Semantic and Language Barriers

Semantic barriers include poor grammar, the use of technical or uncommon words, inclusion of too many topics without a clear transition, or use of words that have different meanings. **Language barriers** may be as simple as the receiver speaking a different language from the sender, but can also include the sender using technical terms with which the receiver is unfamiliar.

Semantic barriers are often encountered in electronic communications that use jargon such as LOL (laugh out loud), IMO (in my opinion), and OMW (on my way). At an EMS incident, an example of semantic barriers would be using radio 10 codes (e.g., 10-98 and 10-19) when the receiver is used to plain text. In this case, instead of using 10-98 and 10-19, the sender should be using plain text such as "assignment completed" and "returning to station." To avoid errors in code usage and understanding, many emergency response agencies have now adopted the practice of "clear text" when communicating with each other. As part of this system, the 10 codes have been replaced with basic language everyone can understand. Using appropriate terminology that both the sender and the receiver understand reduces the likelihood of a breakdown in communication.

If your office is responsible for the oversight of EMS, you may also have nonmedical employees in the office who are not familiar with medical terminology; this difference in employees' backgrounds may create a barrier in communication. In addition, consider the technical language used by emergency care providers, information technology administrators, engineers, and others in technical fields. Errors are likely to occur if not everyone within the organization is familiar with this terminology. Terminology issues among employees can be minimized by ensuring that your staff is trained to understand the technical language within the related field or by agreeing to use a language that all staff members understand.

When speaking with a customer who does not speak the same language or perhaps is not as fluent, you need to have someone available who is fluent in the customer's language.

WRAP-UP

Concept Review

- A managerial leader can expect to spend the majority of his or her time at work being engaged in a conversation with colleagues, team members, senior leadership members, customers, and others.

- The communication process includes seven basic elements:

  - The sender

  - The receiver

  - The message

  - Encoding

  - Decoding

  - Feedback

  - Noise

- Expecting team members to understand what you are telling them without providing them with clear direction and without asking for feedback to ensure that they understand the directive will most likely result in a poor performance outcome.

- Verbal communication must be clear, concise, and to the point, especially if you will not have a lot of time to discuss the message being communicated. Introducing a message and leaving it for someone to interpret with no opportunity for immediate discussion can create confusion.

- Written communication may be the most challenging because the sender cannot see the receiver's body language, the receiver may interpret the tone of the message as being offensive, and the sender will not be readily available to answer any immediate question the receiver has.

- Written evaluations of employees are most commonly done on an annual basis, but verbally acknowledging an employee's performance is essential and should be done more often than once a year.

- Many organizations have appointed media relations specialists or public information officers to deal directly with the media. These representatives most commonly have an established relationship with the media representatives within their local jurisdiction.

- Four types of barriers can prevent effective communication:

  - Personal barriers

  - Physical barriers

  - Process barriers

  - Semantic and language barriers

Managerial Terms

Crew resource management (CRM) A multidisciplinary management system with the primary goal of improving safety and efficiency by focusing on leadership, communication, situational awareness, teamwork, decision making, and use of all resources available to meet the goal.

Decoding How the receiver interprets the message.

Encoding How the sender formats the message.

Feedback The response from the receiver to the sender based on the message received.

Language barrier Use of a particular language or technical terminology with which the receiver of a message is not familiar.

Medium The format through which the sender is trying to communicate.

Message What the sender is trying to communicate.

Noise Any internal or external element that affects the message being received as the sender intended.

Personal barrier A breakdown in communication based on the sender's or receiver's poor communication.

Physical barrier Any environmental factor (including distance) that disrupts the communication process.

Process barrier A breakdown of communication based on failure of part of the communication process.

Receiver The person with whom the sender is trying to communicate.

Semantic barrier Use of confusing wording or sentence structure that keeps the receiver from understanding the message.

Sender The person who is trying to communicate.

Case Review: Impact of Short-Sighted Communication

Captain Thomas had been assigned to the training division for 5 years, but was recently promoted to district chief. District Chief Thomas would now be responsible for the supervision of six EMS crews, which consisted of a total of 12 front-line personnel. Many of the other district chiefs considered District Chief Thomas extremely lucky because he was assuming his leadership role in a district known for its outstanding commitment to the organization. The employees were model employees, their excellent patient care was well recognized by many of the local emergency department physicians, and the district was known for going above and beyond to help the organization become an industry leader.

Upon assuming the new role, District Chief Thomas e-mailed his crews, stating his expectations for all the employees in his district, including that poor performance would not be tolerated and that the crews would be disciplined if they failed to do their job. Several days after sending the e-mail, District Chief Thomas began noticing that the crews were giving him the cold shoulder when he visited the stations, were seeking operational answers from other district chiefs, and would do only the minimum work required to get through each shift. Input from the employees to improve the organization was no longer appreciated, and the district that was once one of the most productive became one focused on maintaining the status quo.

Case Discussion

What caused the once highly productive district to become one in which employees were just doing the minimum work required each shift? After interviewing the crews and asking them what prompted the change, it all came down to the way District Chief Thomas was communicating with his employees. The crews pointed out that he would send e-mails to the district that were considered unprofessional by the crews. Moreover, he would seldom communicate with the crews in person. District Chief Thomas failed to establish a professional relationship with his crews initially, then chose to communicate with them primarily via e-mail, which is rather impersonal. This approach created a void and diminished the opportunity for the crews and District Chief Thomas to begin establishing a professional relationship.

During a staff meeting, District Chief Thomas asked his colleagues for input in getting his district motivated again. He did not understand how such a productive district was now one just doing the minimum work required. During the meeting, the chief of the department recommended that District Chief Thomas meet face-to-face with his crews and asked them the same questions. Taking this suggestion, District Chief Thomas made it a point to meet with each of the crews. He opened each meeting by saying that feedback was encouraged and everyone could speak freely without fear of being disciplined. When the crews began to speak freely, they informed District Chief Thomas that they did not appreciate e-mail being the primary method of communication. The crews felt that communicating in person would be more effective and would demonstrate that he had an interest in what they had to say.

In addition, the crew found the content of the e-mail not only unprofessional but also confusing because it included terms not familiar to many of the crew members. District Chief Thomas was taken aback by this information because his intent had been to come across not as a micro-manager, but rather as a leader who supports his crews. His main reason for using e-mail was to allow the crews the flexibility to review his message on their own time. He explained that by visiting the stations, he believed he was taking up much of the time they needed to get things done. He stressed that his choice to communicate by e-mail in no way meant that he was not interested in meeting with the crews. He did not know that his e-mail messages were confusing to the crews because he was never told so, so he had not made any attempt to change the language used in his e-mails.

It was acknowledged by both District Chief Thomas and his crews that this was obviously a huge miscommunication on both sides. District Chief Thomas apologized to every member in his district, and moving forward he began meeting with crews once per shift. He chose to communicate by e-mail only when he needed to get a message to all team members within his district and time was a critical factor or if he was unable to meet with a crew member or members during the shift.

Soon after District Chief Thomas met with every crew member and all concerns were discussed, the district returned to its high-performing ways. The lesson was clear: E-mail can be an effective form of communication, but it should not replace face-to-face interactions.

Case Review: Message Not Received

Captain Nicks was asked to develop a training session pertaining to customer service. She booked several speakers—experts in the field—to participate in the one-day training session. All the speakers were confirmed to be in attendance on January 10 for the training. A week later, Captain Nicks got a call from the coordinator managing the event, informing her that the event would have to be moved to January 11. Since it was early September and the training had not been advertised to the public, Captain Nicks agreed that this would not be a problem. She sent e-mails to all the speakers informing them of the new date and assuring them that the new date was set in stone. All the speakers received the e-mail except for one. This one speaker arrived on January 10 and was not able to participate in the training session on the following day because he had another commitment. Paying for a speaker who was unable to attend the session was not only costly for the department, but also showed a lack of thorough organization, planning, and communication skills. Needless to say, Captain Nicks's boss was not pleased.

Case Discussion

What should Captain Nicks have done upon receiving the notice of the new date? It was fine to e-mail the speakers if they had been communicating via e-mail in the past, but Captain Nicks should have followed up with a telephone call to each speaker. This not only would have established clear communication between both parties, but also would have ensured that all speakers received the message, and it would have given Captain Nicks an opportunity to answer any questions the speakers might have had as a result of the date change.

5

Creating a Culture of Quality

Learning Objectives

After studying this chapter, you should be able to:

- Define the term *quality*.

- Discuss the history of quality initiatives.

- Discuss the benefits of quality management programs.

- Describe how to introduce quality into an EMS organization.

- Describe the components of quality management.

- Describe how to select a quality management program.

- Describe the tools used for continuous improvement.

Introduction

Recall a positive experience that you have had with a business such as a retail store, hotel, restaurant, airline, or hospital. Your positive opinion most likely resulted from the way you were treated during the interaction and the quality of the goods and/or service provided. Although price is an important factor, it is not the entire reason why we decide to engage with a certain organization. Would you buy goods or services because they were inexpensive if you knew the product would soon break or did not meet your expectations?

As an emergency medical services (EMS) officer, it is important to understand that both tangible and intangible items must be quality driven. Tangible items include goods, such as a stretcher, heart monitor, ambulance unit, or ECG strip; intangible items include services, such as the act of responding to the scene of an emergency or transporting a patient to the hospital. The EMS officer will primarily work with service delivery patient care (intangible), but will certainly be involved with the purchase of numerous goods (tangible) to ensure effective EMS operations.

When providing EMS, quality must be embedded at the very core of the service being provided to ensure it meets—or, even better, exceeds—customer expectations.

To ensure quality service delivery in EMS, it is important not just to look at how other EMS organizations provide quality service, but also to benchmark your organization against non-EMS-related industries. The goal is to learn how successful organizations best serve their customers, remain competitive, and provide a culture of quality across the organization. Benchmarking your organization against EMS industry leaders in the areas of patient care, customer service, marketing, budgeting, employee retention, crisis management, training, and strategic planning will certainly benefit your organization. Every EMS officer or other individual in a leadership role must be committed to a culture of quality and demonstrate the importance of quality to all members across the organization.

Many businesses are known for continuously delivering quality goods and services and excelling at exceeding customer expectations. Elements of the way in which these businesses operate can be adapted to EMS organizations. As the EMS officer, you can share your vision of quality and explain how you expect the team to deliver quality service. Recall that instilling a culture of quality is one of the five business priorities (5 BPs). By clearly describing your expectations for your team, you will ensure that all team members know their roles in delivering quality service.

Team members must embrace the fact that EMS is a business and is delivering a service. They should not assume that patients have no choice when requesting EMS simply because that organization is the sole provider for the community. Customers are very powerful, and they can either support the organization or abandon it. The moment an organization stops delivering quality services and becomes complacent, either the leadership team or the organization will be replaced. As an EMS leader, you must look at your patients as customers and exceed their expectations in the services you provide. Customer service (discussed further in the "Customer Service" chapter) is only one element of quality service.

Definition of Quality

The definition of *quality* may vary depending on who you ask, but a common thread can be detected among definitions. Regardless whether it is a product or service, the outcome must consistently meet or exceed a customer's expectations. Therefore, **quality** entails meeting or exceeding customer expectations by delivering goods or services consistently with minimal to no variation from the expected outcome.

As an EMS officer responsible for the organization's service delivery, why should having a formal quality system in place be at the top of your priority list? Delivering quality service, regardless of the business industry, must be a point of emphasis because it is what sets the organization apart from its competitors and it gives the patients the care they need.

The History of Quality Initiatives

The introduction and use of quality initiatives is nothing new. In fact, the quality philosophy dates back hundreds of years. More recently, during World War II, a surge in quality efforts occurred as part of a drive to ensure the safety of military equipment. Manufacturers used routine inspections and other quality control systems as a form of ensuring quality outcomes. Nevertheless, it was not until after World War II that a quality focus gained significant traction in business. Organizational leaders began to understand the importance of having a quality initiative, and the "total quality" philosophy was born.

Benefits of a Quality Management Program

All organizational leaders must demonstrate their commitment to quality. Numerous benefits can be realized from incorporating a **quality management program** into an organization, including the following:

- Improvements in organizational processes and systems
- Identification of processes that do not add value
- Reduction of operational and administrative waste
- Focus on meeting or exceeding customer expectations
- Detection of underperforming processes before they affect customer satisfaction
- Comparisons of similar processes to determine whether the processes overlap
- Informed decisions about keeping or eliminating processes
- Cost savings and promotion of a lean environment

The intent of a quality management program is to identify variations within current processes that might prevent the organization from delivering quality goods or services and meeting customer expectations. Variation produces a change in the output of a process. When variation occurs within a process or system, the organization will continually miss the intended outcome of quality goods or service. Without a quality management program, quality activities, and tools that make up the quality management program, your organization most likely will experience a loss of customers, increased expenses, duplication of work, poor outcomes, and loss of market share.

Correcting a process can be easy when customers tell you that they are unhappy with a specific product or service. (See the "Customer Service" chapter for more information on gathering customer feedback.) Unfortunately, customers often do not report their complaints to the business. A quality management program can help the EMS officer know whether his or her organization is meeting customer expectations, failing to meet expectations, or even having a detrimental effect on patients. The collection of such information and data is the primary reason any organization needs a quality management program. Many organizations conduct quality assurance reviews pertaining to patient care only. The EMS officer, however, must ensure that the quality management activities go beyond reviewing patient care charts and continuously address a broad spectrum of organizational EMS processes and systems. EMS delivery encompasses patient care, response times, on-scene times, transfer of care, transportation to the appropriate receiving facility, treatment modalities, and more. Given this wide scope of operations, quality assurance reviews are important, but they do not provide the entire picture. In addition to quality assurance, the EMS officer must consider quality control measures, continuous quality improvement, tracking outcome metrics, and more.

Introducing Quality Management to the Organization

To introduce the concept of quality within the organization or division, the EMS officer and those in managerial leadership roles must first understand that if a culture of quality is to exist within the organization, the initiative must begin and be supported by the top leaders of the organization. Establishing a culture of quality is a top priority; however, a culture of quality will be difficult to attain if the managerial leadership team does not have a plan in place to support such a culture on an ongoing basis.

Before implementing a quality initiative, the leadership team may establish a quality management team to ensure that all phases of the organization's new quality initiative have been addressed before it is presented to the organization. These phases may include introducing the desired culture, establishing a quality management program, selecting a quality management program, and identifying continuous improvement projects. Introducing a formal quality management program to the organization must be done slowly to provide an opportunity for all team members to grasp the required material in the program, prevent learning frustration, and avoid resistance to the new program.

The quality management training program must meet the needs of the organization and its members. Regardless of which program is chosen for the organization's quality initiatives, all members assigned to quality improvement projects must be trained to follow the organization's quality management program and be provided with the tools necessary to achieve the desired results (**Figure 5-1**).

Establishing a culture of quality will set the organization on a path to achieve operational effectiveness and efficiency, leading to excellence in service delivery. The success of a quality result-driven organization is directly related to the commitment by the organization's leadership team and its team members in embracing a culture of quality. Put simply, a culture of quality must be supported across the board—by the top leadership members, middle managers, supervisors, and front-line employees. To establish a culture of quality, the EMS officer must share a clear message regarding the importance of quality with all team members and must show his or

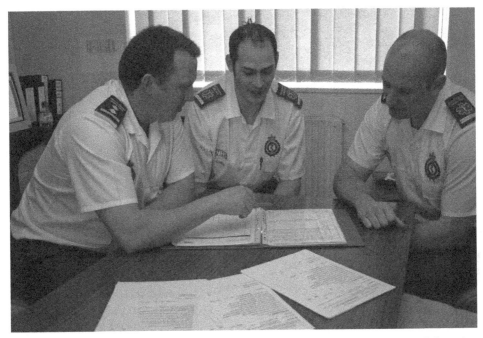

Figure 5-1 All members assigned to quality improvement projects must be trained to follow the organization's quality management program.

© Jones and Bartlett Publishers. Photographed by Kimberly Potvin.

her own commitment to the initiative. In addition, the quality initiative must have buy-in from team members and those at the top of the organization, who must make continuous quality improvement an organization-wide initiative.

Establish Leadership's Commitment to Quality

First, the EMS officer must demonstrate his or her own commitment to the organization-wide quality initiative. Although it is imperative to obtain buy-in from the team members, the initiative starts with those in the leadership role. That leadership team must be fully committed to the quality initiative before introducing it to the organization as a whole, and must demonstrate that all organizational leaders stand behind a culture of quality. It is paramount that the organization's leadership team not only introduce the quality management program and specific quality projects, but also demonstrate an ongoing commitment to quality outcomes across the organization. Unless the senior leadership team publicly embraces a new culture of quality, the new initiative is likely to fail. Thus the quality initiative must start at the top.

The EMS officer can demonstrate commitment to the organization's quality initiatives by being trained in quality management, providing opportunities for the team members to learn about continuous quality improvement, providing the team members with the tools necessary to achieve quality outcomes, asking questions and seeking input from the team members, and making it a point to celebrate successful quality outcomes with the team members.

Establish a Clear Message About Quality

The second step in establishing a culture of quality is to send a clear message about embracing a culture of quality and defining what the results of being a quality-driven organization will look like. The message must demonstrate how this initiative will impact the organization, its members, and its customers. The EMS officer cannot simply promote a culture of quality without taking action. If the quality initiative is to have a chance of being successful, quality must be deeply rooted in the organization and be embraced by every team member. The team members must understand the EMS officer's vision and appreciate why a culture of quality is important in getting the organization to a level where it is delivering quality outcomes.

Introduce Quality Across the Organization

Third, the total quality management approach must be an organization-wide effort that obtains buy-in from the team members. Quality management may be new to many of the team members, and as an EMS officer you must be prepared to work with any employees who are resistant to change. To achieve buy-in from the team members, the EMS officer must include the team members as part of the total quality decision-making process. The team needs to see that tangible results are possible within a quality result-driven organization and to understand that commitment from the team is invaluable in realizing the desired goals. In addition, the EMS officer should seek input from the team when attempting to identify quality improvement opportunities and then make the team part of the quality initiative.

EMS officers, as well as other organizational leaders, must be prepared to empower their team members and allow them to be part of the quality movement. The employees must feel that their role will be directly tied to the success or failure of the organization. It is important that all members understand what the organization plans to achieve through the quality management program, why it is important, and how they plan to get there. Also, the leadership team must provide mission and vision statements to help every member of the organization understand where the organization is heading (see the "Strategic Planning" chapter) and what role total quality management will play in helping the organization achieve its goals.

In some cases, the EMS officer may consider implementing a reward or incentive program to motivate employees when introducing the total quality improvement approach. This approach may pose some challenges, but, if done correctly, may be very effective. For example, the EMS officer may choose to recognize an individual or an entire team by giving them gift cards, paid time off, additional paid training of the individual's or team's choice, or some other token of appreciation. Many organizations celebrate their accomplishments as a team—a strategy that not only acknowledges the great work in successfully completing a project, but also fosters unity across the team and the organization.

When working with an incentive or rewards program, you must know what motivates your employees and make sure that employees are not rushing through a project just to get an award. Moreover, the EMS officer must ensure that all members have an equal opportunity to participate in continuous quality improvement projects and to receive rewards for the successful completion of projects. Any rewards must be truly earned; therefore, the project improvement outcomes must be measurable, key performance indicator benchmarks must be achieved, and the project must provide a real benefit to the organization and its customers.

Some organizational leaders have asserted that having a job and receiving a paycheck are enough reward and recognition for completing a project. Other managers express concerns about rewards and incentive programs because they create an additional expense for the organization and further limit the financial resources available for service delivery. However, it is imperative that every organizational leader take the first of the 5 BPs—people—seriously and remain committed to supporting the organizational members when introducing a quality management program for the first time.

Regardless of whether the organization chooses to establish a rewards or incentive compensation program, a total quality management approach cannot exist without continuous improvement; therefore, people (teams) must be your most valued asset. The team members are the driving force behind every organization's total quality management and continuous improvement process; organizational leaders, in turn, must let every team member know how much his or her role means to the organization and find ways to keep the team members engaged with the quality management approach. Consider partnering with a quality leader of a similar type organization who can share his or her quality experiences.

Ensure Quality Is Ongoing

Fourth, the EMS officer must ensure that the total quality approach is ongoing and not a one-time event. An effective quality management program will serve as the foundation and resource for every quality project and must be in place before tackling any project. Once the senior leadership team and the employees have made a solid commitment to quality management, a culture of quality is interwoven into the organization, and a quality management program is firmly in place, then the organization can begin addressing underperforming processes or systems. When deciding what will need improvement, if anything, the EMS officer must review the organization's (or division's) quality assurance (QA) outcomes, conduct a quality improvement survey that includes all members of the organization, and seek customer feedback pertaining to the organization's service delivery. With these data in hand, the EMS officer and team members must prioritize the quality initiatives, execute the improvement strategy, and evaluate the outcomes.

The steps for executing a process or system improvement initiative must be part of the organization's quality management program. This system should also incorporate a quality plan specific to the improvement of the underperforming processes or systems. In addition, the EMS officer must consider creating a **project charter**, a document that is commonly prepared by a senior leadership team member or the project manager and contains information about how the project will be managed. This project charter is subsequently shared with all participating team members, thereby ensuring that everyone knows what is expected and what his or her roles and responsibilities are throughout each phase of the project.

Once an underperforming process or system resulting in poor outcomes is identified using the QA process, the EMS officer must take action to either improve the underperforming process or system or eliminate it completely if it does not add value. If the EMS officer decides to improve the process or system, he or she must determine which quality tools and activities would best help remedy the underperforming process or system. The goal of using quality program tools and activities is to identify the root cause of the underperforming process or system, analyze why the problem is happening, take action to correct and improve the process or system, and ensure that the corrected process or system performs to the expected standard.

The implementation of a quality management program and the use of its tools and activities require training. Quality initiatives should be managed by someone who has experience in dealing with quality programs.

When initially rolling out a quality management program, start small, especially if the organization is new to working with continuous quality improvement methodologies. As the organization team members become proficient with quality improvement initiatives and their application becomes part of the organization's daily operational business, the EMS officer must support the quality movement by doing the following:

- Routinely evaluate the organization's strategic quality objectives and ensure that they are clearly defined
- Provide the necessary tools and training to maximize quality outcomes
- Ensure that the quality initiatives align with the organization's vision and the organizational performance measures are reflective of a quality-driven organization
- Ensure that continuous quality improvement initiatives are taking place at all levels of the organization
- Gather feedback from external customers to ensure that the organization is meeting or exceeding their expectations
- Gather feedback from internal customers and continue to empower the team members when making quality improvement decisions

Components of Quality Management

For a culture of quality to exist within an organization, the organization's senior leadership team must promote and continuously support a quality philosophy within all aspects of the organization. Within an EMS organization, the EMS officer must ensure that a quality system is in place to achieve administrative and operational (patient care) process excellence and to support a total quality management commitment. For a quality management program to thrive within an organization, the organizational leaders must choose the most appropriate quality management program and must have clearly defined quality objectives, well-understood policies, sufficient employee training for the activities, the tools necessary to achieve quality outcomes, and a commitment across the entire organization for continuous improvement.

As part of every quality management initiative, organizational leaders must select the quality management program that will best fit their organization's goals for achieving quality outcomes. Although each quality management program will have its pros and cons, all share similar goals focusing on achieving a level of performance excellence that will benefit the organization and its customers. Many EMS organizations already use quality management activities—for example, during patient care chart reviews. Quality planning, quality assurance, quality control, and continuous quality improvement are all activities that can help the organization when monitoring or correcting quality outcome issues.

Quality Planning

Quality planning is a critical component of quality management that is used when preparing to work on a specific project or when attempting to improve other organizational performance outcomes. Ultimately, the scope of the project will dictate what must be included within the plan. Therefore, a quality plan can be short or very long depending on the size of the project. The EMS officer must consider the following elements when creating a quality plan:

- Description of the project improvement initiative
- The project baseline (current) and benchmark (desired outcome)
- Who is responsible for the project (project manager)
- Which participants are assigned to the project
- Measurable objectives
- Evaluation of quality assurance, quality control, and quality improvement outcomes
- Which quality management tools will be used
- Which operational and administrative resources will be needed
- Feedback from stakeholders during and after project completion

The plan must be clear and concise, but adjustments should be anticipated as the program evolves. Only the items that will have a direct impact on the project and contribute to performance improvement should be included in the quality plan. Therefore, the EMS officer must become familiar with the scope of the project, determine what must be included in the plan, and then assign the project to the appropriate team members.

Regardless of which quality management program is used, the goal must always be to improve the organization's processes and systems, remove processes that do not add value, meet the organization's strategic and financial objectives, and deliver quality outcomes that meet or exceed customer expectations. Thus, four of the 5 BPs are impacted by implementation of a quality management program: people, strategic objectives, financial management objectives, and culture of quality.

The EMS officer must create a quality management program that will support the implementation of the organization's quality management plan. He or she must consider whether the following components are in place when building a quality management program:

- Senior leadership's commitment to quality management
- A quality management program that meets the needs of the organization and its customers
- Policies, procedures, and resources that are aligned with the quality management program and that support the organization's quality management movement
- Quality management training available to team members
- Quality tools available for team members to use
- Continuous improvement of processes and systems

Ultimately, the reason for implementing a quality management program is to ensure that the organization is well positioned to achieve the desired quality outcomes when delivering goods and services. If the organization has no operational or administrative support dedicated to quality management initiatives, it will be nearly impossible to achieve the desired quality outcomes. The EMS officer and those in managerial leadership roles must develop a quality management program that will support the organization's mission and vision.

When deciding which policies and procedures to put in place, it is important to seek input from the senior leadership team, because those managers will need to support the initiative to ensure its success. The individuals responsible for establishing a quality management program must keep in mind what they are trying to accomplish concerning service delivery quality outcomes. Why is delivering quality service a priority? How can the organization get there? Those individuals responsible for implementing a quality management program framework must also dedicate uninterrupted time to completing this project. This time might consist of 2 hours per week or a 3-day retreat; there is no rule as to how much time is needed. You simply keep going until the framework has been completed and is ready to be shared with the rest of the organization. The goal when implementing a quality framework that is supported by standard operating procedures (SOPs) is to ensure that any current and future members of the organization understand what is expected of them as part of the organization's quality management program.

After the quality management program is in place, the senior leadership team or those assigned to oversee quality management initiatives can add or remove policies, barriers, or processes that do not add value to the quality outcomes. In addition to gathering input from the senior leadership team, it is equally important to seek input from the team members. They are the individuals "in the trenches" who will be dealing with the future quality management policies and procedures on a daily basis. They, too, can answer many questions as to what will work and what will not. Obtaining their input can be accomplished by holding one-on-one meetings with the team members, walking around the work areas, and visiting EMS stations and speaking with the crews. The employees need to know that what they say is important and that their contributions to the organization's quality management movement are welcomed. As the organization begins to feel the quality buzz, a culture of quality will also begin to grow, as will the confidence needed to embark on quality management initiatives.

If someone within your organization has experience with quality management initiatives, ask that individual for help. If there is no one to offer guidance, you should get involved in a quality training session and not be afraid to jump in, rally the team, and determine where service delivery improvements can be made. Learn as you go along and continue to move the quality initiative forward. Having a thorough and well-organized quality management program in place is what will lead to the sustainability of current and future quality management initiatives. As the organization moves forward with current and future quality management initiatives, the organization's service delivery outcomes will be directly related to the senior leadership team's commitment to quality and the extent to which the employees embrace the quality management initiative.

Quality Assurance

Quality assurance (QA) is a quality management activity that monitors (audits) organizational standards and detects any variation from the expected delivery of quality goods or service. QA activity is required to ensure that the organization's quality objectives are being met. When it is used during EMS patient care chart review, for example, the reviewer attempts to identify any variation in the care rendered by the EMS providers from the organization's medical protocols (**Figure 5-2**). That is, the reviewer looks for treatment modalities, the completion of a head-to-toe assessment, proper documentation, documentation of all vital statistics in the report (including the time of patient assessment), electrocardiogram (ECG) tracings, and inclusion of any other medical directives within the patient's chart. Although each organization will conduct its QA review differently, it is essential to have a process in place that will monitor any variation from the desired outcome or from the organization's medical protocols.

The organization's medical director must determine what would be considered a variation from a protocol and must then share his or her expectations with the QA review committee. This step will ensure that all parties participating in the QA review process have clear direction regarding what is considered a protocol violation and understand what is expected of them.

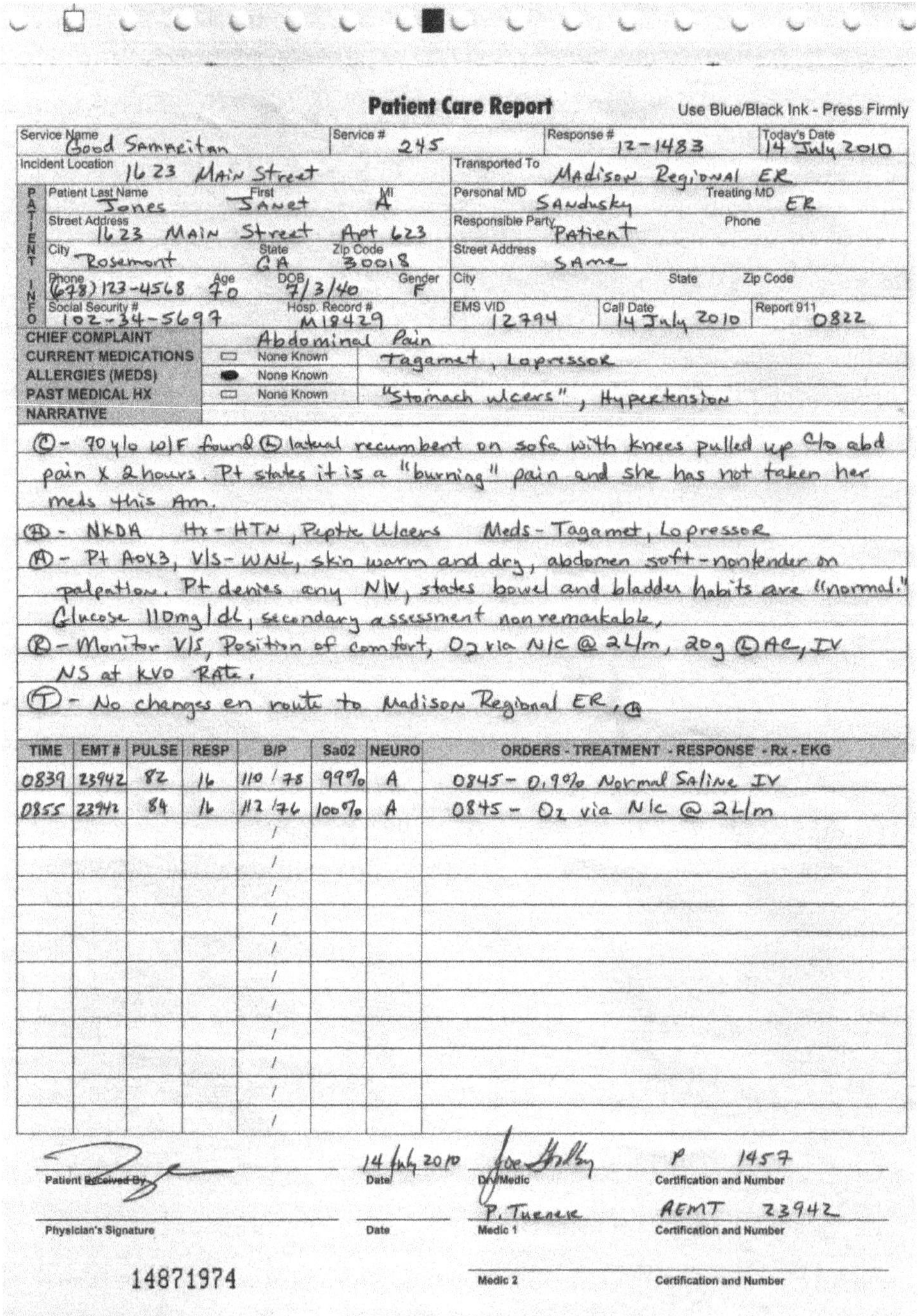

Figure 5-2 One element of quality assurance involves review of patient care reports to ensure they meet the organization's requirements.

Courtesy of Rhonda Beck.

The QA committee may comprise the organization's medical director, EMS officer, senior paramedics, and emergency medical technicians (EMTs). The goal is to provide balance and experience evenly throughout the committee, as the chart review process must be peer driven. This review process must not be confused with an investigation of wrongdoing; it is used merely to identify whether any variation from the organization's protocol has occurred and to determine whether the organization is meeting its target quality objectives.

Quality assurance is often confused with quality control, but they are actually different quality activities. Quality assurance is an audit or an evaluation of a business activity, such as patient care, whereas quality control is a specific activity within the quality management program set in place to ensure quality service is being delivered. Quality assurance is process oriented, ensuring that things are being done correctly; quality control is product oriented, ensuring the desired outcomes occur.

Quality Control

Quality control (QC) is a quality management activity that seeks to ensure necessary procedures are in place to support a quality outcome. If a violation of protocol is detected during the QA process, the first action must be to review the quality control mechanisms and determine which activities are in place to prevent the deviation in protocol. For example, the EMS officer must determine whether the medical protocols are concise and easy to follow, whether there is a protocol specific to the care in question, whether the organization has provided the required training pertaining to the care in question, and whether the crew member(s) had the necessary tools to provide the care required by protocol appropriately. These considerations, among others, will help the EMS officer determine whether the necessary quality control procedures were in place to prevent the variation from protocol.

As the EMS officer, you must ensure that you implement a quality control process so there is constant evaluation of the division's systems and processes prior to and after implementation of any operational or administrative activity. For example, quality control measures should be in place prior to care of a patient being conducted by prehospital personnel. This is done through protocols, training, providing the necessary tools, and so on. Then, through the quality assurance process, you will be able to determine whether the quality control processes are effective, need adjustment,

Managerial Leadership BRIEFCASE

Commitment Is Key

Every organization manages quality differently and uses different tools to achieve quality, depending on the quality management program used. The key for every organization, however, is a continued commitment to quality management.

or should be eliminated. Any process or system that does not align with the organization's quality plan and is not meeting or exceeding customer expectations must be addressed immediately. Subsequently, by using the continuous quality improvement process, you have the option to improve any underperforming activity or eliminate the activity if it does not add value.

Continuous Quality Improvement

Continuous quality improvement (CQI) is an ongoing quality management activity pertaining to continuous process and/or system improvements. First and foremost, those participating in the quality improvement activity must have a thorough understanding of the organization's processes and systems. The continuous quality improvement activity focuses on the use of tools that will lead to improvements in organizational internal and external outputs. These tools will be directly related to the quality management program adopted by the organization (e.g., total quality management [TQM] or Six Sigma). Therefore, it is important to become familiar with the tools included within the organization's adopted quality management program. The quality management program will set the standard for the quality tools used during continuous quality improvement initiatives. Examples of these tools include define, measure, analyze, improve, control (DMAIC); critical to quality (CTQ); cause and effect (fishbone) diagrams; process charts; and brainstorming.

Once a system or process has been identified through the quality assurance process as not meeting the organization's objectives, and the quality control measures are not ensuring quality outcomes, the organization must have a quality improvement activity in place to ensure that the variation is corrected. Furthermore, CQI should not be used solely when a process or system has been identified as underperforming during the quality assurance or quality control activities. Using the example of a medical protocol violation identified through the quality assurance process, the EMS officer, after reviewing the quality control procedures, must determine why the violation of protocol occurred and what can be done to ensure that a repeat occurrence is unlikely. If the reason for the violation is a lack of clearly defined protocols, minimal training to appropriately manage the patient, not having the tools available to provide the care, or negligence on the part of the provider, the EMS officer must make the necessary improvements to address the root cause of the problem and ensure that the protocol violation is not repeated.

Quality improvement is not a one-time event, but rather must be part of every quality management program and initiated quickly when a process or system is identified as underperforming—or even performing optimally. Improvements must be continuously evaluated. Organizational leaders must provide the necessary tools and empower their teams so they can improve processes and systems on an ongoing basis. These changes and continuous improvements must take place on the front lines, where service delivery meets the customer.

Sample Use of a Quality Management Program: Jones EMS

The Jones EMS Department, consisting of approximately 500 employees, realized that many of the EMS patient care reports were incomplete or never submitted to headquarters by the crews after completing an emergency response. This issue came to light when an administrative

Managerial Leadership BRIEFCASE

Resistance to Change

EMS officers and other organizational leaders must anticipate resistance from employees during the introduction of additional responsibilities, including those associated with a new quality management program. Resistance often results from the employee's uncertainty, in addition to the increased workload of learning new skills and taking on additional responsibilities and work duties. Also, if the organization has a collective bargaining agreement (union contract), the EMS officer will have to abide by the terms within the mutually agreed contract (between management and the labor force) regarding specific training.

How, then, as an EMS officer and managerial leader, can you overcome team member resistance when introducing a quality management program? If implementation of the program is within the scope of the bargaining contract, the following steps should help ensure success:

1. Be transparent and explain what the quality program will entail, the goals the organization is hoping to achieve, and the expected role for each member involved in the total quality management approach.

2. Seek input from the members of the organization. Make every effort to spend time with the front-line crews. Ride with the crews, spend time with them at the station, ask questions about what they would improve, and discuss why total quality management is important.

3. Explain any training that will be required and promote an environment of learning (one of the 5 BPs). Reinforce the idea of training as a lifelong process.

4. Demonstrate a commitment to quality, address any quality improvement process adjustments, report quality improvement outcomes, and continue to promote continuous quality improvement.

5. Celebrate the team's success with any quality improvement projects that have been completed. Provide recognition for members involved in the project to bring the organization's members together as you continue to promote a community of quality.

employee could not find a report that was requested by a local hospital a week after the incident had occurred. The organization did not have a quality management program in place; therefore, it was difficult to determine how long the organization had been experiencing this underperforming process. The Jones EMS director ordered an investigation to determine how many reports were incomplete or missing during the previous year. The EMS director immediately implemented a quality management plan that consisted of the following elements:

- The EMS director obtained senior leadership team support for the project and introduced a quality management program across the organization.
- The EMS director's vision was shared with all employees.
- Policies and procedures were implemented to provide guidance to all employees regarding the concepts and activities included in total quality management. The plan consisted of the following quality activities:
  - Quality assurance: To identify the variation from the expected outcome
  - Quality control: To ensure that the desired quality outcomes are achieved
  - Quality improvement: Consisting of tools to make the necessary improvements to the current process or systems
- The EMS director provided the team with direction and tools to accomplish the project.

Jones EMS Quality Plan in Action

The Jones EMS director created an action plan to address the underperforming process of completing patient care reports. The EMS director included the following actions as part of the quality action plan:

- Determining the root cause. Supervisors were not providing any oversight to ensure that patient care reports were completed prior to filing the report to headquarters. Also, many of the employees were not well trained in report writing and were unfamiliar with many of the functions that were part of the patient care report writing software.
- Determining why the underperforming process was not identified sooner. No quality management program was in place, which led to no quality planning, quality assurance, quality control, or continuous quality improvement activities. In the absence of a quality management program, many of the organization's activities, including patient care report writing, were not routinely evaluated for performance outcomes.
- Implementing a corrective measure and setting benchmarks. The EMS director requested that patient care report writing be part of the organization's quarterly in-service EMS training. The patient care report training would consist of a general review of patient care report writing management and instruction on how to troubleshoot the patient care report writing software. Information technology (IT) specialists were available during the training to answer any

technical software questions. In addition, an SOP was created, stating that all front-line supervisors were responsible for reviewing patient care reports prior to filing the reports to headquarters. As part of the quality management initiative, when a report was submitted for filing but was identified as being incomplete, the report was automatically returned to the employee for completion, and the employee was given 5 days to resubmit a completed report. Offenders were tracked for habitual patterns. Habitual offenders (employees writing the reports and officers responsible for reviewing reports) were not disciplined, but rather retrained to ensure they recognized the errors.

- The EMS director implemented a zero-tolerance policy for incomplete patient reports and expected 100 percent of reports to be thoroughly completed and ready for filing after the report had been completed. This quality initiative was evaluated for 30, 60, and 90 days post implementation for consistency. As part of the organization's commitment to quality management, moving forward, all of the organization's systems and processes would routinely be evaluated for variation from the expected outcomes.

As part of the action plan, the EMS director not only made every effort to correct the under-performing patient care report writing process, but also made a commitment to the implementation of the TQM philosophies and concepts on an organization-wide basis.

During the Quality Assurance Phase

Every morning, several team members would cross-reference the calls for service from the previous day with the patient care reports that had been completed and submitted to headquarters from that shift. This process would take approximately 2 hours, depending on the number of requests for service handled during the previous shift. If this process revealed that a report was missing or incomplete, the crew members would be notified and required to complete the report immediately.

During the Quality Control Phase

Initially, there were no quality control measures in place. Once the issue was identified, however, the following control measures were put into place:

- EMS field supervisors were required to review each completed patient care report before the report was submitted to headquarters.
- Increased emphasis was placed on documenting, completing, and submitting patient care reports to headquarters in all new-hire orientation classes and with senior employees.
- Every Monday morning, an e-mail was sent to all members of the organization providing an update on how many reports were missing or incomplete during the previous week.
- The organization acknowledged the continued improvements and celebrated the accomplishments across the organization.

Quality Improvement Phase

The organization implemented a policy that reinforced the importance of completing and submitting patient care reports after every emergency response. In addition, a brochure was created and disseminated to all field stations that outlined the proper procedure for submitting the patient care reports. This brochure also included instructions on how to submit a report in the event that technical issues with the computer arose, considering that all patient care reports were being submitted electronically. If a report was identified as being either incomplete or not submitted, the crew member would be notified electronically via e-mail and would receive a second notification when logging into the patient care report writing system. Lastly, a tracking system was implemented to detect habitual offenders who routinely did not complete their reports or did not submit them to headquarters after a duty-day. These individuals would be required to attend a short one-on-one in-service program to review the proper procedure for completing and submitting patient care reports. If the pattern continued, the employee would be issued a verbal counseling.

The EMS team was able to identify how many patient care reports were missing or incomplete during the previous year and used these data as a measurable starting point prior to beginning the quality improvement activity. The team then tracked improvement outcomes after the implementation of the continuous quality improvement activity. A total of 378 reports were either missing or incomplete prior to implementation. A total of 126 reports were identified as incomplete or not in the system after implementation of the quality management plan. Thus the organization achieved a 67 percent improvement within 6 months after initiating the improvement initiative.

There is no doubt about the importance of implementing a quality management program within every organization. The success of the Jones EMS Department clearly demonstrates what can be achieved if an organization has an organized and systematic quality management program that it can rely on when addressing underperforming processes or systems. The improvements in this case did not require in-depth or advanced quality tools or activities. Indeed, the Jones EMS Department kept the quality improvement process fairly basic, because it was the organization's first project and primarily focused on improving the report writing process. However, moving forward, the Jones EMS Department knew it was important to identify when any variations occurred from the expected outcomes for all organization-wide processes and systems, to ensure that quality control measures were in place to prevent variations from the expected outcomes, and to sustain the new quality management program. The organization, within a very short time, improved its outcomes by two-thirds, and there was potential for further improvement.

Selecting a Quality Management Program

The information included in this section is intended to serve as an introduction to commonly used quality management programs. EMS officers and other organizational leaders are encouraged to get involved and adopt a quality management program for their organization. When discussing quality management programs, similar programs may be referred to by different names. For example, several quality management programs use a total quality approach; however, the specific name of the program is likely to vary depending on the philosophy, quality tools, and the pioneer credited for creating the program. The quality philosophies are similar in that they aim to achieve total quality throughout the organization; meet or exceed customer expectations; increase revenue; reduce waste (materials and processes that do not add value); ensure continuous improvement of the organization's processes and systems; promote a culture of quality throughout the organization, starting with the leadership team; and ensure that all team members have the necessary tools and training to achieve quality outcomes.

The key for every organizational leader is choosing the program that will best fit the organization's needs. Options include total quality management (TQM), Six Sigma, ISO 9000, and Baldrige National Quality Program, among others. These quality management programs all share a similar philosophy about quality and a commitment to continuous improvement. Many quality programs share at least some of the same statistical tools, continuous improvement approaches, quality processes, and the total quality philosophy. **Table 5-1** lists seven prominent leaders of the quality movement and summarizes their philosophies.

Table 5-1 Total Quality Leaders	
Leader	**Philosophy**
W. Edwards Deming	Deming was invited by Japanese leaders to give lectures and provide guidance about quality in the post–World War II country. Although Walter Shewhart conceived the plan–do–check–act (PDCA) model, Deming was an influential advocate of the model, used statistical methods for process control, and was known for his 14 principles (presented in his book *Out of the Crisis*) used to make organizations highly effective. The introduction of Deming's 14 principles marked the beginning of the TQM movement.
Joseph M. Juran	Juran was a quality leader sought out by Japanese organizational leaders, in 1952, to give lectures and provide consulting on quality management. According to Juran, managing for quality consists of quality planning, quality control, and quality improvement—collectively known as the Juran trilogy.
Kaoru Ishikawa	Ishikawa, the so-called "father of Japanese quality control efforts," developed the concept of company-wide quality control (CWQC), quality circles, and quality education. He emphasized company-wide participation and seven basic quality tools: ■ Flow charts ■ Check sheets ■ Pareto charts ■ Cause and effect diagrams ■ Scattered diagrams ■ Control charts ■ Histograms

(continues)

Table 5-1 Total Quality Leaders (continued)	
Leader	**Philosophy**
Armand V. Feigenbaum	Feigenbaum is credited with developing total quality control (TQC) in an attempt to achieve quality. His basic principles emphasized serving internal and external customers and ensuring competitive advantage, market share, and productivity.
Genichi Taguchi	Taguchi was an engineer and statistician who is credited with developing specific quality techniques, known as the Taguchi Methods, to improve quality and reduce cost. One of these methods, quality loss of function, is a tool (an equitation) used to quantify customers' diminishing perception of value as production variation occurred, resulting in poor quality outcomes. Taguchi's methods focused on improving products and processes. Taguchi is credited with being the first person to identify the relationship between quality outcomes and cost.
Philip B. Crosby	Crosby concluded that quality performance issues could be addressed within the current management structure of an organization. His quality philosophies included the following: ■ Do it right the first time (DIRFT) and prevent multiple attempts to achieve quality outcomes of the same product or service. ■ Understand the process of manufacturing goods or delivering service. ■ Include the concept of "zero defects" as a performance measure and encourage managers to determine the price of not delivering quality goods or service.
Frederick Taylor	Taylor was an engineer and scientist credited with the development of industrial efficiency. Taylor conducted workplace experiments to find ways to achieve maximum performance efficiency, leading to what is known as Taylorism. Taylorism consists of the following basic scientific management principles: ■ Determine the most efficient way to get the work done. ■ Managers should spend time planning and training employees, while allowing the employees to complete the work tasks. ■ Evaluate employee performance and implement instructions to ensure that the most efficient methods of achieving the set tasks are being achieved. ■ Employees must be aligned with the jobs that match the employees' skill sets to achieve optimal performance efficiency.

Once a quality management program has been selected, the EMS officer will need to determine which activities and tools are part of the adopted quality management program. It does not matter which tools or which quality program is selected; the key point is to create a culture of quality (one of the 5BPs) throughout the organization and to determine which quality management program and tools will most benefit the organization in achieving the desired quality outcomes. As long as quality initiatives are taking place throughout all levels of the organization, the organization is on the path to achieve total quality management.

Prior to the selection of any quality management program, the EMS officer or organizational leader responsible for introducing a quality program must have formal quality management training. Having someone who is well trained in the quality concept, language, activities, and some of the tools is beneficial when it comes time to explain the quality philosophy to the rest of the organization and select the program that will be most beneficial to the organization. Although many quality management programs are used primarily by members of the manufacturing industry, they can actually be used within any type of business organization, such as EMS.

Several of the quality management programs in use today were created by highly regarded quality and management leaders of the past. One quality management leader in particular was regarded as a quality guru: Dr. W. Edwards Deming was credited with promoting quality improvement methods in the United States after World War II. His quality management programs were credited with contributing to the success of many well-known organizations—for example, the Toyota Motor Company, Allied Signal (now Honeywell), Motorola, and General Electric.

Although several quality management programs might potentially serve an EMS organization well, choosing the quality management program that will *best* fit the organization, its employees, and its customers is critical. When selecting a quality management program, you should not choose one program over another based on the fact that some other organization is using it. What works for one organization might not work for your own organization. Ask yourself what you are trying to accomplish, why you are trying to accomplish it, and how you can get there. Quality management is not a "one size fits all" proposition; rather, it must be tailored to the organization's desired outcomes. When determining whether your organization or functional workgroup can benefit from a particular quality management program, consider the following questions:

- Why should the organization implement a quality management program?
- Does a current process or system need improvement?
- Are there mechanisms in place to identify and correct variations and prevent defects?
- Are continuous improvement activities currently taking place throughout the organization?
- Is a new process needed?
- What will be needed to redesign a current process or design a new process?
- Who will be the project manager and team members if improvements need to be made to a process or system or when working on a new project?

Managerial Leadership **BRIEFCASE**
Quality for Business Survival

Quality is essential for the survivability of every organization, and ensuring that a culture of quality exists within an organization must be a priority for all organizational leaders. Choosing *not* to use a total quality management approach will result in decreased profits, a smaller market share, falling behind competitors, and a diminishing customer base.

Success in the BUSINESS WORLD

Copa Airlines

When introducing a quality management program to the organization, it is important to convey the message that quality management can exist only if the organization's members firmly support it. Quality management cannot exist without buy-in from members of the organization. Copa Airlines, for example, demonstrated that an essential component of its quality initiative was ensuring that every member understood the organization's vision and that the necessary resources were aligned appropriately to achieve the organization's goals.

Copa Airlines began as a small regional airline, but grew into one of the most highly ranked airlines in Central America and the Caribbean. In addition, the airline was recognized as having the best cabin crew and airport support in Central America and the Caribbean by the SkyTrax research group. Copa Airlines went from having 3 aircraft in 1991 to having a fleet of more than 90 aircraft in 2014. In the same time period, its flight destinations increased from 8 to 69. Prior to these remarkable improvements, Copa Airlines' arrivals and departures were on time only about half the time. After implementing a clearly defined vision—to be on time—as the company goal across the organization, Copa Airlines began to notice improvements.

Senior leadership members were committed to learning what airline industry leaders were doing successfully, and they observed that a high priority for the most successful airlines was to meet their arrival and departure schedules. Realizing how many passengers valued the on-time arrival and departure commitment from airlines, Copa Airlines made it a benchmark within its own organization. Company leaders vowed to do whatever it took to be on time. They were so committed to this benchmark that organizational leaders even videotaped how other organizations conducted their process flow and activities to meet the on-time departure and arrival goal. All processes and activities were measured to determine performance outcomes. If it was not being measured, the leaders figured, then it was not getting done.

The senior leadership team at Copa Airlines began to empower the front-line personnel to meet or exceed customer expectations; such decision-making power had previously belonged only to supervisors and pilots. Also, Copa Airlines made a commitment to reward all of its employees whenever the organization met a set benchmark. The organization celebrates these accomplishments on an organization-wide scale, even when the success occurred in just one division. Promoting a philosophy of teamwork and recognizing every team member for his or her contributions has paid handsome dividends for this growing airline.

- Does the team understand the goal of the project?
- Who will champion the project?
- How soon can employees start training?

All of these questions can be answered when an organization or functional workgroup has finally made a commitment to adopting a quality management program.

A few quality management programs are described in the remainder of this section. Only a brief introduction to each of these programs is provided here; if one of these programs will be adopted, additional research into its specific components will be required. Regardless of which program is ultimately selected, training must be a key priority for any quality initiative.

Total Quality Management

Total quality management is a management philosophy and program that emphasizes the importance of continuously improving processes and systems so as to deliver quality products and service. In addition, TQM strives to meet and exceed customer expectations by eliminating variations within the organization's service delivery outcomes. TQM is not just about data, charts, and measuring outcomes, however; it is also about people, both internal and external to the organization. Allowing the members of the organization to be part of the TQM initiative is just as important as collecting data.

The statistical charts that led to TQM were developed in 1923 by Walter Andrew Shewhart, an American engineer, physicist, and statistician. Shewhart is considered the father of statistical quality control, but other quality management theorists also played a critical role in promoting the importance of TQM, including W. Edwards Deming, Joseph M. Juran, and Armand V. Feigenbaum.

As manufacturers in Japan transitioned from production of military equipment to production of civilian goods after World War II, the quality of those companies' products often failed to meet customer expectations, resulting in a decreased demand for Japanese export goods. This trend, in turn, threatened the viability of Japanese manufacturing organizations. Japanese business leaders acknowledged that something needed to be done if they were to remain in business, so they sought assistance from several quality experts and other industry leaders as they worked to improve their production outcomes. Working independently of each other, Japanese manufacturing leaders and engineers invited the quality experts Deming and Juran to assist them in establishing the foundation for quality initiatives within their organizations.

The plan to turn around Japan's poor quality outcomes was embraced by Japanese business leaders; however, the plan included a different quality approach to doing business. Japanese business leaders acknowledged the importance of quality, but this new approach was based on "total" quality. In other words, quality needed not only to be in place to address certain products or services within the organization, but also to be present at all levels within the organization and with all team members. **Total quality** is a commitment to creating a culture of quality across all levels of the organization, ensuring that the goods and service meet or exceed customer expectations and that continuous improvement is at the center of every quality initiative.

Within about 20 years, the transition to "total" quality was achieved. Japan soon became recognized as the world's leader in quality, surpassing its international competitors. American organizations, for their part, often focused on the price of a product rather than its quality, and this approach ultimately led U.S. manufacturers to fall behind their Japanese competitors' quality approach of doing business. U.S. companies attempted to compete with Japan's quality improvement by adjusting their prices downward, but they soon realized that the better quality was at the very core of Japan's market success.

Quality was not completely absent from all U.S. businesses during the middle to late 1970s; in fact, many American organizations did use statistical tools for product inspections and identification of poor product outcomes. Nevertheless, quality remained a low priority for many American businesses. During the 1980s, however, U.S. business leaders realized that they had no choice but to address quality concerns within their organizations if they were to remain competitive in the world market. It was through Deming's guidance that American organizations began to understand the importance of total quality and to adopt this approach.

If TQM is the quality program adopted by the organization, training must be provided to all personnel on appropriate use of the tools that are part of the TQM program. Selecting, being familiar with, and using the tools necessary for continuous improvement is as important as selecting the quality management program that will best fit your organization. The following are key activities that support the TQM philosophy:

- One hundred percent customer satisfaction (internal and external)
- Prevention of variation from the desired outcome by committing to continuous improvement of processes and systems
- Leadership-driven program
- Corporate-wide initiative (e.g., finance, operations, training, fleet, communications, logistics)
- Continuous improvement, elimination of waste, zero defects, and setting best practice benchmarks
- Establishing performance measures
- Employee buy-in
- Culture of quality
- Quality training
- Celebrating success
- Employee empowerment

When working with TQM, all participants must have a clear understanding that customer satisfaction is paramount and that quality improvement must be involved in every step of the value chain, from the start of the process to the end. For TQM to work in your organization, everyone must be on board and willing to support the quality initiative.

Six Sigma and Lean

The **Six Sigma** quality management program focuses on achieving near-perfect outcomes. The goal with this program is to measure outputs, thereby identifying variations within a process or system, allowing the organization to make necessary improvements, and ultimately delivering a defect-free product or service. Six Sigma uses several tools (methodologies) for continuous improvement, including DMAIC, critical to quality definitions, cause and effect (fishbone) diagrams, and process flow charts. These tools are applied to improve processes or systems when working with the Six Sigma quality management program.

It is not uncommon to hear the terms *Lean* and *Six Sigma* used in the same sentence. The **Lean** quality program is based on the Toyota Production System (TPS). Although Lean and Six Sigma are slightly different in their approach to continuous improvement, they complement each other. The Lean quality approach focuses on eliminating waste (i.e., doing things over because of errors), eliminating excessive inventory, and using the necessary resources to ensure continuously flowing activities that add value to quality outcomes and enhanced speed of completing processes to meet or exceed customer expectations.

When working within the Lean philosophy, the members of the organization identify the steps in each of the organization's processes and systems that add value and those that do not add value. By eliminating waste, the organization is able to save money, have higher profits, and be more efficient with its internal and external operations. Waste is any step within a process or system that does not add value to the internal and/or external customers. Waste can also take the form of excessive inventory, poor continuous improvement flow, and poor outcomes. From an EMS perspective, waste is apparent when the organization purchases equipment that is seldom used, resulting in increased inventory; when poorly trained personnel translate into detrimental outcomes; and when having an increased number of units in service during non-peak times leads to increased costs to the organization.

Six Sigma, by comparison, focuses on identifying the variation (root cause) within a process and improving outcomes. Its goal is to deliver an error-free product or service. Lean and Six Sigma work well together because an organization should ideally make a concentrated effort both to prevent waste (Lean) and to deliver an error-free product or service (Six Sigma). Both of these quality activities can lead to a more profitable organization that exceeds internal and external customer expectations.

Success in the BUSINESS WORLD

Six Sigma at General Electric

Six Sigma has been adopted by many well-known organizations. In the late 1980s, General Electric (GE) began laying the groundwork for quality initiatives by implementing a quality program referred to as Work-Out. The goal for the Work-Out program was essentially to empower the organizational members, remove organizational barriers between departments, eliminate waste (non-value-added activities), and realign the organization's resources to achieve the desired outcomes. However, after the implementation of the Work-Out program, employee surveys indicated that the organization was still not doing enough to improve quality outcomes.

Chief executive officer Jack Welch decided to adopt a more robust quality program—Six Sigma—in an effort to transform GE. In implementing the program, Welch required that organizational projects and continuous improvement initiatives be managed through the use of the Six Sigma methodology tools. In addition, it became a corporate policy that all quality issues would be addressed using the Six Sigma program by 2000. GE's success depended on the following steps:

- Six Sigma was deemed a corporate-wide initiative and needed to be supported by all members of the organization, not just the leadership team.
- Six Sigma has different levels of mastery for those choosing to adopt the Six Sigma tools (e.g., green and black belts). GE used Six Sigma black belts to train members of the organization on the Six Sigma methodology and its many tools, which played a critical role in making Six Sigma part of GE culture.
- After the initial corporate Six Sigma training, GE used its own employees trained as Six Sigma black belts to serve as project leaders throughout the organization.
- Welch's commitment to the Six Sigma program was evidenced by the resources allocated to the program. Moreover, he incentivized employees financially with bonuses as well as promotions for successful Six Sigma project outcomes.
- Welch took a hands-on approach, stopping in during Six Sigma training sessions, answering questions, and visiting front-line team members and the organization's master black belt teams.
- Welch focused on the bottom line, stressing the importance of identifying variations, eliminating product defects, and ensuring that everyone understood that delivering quality outcomes was a corporate-wide initiative. Every team member needed to be involved if Six Sigma would stand a chance.
- GE depended heavily on its suppliers. The goal was to involve suppliers so they would be heavily invested with GE's Six Sigma initiatives.

General Electric's adoption of the Six Sigma quality management program not only promoted a culture of quality throughout GE, but within 2 years of its implementation at GE contributed to approximately $700 million in corporate benefits. It was the commitment from the organization's leadership team and all members across the organization that made Six Sigma work.

ISO 9000

Like other quality management programs, the one set forth by the International Organization for Standardization (ISO) has its primary focus on delivering quality products and services. ISO is an organization comprising members from different countries that publish standards intended to ensure products and services are safe, reliable, and meet specific quality levels. The ISO standards are geared toward a variety of industries:

- ISO 9000, *Quality Management*
- ISO 14000, *Environmental Management*
- ISO 22000, *Food Safety Management*
- ISO 31000, *Risk Management*

Although ISO 9000 (*Quality Management*) standards were published in the late 1980s, the ISO concept actually first began to gain traction in the 1940s, when delegates from several countries decided to create a new international organization to establish industrial standards (primarily in the manufacturing sector) that would ensure all products met the same quality specifications no matter where the products were sold. Organizations that adopted these quality standards as part of doing business, it was thought, would send the message that their products and services could be trusted by customers all over the world. ISO 9000 was created to ensure quality standards across all types of business sectors. This umbrella standard provides the framework for the ISO quality standardization program and includes terminology pertinent to ISO standards, but several subsections have since been formed to explore the individual components of the quality management program. For example, ISO 9001 includes quality management program requirements, ISO 9004 includes guidelines for making a quality management program more efficient and effective, and ISO 19011 includes guidelines for internal and external audits of quality management programs.

If an organization chooses to adopt ISO 9000 as its quality management program, it can either informally use the standards as guidelines to ensure quality outcomes or, more formally, seek to become a certified ISO organization. The ISO 9000 standards and guidelines can be applied in any business organization because they promote the use of quality management and continuous improvement activities and stress the importance of closely monitoring all organizational processes, not just a few of the processes within the organization.

As consumers, regardless of where we are in the world, it is important to know that when we purchase a product or use a service, the organization providing that product or service has implemented a set of standards that ensure its reliability and safety and its ability to meet our expectations. As medical practitioners, we have been taught to deliver, at a minimum, the "standard" of care when caring for our patients. If organizations are to remain competitive and strengthen their market share, they must adhere to a set of quality standards that provides a sense of security and consistency for their customers while reducing the organization's liability. When an organization demonstrates a commitment to quality, that commitment will both set it apart from its competitors and send a message to customers that the organization's product and service has met a set of quality standards that are continuously evaluated and improved. Furthermore, when organizations elect to do business in other countries, they may be required to show proof of their organization's quality standards. ISO 9000, like many other quality management programs, is used to ensure quality outcomes, and it achieves this goal by ensuring standardization of products and services.

The Baldrige National Quality Program

During the mid-1980s, many organizations in the United States were struggling both to compete with their international rivals and to stay viable within their local area. One of the major reasons why U.S. businesses struggled in this era was because they had made few investments in quality management programs. When U.S. companies started losing market share to international competitors, they had to adjust their business models and reexamine the importance of quality in their products or services.

In 1987, the U.S. Congress passed a bill, which was subsequently signed by President Ronald Reagan, geared toward recognizing organizations that demonstrated performance excellence by meeting a set of performance criteria. The award established by this legislation, named after deceased Secretary of Commerce Malcom Baldrige, identifies U.S. organizations that have demonstrated performance excellence within their organization as well as in their products and services. More than simply being an award, the Baldrige National Quality Award criteria serve as a framework for the foundations of performance excellence. Malcom Baldrige National Quality Award recipients have met all seven categories demonstrating that they are truly performance excellence organizations:

1. Leadership
2. Strategic planning
3. Customer market focus
4. Measurement, analysis, and knowledge management
5. Workforce focus
6. Operations focus
7. Business results

Organizations seeking to adopt the Baldrige Performance Excellence Program must incorporate this framework into their core values and culture and answer the Baldrige Performance Excellence Program questions specific to each criterion. To achieve the performance results the organization is seeking, it is important to understand what drives the quality management process. The seven criteria can be divided into three sections: leadership, system foundation, and results processes. The leadership section is responsible for oversight of the organization's strategic planning and customer focus (criteria 1–3). The link between the leadership and the results activities is criterion 4: measurement, analysis, and knowledge management. That is, the desired quality outcomes could not be achieved without measuring, analyzing, and knowledge management, which represents a commitment to continuous improvement. The results section (criteria 5–7) focuses on the workforce, operations, and ultimately delivering the results. The interrelationships of the criteria are shown in **Figure 5-3**.

Organizations may choose to use this program as a framework to ensure total quality throughout the organization or even apply for the Malcom Baldrige National Quality Award. Like other quality management programs, the Baldrige Performance Excellence Program stresses the importance of continuous improvement.

Leaders choosing to adopt the Baldrige Performance Excellence Program as the framework for total quality within their organizations must seek assistance from other Baldrige organization

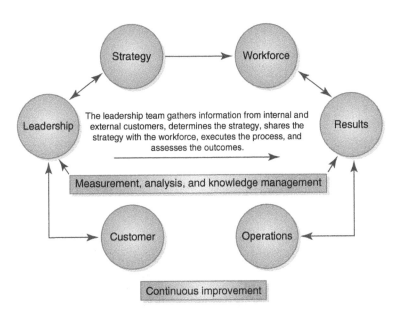

Figure 5-3 Baldrige Criteria for Performance Excellence.

leaders, learn the key components that make up the Baldrige Performance Excellence framework, and thoroughly understand what it takes to be a Baldrige Performance Excellence organization before rolling out such a program. As an organizational leader, team members will look to you for guidance after the program has been implemented within the organization. The commitment to quality and continuous improvement starts with you.

Quality Tools for Continuous Improvement

When working toward implementing a quality management program, the leadership team must learn the requirements and tools that are part of the program. Numerous tools have been developed, and many are used in multiple quality management programs. If a specific quality tool has proved beneficial when team members are working with continuous process improvement activities, then it should be used regardless of which quality management program has been adopted. Organizational leaders must keep in mind that the goal is to achieve total quality across the organization; therefore, using tried-and-true tools must be the priority. This section describes several quality tools used in quality management programs to improve the organization's quality outcomes.

DMAIC

DMAIC is a Six Sigma methodology tool that can help identify a process or system that should be improved. DMAIC—which stands for "define, measure, analyze, improve, and control"—can give the team a roadmap to ensure that everyone stays on track.

- *Define:* The EMS officer clearly defines set goals and objectives for organizational processes and systems under his or her responsibility. The EMS officer must routinely ask himself or herself whether the current organizational processes and systems are performing at optimal efficiency and effectiveness. This is done by reviewing key performance indicators (KPIs) and defining the goals that must be met to achieve the desired outcomes in meeting or exceeding customer expectations.

- *Measure:* Metrics are set to evaluate performance outcomes. Each measure must be specifically defined to include what is being measured and how it must be measured, to maintain consistency. The EMS officer must review the functional unit's or organization's processes and systems and collect data to determine whether the functional unit or organization is achieving the set goals. If the organization is not tracking performance outcome data, it will be difficult to identify underperformance of its processes and systems. For example, how will the officer know how long it takes the crews to get on scene after being dispatched, how long they are on scene managing the patient, how long the transport times are from the scene to the hospital, how long hospital turnaround times are, or how successful the crew members are when initiating intravenous access or performing endotracheal intubation? If the process or system is not measured, there will be no way of knowing how well the actual performance outcomes are measuring up to the expected outcomes.

- *Analyze:* The EMS officer gathers all data that suggest the presence of a problem (not meeting KPIs) and begins to uncover the root cause of the variation in the desired outcome. The EMS officer continuously analyzes current processes, technology, customer needs, and external forces that are continuously changing. What was once a quality process may, however, be outdated 6 months or a year later.

- *Improve:* The EMS officer removes the root cause of the underperformance by either implementing a new process, improving the current process, or eliminating the process if it does not add value. The EMS officer must also empower team members across the organization to make the necessary adjustments to improve the process.

- *Control:* The EMS officer monitors the new processes to ensure that the root cause of the problem has been removed and that the problem/variation will not recur. The officer must be diligent to eliminate variations from quality production.

Critical to Quality Tree

Another tool used to measure quality outcomes is the critical to quality (CTQ) tree, which is often used as part of the Six Sigma quality program (**Figure 5-4**). The CTQ tree is used to identify the critical components for achieving a desired outcome. It can be used in many different business sectors, including EMS. Steps taken when creating a CTQ tree include the following:

- The EMS officer first identifies those components that are critical in delivering quality goods or service (e.g., training, equipment, staff, customer service).

- After the EMS officer or quality team identifies a need for a process or system improvement, they must determine the key drivers in achieving the desired outcomes. Drivers are designed to move the improvement process toward the goal of delivering quality goods and services.

- When the drivers are in place, the team determines whether the drivers have been effective by measuring and assessing the outcomes. Are the desired outcomes being achieved? Are the outcomes meeting or exceeding internal and external customers' expectations? Such questions must be answered before accepting that the critical components for quality have been achieved.

Value Stream Mapping and Process Flow Chart

Part of any continuous improvement process is a clear delineation of the steps required to evaluate the activities and to improve the flow of production or service delivery. Recall that

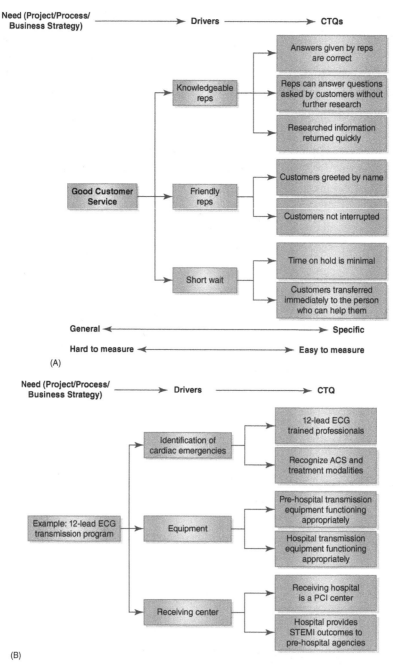

Figure 5-4 A. Sample CTQ tree. **B.** A 12-lead ECG transmission project set in a CTQ tree.

speed was one of the critical components within the Lean quality approach; in turn, value stream mapping and process flow charts are two quality tools regularly used within the Lean quality program. However, they could also be used on their own (without Lean) to improve processes.

Value stream mapping (VSM) is a technique that is used to illustrate the steps in a process or system and that can be extremely beneficial for an EMS officer who is attempting to track the flow of EMS activities. In addition to tracking each step in a process or system, VSM requires analyzing each step in detail to provide information that will allow the quality management team to determine which improvements need to be made to ensure quality outcomes (**Figure 5-5**). For example, a value stream map may focus on the activities involved from the time an emergency request for service is received at the dispatch center until the unit has completed its assignment. However, the value stream map should not include only those activities that make up the process or system, but rather should also include details about each segment of the process and the time it takes to move from one activity to the next—for example, the time it takes a dispatcher to process the request for service, the time it takes a crew to acknowledge the call, the on-scene time spent managing the patient, the time spent transporting the patient to the hospital, and the time spent transferring patient care to hospital staff.

Each of the components of the value stream map must be dissected and analyzed to determine whether each activity is functioning effectively and efficiently. The EMS officer, along with the quality management team, must evaluate the activities that go into each step of the value stream and determine the time it takes to move to the next step. The goal is to have the entire process or system be as efficient and effective as possible and to eliminate wasted activities that add no value in meeting or exceeding customer expectations.

If analyzing each step in a process is not required, but a general overview of a process or a system is needed, a **process flow chart** will be extremely helpful. Such a chart includes the start and finish points within a process and the tasks that make up the process. When creating a new process flow chart, it is important not to make the chart too complicated and to thoroughly review each step to ensure the activities have been clearly delineated.

Creating a process flow chart also requires familiarity with a few symbols that are important for process mapping (**Figure 5-6**). There are three main symbols (oval, rectangle, and diamond), but use of many additional symbols can contribute to the utility of the chart (**Figure 5-7**).

Cause and Effect (Fishbone) Diagram

After discovering a variation in a process or system, determining the root cause of that variation is critical to eliminating it, and selecting the right cause and analysis tool is a priority. The cause and effect (fishbone) diagram shown in **Figure 5-8** is an effective tool for this step. With this tool, you can move backward from the ultimate effect and determine which causes and effects in different areas helped lead to the ultimate effect.

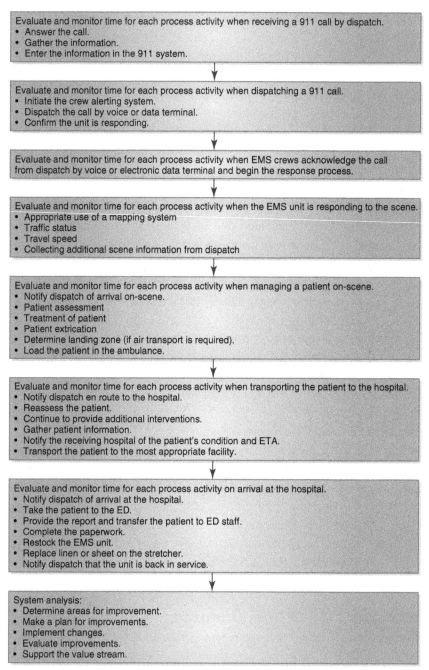

Evaluate and monitor time for each process activity when receiving a 911 call by dispatch.
• Answer the call.
• Gather the information.
• Enter the information in the 911 system.

Evaluate and monitor time for each process activity when dispatching a 911 call.
• Initiate the crew alerting system.
• Dispatch the call by voice or data terminal.
• Confirm the unit is responding.

Evaluate and monitor time for each process activity when EMS crews acknowledge the call from dispatch by voice or electronic data terminal and begin the response process.

Evaluate and monitor time for each process activity when the EMS unit is responding to the scene.
• Appropriate use of a mapping system
• Traffic status
• Travel speed
• Collecting additional scene information from dispatch

Evaluate and monitor time for each process activity when managing a patient on-scene.
• Notify dispatch of arrival on-scene.
• Patient assessment
• Treatment of patient
• Patient extrication
• Determine landing zone (if air transport is required).
• Load the patient in the ambulance.

Evaluate and monitor time for each process activity when transporting the patient to the hospital.
• Notify dispatch en route to the hospital.
• Reassess the patient.
• Continue to provide additional interventions.
• Gather patient information.
• Notify the receiving hospital of the patient's condition and ETA.
• Transport the patient to the most appropriate facility.

Evaluate and monitor time for each process activity on arrival at the hospital.
• Notify dispatch of arrival at the hospital.
• Take the patient to the ED.
• Provide the report and transfer the patient to ED staff.
• Complete the paperwork.
• Restock the EMS unit.
• Replace linen or sheet on the stretcher.
• Notify dispatch that the unit is back in service.

System analysis:
• Determine areas for improvement.
• Make a plan for improvements.
• Implement changes.
• Evaluate improvements.
• Support the value stream.

Figure 5-5 Value stream mapping (EMS response).

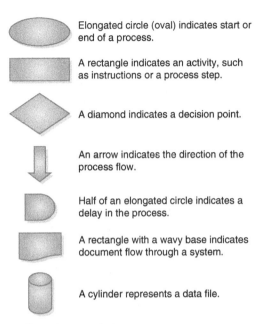

Elongated circle (oval) indicates start or end of a process.

A rectangle indicates an activity, such as instructions or a process step.

A diamond indicates a decision point.

An arrow indicates the direction of the process flow.

Half of an elongated circle indicates a delay in the process.

A rectangle with a wavy base indicates document flow through a system.

A cylinder represents a data file.

Figure 5-6 Common process flow chart symbols.

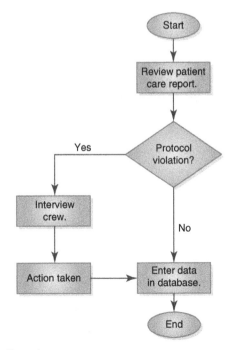

Figure 5-7 Sample process flow chart.

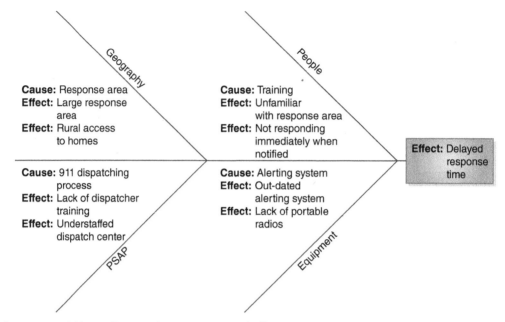

Figure 5-8 Fishbone diagram showing cause and effect.

Plan-Do-Check-Act

Plan–do–check–act (PDCA) is a cycle used as part of the continuous improvement process. The PDCA cycle is included in many quality management programs, such as ISO and the Baldrige Performance Excellence Program, but it can certainly be part of any organization's continuous improvement business activity. Also known as the Deming cycle (after its creator), the Shewhart cycle, or plan–do–study–act (PDSA), PDCA is used to control and manage continuous improvement. When attempting to eliminate a quality control issue, you may consider this plan, which consists of the following elements:

- *Plan:* Design or redesign a business process by setting goals that will meet or exceed internal and external customer expectations.
- *Do:* Execute the plan to achieve the goals set in the plan phase.
- *Check:* Determine how well the plan is working by measuring its performance.
- *Act:* Support the plan if it is successful. If changes are required, then the cycle starts over with planning the necessary adjustments to improve the process, then moves through the do–check–act phases again. The cycle repeats until the desired outcomes are achieved.

The PDCA cycle is effective and easy to follow when attempting to improve your organization's processes (**Figure 5-9**).

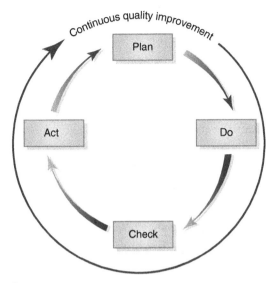

Figure 5-9 The PDCA cycle.

Benchmarking

To evaluate how well the EMS organization or division is performing, the EMS officer must have a thorough understanding of the organization's practices, processes, systems, products, and services. In addition, the EMS officer must review the performance outcome data pertaining to the processes and systems. Only then will he or she have the opportunity to make truly beneficial improvements. The question becomes, "What is acceptable or best in the business performance outcome?" Organizational benchmarking is extremely valuable because it requires the EMS

Managerial Leadership BRIEFCASE

Quality Training

Continuous quality improvement can be labor intensive and overwhelming. Therefore, quality training must be a requirement for all team members who will be dealing with quality improvement initiatives. Learn from other organizations and industries, and then choose a program that will add value when improving your own organization's processes and systems. Your competition is striving to outperform you, and quality is a critical component in determining the leader in any market segment. It is especially important in the healthcare business, where providing the most up-to-date EMS care can have life-saving consequences.

officer to gather information from other organizations. These data can be captured by calling other organizations or networking with other professionals during seminars, by reading posted information about the organization on its website, and through electronic surveys. The data gathered in this way can then be compared to your organization's performance data to determine how well your organization matches up with its competitors.

When working on a benchmark plan, the EMS officer should do the following:

- Consider whether an identified service delivery component is underperforming as compared to the competitors. Is a process or system not meeting best practice standards? Are any performance outcomes resulting in dissatisfied customers?
- Determine how the organization can ensure that it is using best practices with its processes and systems and how it can become a leader within the EMS industry.
- Assess and survey industry leaders within and outside the industry for performance-improvement practices.
- Continuously monitor the organization's processes, systems, and service delivery outcomes to ensure the organization exceeds customer expectations and stays ahead of its competitors.
- Determine whether the organization has a quality management program in place.

Benchmarking means comparing your business processes, practices, and metrics to those of organizations that are industry leaders. Several types of benchmarking should be considered when creating a benchmarking plan:

- *Competitive benchmarking:* In competitive benchmarking, you assess how well your organization is performing compared to the competition. How do your customer loyalty, customer satisfaction, and branding compare to your competitors'?
- *Functional benchmarking:* This type of benchmarking focuses on the product or service provided by the organization. For example, if you are in the healthcare business and provide emergency care, then you will compare your services to those offered by a leading healthcare organization.
- *Internal benchmarking:* This form of benchmarking compares the internal units (divisions) of the organization to those of industry leaders. For example, how long does it take from the time a patient is dropped off at the hospital until a report is completed? How long does it take for the report to be approved for quality assurance and then sent to a billing agency? Internal benchmarking compares the internal processes of the organization to the best practice processes within the industry.
- *Strategic benchmarking:* This form of benchmarking observes the practices, processes, products, and services of industry leaders not necessarily within the same industry as your organization. It allows your organization's leaders to look outside their industry and learn from other best-practice organizations. For example, when Motorola was developing its pager system, Motorola representatives traveled all over the world to observe how retail companies used a notification system for product deliveries. To improve the processes, practices, products, or

services of your organization, you should focus not only on best-practice organizations within your industry, but also on all industries' practices.

Performance measures and benchmarking must be part of every organization's continuous improvement plan. The EMS officer must have a system in place to evaluate EMS performance outcomes, evaluate and implement new benchmarks, make improvements, and ensure that the organization is exceeding customer service expectations. The ultimate goal for the EMS officer when working with performance measures, benchmarking, quality management, continuous improvement objectives, and exceeding customer expectations is to align the organization's resources to meet the operational and administrative demands and achieve the desired service delivery outcomes.

Balance Scorecard

A **balance scorecard** is a management tool that focuses on aligning key business practices and processes with the vision, mission, and strategy of the organization. It is used by numerous service industry organizations, and its goal is to ensure that the organization is well balanced to provide quality products and services. The balance scorecard, which was developed by Drs. Robert Kaplan and David Norton as a performance measurement framework, assesses the organization from four perspectives:

1. *Learning and growth perspective:* Make sure your employees are learning and growing with the organization. Implement new training programs so they can stay informed of the latest practices.
2. *Business process perspective:* Implement metrics to monitor the performance of your business, and continuously monitor and benchmark your practices, processes, products, and services. Consider new service delivery or product opportunities.

Managerial Leadership BRIEFCASE

Performance Measures

EMS officers must routinely evaluate the quality of services rendered by personnel working under their supervision. Given this need, implementing a system that will track performance outcomes is critical. If no performance metric plan is in place, the EMS officer will be unable to determine the quality of service being delivered. If the service delivery is not being measured, the officer cannot manage it appropriately.

Performance measures are usually stored and displayed in a spreadsheet or project management software system described as a cockpit or dashboard (**Table 5-2**). This system allows organization leaders to quickly review the compiled data and detect underperformance.

Table 5-2 Sample Chart Template for Performance Measures

Dept.	Strategic Goal	Strategic Obj(s).	Performance Benchmarks	Target	1st Quarter (ends 12/31/2015)	2nd Quarter (ends 03/31/2016)	Owner
EMS	Maintain a high-performing EMS system	Ensure that the organization's ambulance units consistently achieve a quick turnaround time upon arriving at the hospital	Ambulance units will not exceed a 15-minute turnaround time from arrival at the hospital to back in service	Ambulance units will achieve hospital turn-around times within the 15-minute benchmark 95% of the time	Ambulance units achieved 90% of hospi-tal turnaround times within the 15-minute benchmark.		

Table 5-3	Sample Balance Scorecard		
Perspective	**Goal**	**Measure**	**Target**
Learning perspective	Train department paramedics in critical care paramedicine	CCEMT-P certification	50% of department paramedics must be certified
Financial perspective	Decrease budget expenses	Organization's master budget	10% overall annual reduction in expenses
Customer perspective	Achieve a customer satisfaction survey score > 4.5	Customer surveys	Achieve > 4.5 on a 1–5 Likert scale (1 = lowest score; 5 = highest score)
Business perspective	Add one EMS station each year for the next 5 years	New EMS station being operational by providing service delivery to the community	Completion of one EMS station each year for the next 5 years and completed within the 1-year time frame from the start date

3. *Customer perspective:* Survey your customers. Remember that customer satisfaction is critical to staying in business.
4. *Financial perspective:* Every organization must be fiscally healthy to remain in business. Every EMS officer must understand funding, revenue, and expenditures.

These four perspectives are essential in ensuring that the organization is balanced to achieve the desired outcomes. They are not just part of the 5 BPs, but must also be part of the organization's strategic plan. With these perspectives in mind, the next step is to determine the goals, measures, and targets specific to each of the four perspectives (**Table 5-3**).

Basic Statistical Tools
In addition to other quality management tools, statistical tools are used to measure outcomes. Although many of the statistics can be computed using a calculator, it is advisable to explore the wide variety of statistical functions found in Excel and similar spreadsheet programs. They can prove highly beneficial when you are working with large numbers and multiple data sets.

Although quality management programs include many statistical elements, you do not need to be a statistician to implement the program; basic math skills are typically sufficient. Training that includes more advanced math skills, however, may enable the team to have deeper understanding and wider use of the quality management tools at their disposal. It is a good idea to complete practice assignments with the quality tools prior to full implementation of a quality improvement project. By conducting training drills, the EMS officer and other organizational leaders will have an opportunity to address areas of weakness and ensure that team members have the necessary training.

Several basic statistical terms, measurements, and charts can help when working with process improvement management:

- **Mean**: The sum of the values divided by the number of values; the average.

  Example: The Jones EMS Department wanted to know the average number of EMS transports per ambulance during a specific year. To provide this value, the team took the number of transports for the year, and then divided that number by the number of Jones EMS ambulance units (**Figure 5-10**). Bear in mind that an average can be misleading when compared to the actual transports done by each of the ambulance units.

- **Mode**: The value that occurs most often.

  Example: The Jones EMS Department was analyzing the number of minutes it was taking to transfer patient care to a local emergency department during peak time and identified the most common transfer time (the mode) (**Figure 5-11**).

- **Median**: The midpoint in a series of values.

  Example: Using the same data for patient transfer times, the Jones EMS Department wanted to obtain the median, which is the center point of the data. The median represents the

EMS Units	Number of Transports	EMS Units	Number of Transports
Med 1	1225	Med 12	908
Med 2	1449	Med 13	1933
Med 3	1404	Med 14	2272
Med 4	1063	Med 15	492
Med 5	1683	Med 16	891
Med 6	1430	Med 17	1825
Med 7	1710	Med 18	1439
Med 8	1918	Med 19	2388
Med 9	825	Med 20	993
Med 10	1667	Med 21	1229
Med 11	765	Med 22	695
		Mean	**1373**

Add the number of transports for all units (30,204) and divide that total by the number of EMS units (22) to find the mean transports per EMS unit (1373).

Figure 5-10 Sample mean calculation.

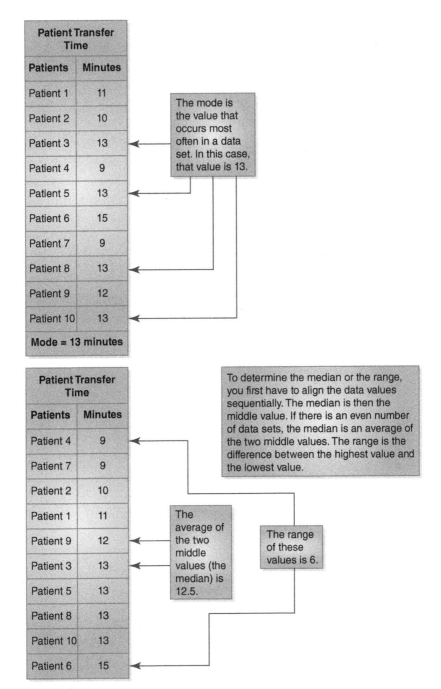

Figure 5-11 Sample mode, median, and range calculations.

halfway point of the entire data set. The data must be placed in ascending order and then the number in the middle is selected. For example, if the data values are 2, 4, 7, 8, 10, the median is 7. If the number of data sets is an even number (as in the example of patient transfer times), take the average of the two center numbers (12 + 13 = 25; 25 ÷ 2 = 12.5). The median in this case is 12.5 (Figure 5-11).

■ **Range**: The difference between the highest and lowest numbers in a set of values.

Example: Using the patient transfer data, the Jones EMS Department wanted to know the range of the data, which would provide insight as to the spread from the lowest data set to the highest (Figure 5-11). However, this statistic should be used only to support additional data research because it does not give an overall picture of the activities being captured.

■ **Trend**: A movement of a series of data points in a specific direction over time. In the Six Sigma quality methodology, six or more points continuously increasing or decreasing from the median and in the same direction indicate a trend.

Example: The Jones EMS Department was exploring the addition of a peak ambulance unit and needed to determine an in-service time frame. The department conducted a year-long analysis of the number of responses at different times of day (**Figure 5-12**). It determined that the trend of increasing demand for service delivery began at around 6:00 a.m., with the busiest time of the day being between 10:00 a.m. and 11:00 a.m.

■ **Variation**: A value or data point that differs from the mean.

■ **Standard deviation**: The amount of variation or distance from the mean. Knowing the standard deviation gives a clearer picture of the data being analyzed.

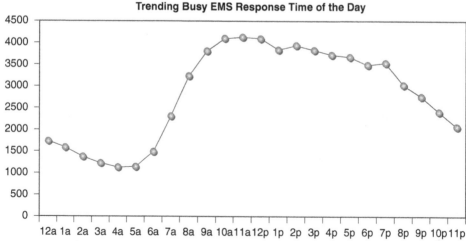

Figure 5-12 Sample trend graph.

Example: Jones EMS Department has an average on-scene trauma time of 8 minutes, which meets its on-scene performance benchmark of less than 10 minutes. Initially, it seems Jones EMS is meeting its goal. When analyzing all data points, however, the following on-scene times are observed: 5 minutes, 8 minutes, 13 minutes, 6 minutes, 12 minutes, and 5 minutes. Thus two data values not only exceed the organization's benchmark, but exceed it by at least 50 percent. In this particular case, it is easy to identify the outliers because there are not many data sets. By obtaining the standard deviation, you can determine how close or "tight" the on-scene numbers are to the mean and the normal range for most of the data. The following steps will help you calculate the standard deviation, but software programs (such as Excel and MINITAB) can also calculate it for you (**Figure 5-13A**).

1. Find the mean (i.e., average) of the data.
2. Calculate the variance. The variance is the squared difference from the mean. The variance calculation must be done for each value individually. First, subtract the mean from the data value. Second, square this difference (multiply it by itself). Once all the differences have been squared, calculate the mean of these new values. This is the variance for the entire data set.
3. The square root of the variance is the standard deviation. A small standard deviation indicates that the values are close to the mean, whereas a large standard deviation indicates that the values are away from the mean.

The standard deviation is usually illustrated by plotting a normal distribution curve (**Figure 5-13B**). With a unimodal (one-peak) symmetrical bell-shaped curve, it is easier to note how much variation exists between specific data points and the mean. The farther away from the mean the data point is, the higher the likelihood that there is a defect that must be corrected. In looking at Figure 5-13B, with the mean, variance, and standard deviation calculated in Figure 5-13A, you will find the mean (8) at the center. Adding (moving toward the right) and subtracting (moving toward the left) the standard deviation of 3.24 yields the numbers under the chart. For example, 8 (mean) + 3.24 (standard deviation) is 11.24 at 1 standard deviation, 11.24 + 3.24 = 14.48 at 2 standard deviations, and so on. This spread encompasses all the times captured by the EMS department. In this case, most of the data fall within 1 standard deviation. The two data values of 12 and 13 minutes that fall within 2 standard deviations require further investigation because the greater the variation, the poorer the outcome.

- **Control limit chart**: A chart with upper and lower limit specifications that pertain to a process or system (**Figure 5-14**). Control charts are beneficial in detecting variations and can be used within any business organization.

Example: The Jones EMS Department began measuring many of its processes and tracking some of the EMS activities. Variations from the expected quality outcomes were identified. Working with the local hospital administrative team, EMS team members discussed EMS to

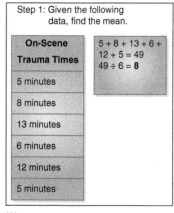

Step 1: Given the following data, find the mean.

On-Scene Trauma Times	$5 + 8 + 13 + 6 +$ $12 + 5 = 49$ $49 \div 6 = 8$
5 minutes	
8 minutes	
13 minutes	
6 minutes	
12 minutes	
5 minutes	

Step 2: Calculate the variance.

(Value – Mean)²

$(5 - 8)^2 = 9$

$(8 - 8)^2 = 0$

$(13 - 8)^2 = 25$

$(6 - 8)^2 = 4$

$(12 - 8)^2 = 16$

$(5 - 8)^2 = 9$

$$\frac{(9 + 0 + 25 + 4 + 16 + 9)}{6} = 10.5$$

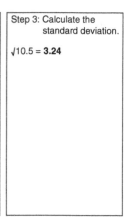

Step 3: Calculate the standard deviation.

$\sqrt{10.5} = 3.24$

(A)

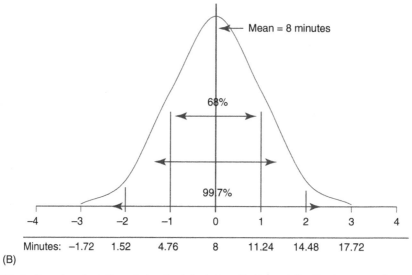

Mean = 8 minutes

68%

99.7%

	-4	-3	-2	-1	0	1	2	3	4
Minutes:		-1.72	1.52	4.76	8	11.24	14.48	17.72	

(B)

Figure 5-13 **A.** Sample calculation of standard deviation. **B.** Normal distribution curve for sample data.

balloon times (E2B). They acknowledged that the more quickly EMS crews identified that the patient was experiencing an ST-segment elevation myocardial infarction (STEMI) and alerted the hospital, the more prepared the hospital would be in managing the cardiac emergency. After setting a benchmark of sending a STEMI alert to the receiving emergency department, the ED team achieved door-to-balloon (D2B) times of less than 90 minutes 100 percent of the time (average time 57.5 minutes). Using a control limit chart, each STEMI response was tracked and crews were given 2 minutes to conduct a rapid assessment upon arrival at the scene (lower limit); 8 minutes was the threshold (upper limit) to transmit the ECG to the receiving emergency department upon STEMI identification on the ECG.

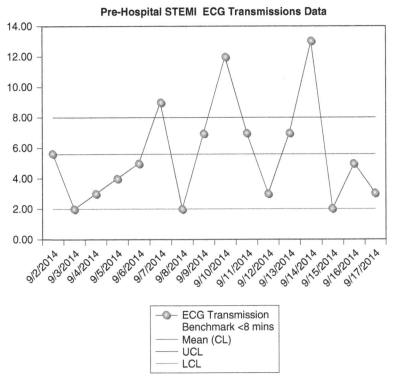

Figure 5-14 Sample control limit chart.

■ **Scatter plot**: A graph in which individual data points are plotted in two dimensions to show their relationship.

Example: An EMS organization was considering the implementation of several peak-time response units and wanted to identify the busiest times for service delivery requests. The quality management team captured response data and placed it in a scatter plot for discussion and strategy planning (**Figure 5-15**).

■ **Histogram**: A group of vertical bar graphs illustrating data points and the frequency of each data point.

Example: The Jones EMS Department wanted to review the time it took crews to identify a stroke patient. The quality team observed, by using a histogram, that most medical emergencies were being identified as strokes within 6 minutes (**Figure 5-16A**). The stroke alert benchmark was set at less than 8 minutes, just like the STEMI performance measure. The EMS director was also interested in monitoring customer service and requested that customer surveys be provided to customers and their feedback be represented in a quarterly report. The customer survey results were set in a bar graph (**Figure 5-16B**). In a

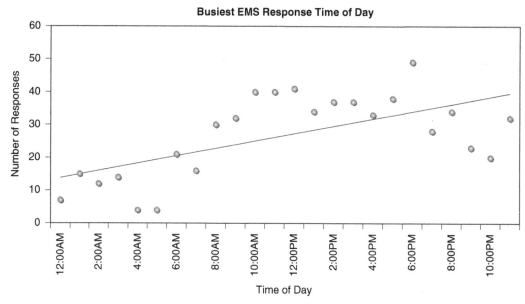

Figure 5-15 Sample scatter plot chart.

histogram, the bars are clustered together and the independent variables are quantitative in nature; in a bar graph, the bars are separated and the independent variables are qualitative in nature.

- **Pie chart**: A circular graph divided into sections containing specific data assigned to each section (**Figure 5-17**).

  Example: The medical director requested a review of pain relief provided to patients with chest pain. The goal was to identify how many of these patients achieved relief after one administration of nitroglycerin sublingual (spray) versus how many required additional medication for pain relief. For those patients who did not achieve pain relief from nitroglycerin, the quality management team would then obtain the patient's hospital discharge diagnosis to see whether the chest pain was cardiac in origin. If the chest pain was not cardiac in origin, the EMS quality team, the training division, and the medical director would work together to determine whether the patient's initial presentation provided any clues to the patient's true underlying condition. This information would then be shared with the EMS crews as part of the organization's EMS medical training in-service program. The initial data was observed over a 3-month period and placed in pie charts for review.

- **Pareto chart**: A graphical bar view, where bars are in descending order, representing the greatest issues affecting an organization (**Figure 5-18**). It helps identify where improvements should be made, based on the principle that 20 percent of sources are creating 80 percent of the problem (80/20 rule). It is one of the most commonly used quality tool to help identify areas of the organization that are underperforming and prioritize which areas to tackle first.

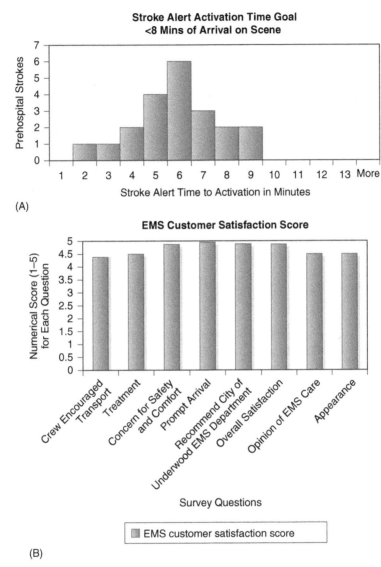

Figure 5-16 A. Sample histogram. **B.** Sample bar graph.

Example: The City of Underwood EMS chief wanted to address what areas of EMS service delivery could be improved. The EMS chief reviewed 6 months' worth of complaints and shared the information with the rest of the organization by placing the data on a Pareto chart, which organized the complaints from most to least common. It was noted that 80 percent of the complaints were related to delays in response and refusing to take patients to a hospital of choice. With this data, the EMS chief decided to focus on improving response times and revisiting hospital choice protocols.

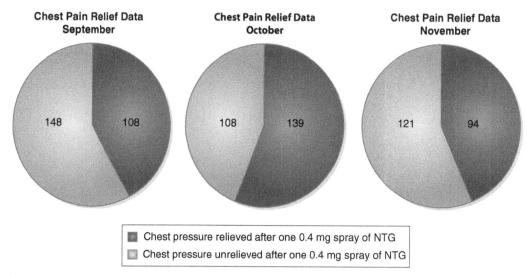

Figure 5-17 Sample pie charts following data over a 3-month period.

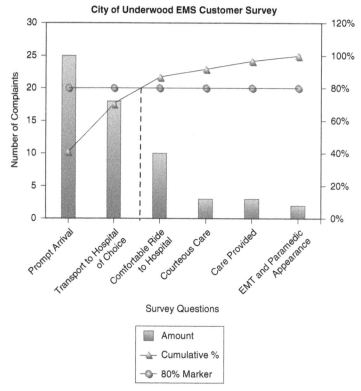

Figure 5-18 Pareto chart.

Frequent use of these tools will improve your proficiency with them and allow you to learn more about data processing and how it can facilitate some of your managerial duties. Setting up the analysis accurately and inputting the appropriate data will produce a clear picture that will help you make better business decisions.

Managerial Leadership **BRIEFCASE**

Standard Deviation and Sigma

The standard deviation is also known as sigma—the same *sigma* discussed in conjunction with the Six Sigma quality program. The Six Sigma quality management program strives to reduce variation by continuously improving processes, and sigma (standard deviation) indicates how much variation or distance exists from the mean or intended target. Six Sigma attempts to reduce the variation to the point where customers seldom receive defective products by reducing the sigma spread and keeping that target product or service within the specification limits. If an organization uses a Six Sigma approach to quality, it hopes to produce only 3.4 defects per million opportunities (DPMO). Many industries are committed to performing at a Six Sigma level or higher.

WRAP-UP

Concept Review

- For an EMS officer, it is important to understand that both tangible and intangible items must be quality driven.

- *Quality* is meeting or exceeding customer expectations by delivering goods or services consistently with minimal to no variation from the expected outcome.

- The use of quality initiatives dates back hundreds of years.

- The intent of a quality management program is to identify variations within current processes that prevent the organization from delivering quality goods or service and meeting customer expectations.

- Establishing a culture of quality is a top priority; however, a culture of quality will be difficult to achieve if the managerial leadership team does not have a plan in place to support such a culture.

- A quality management program encompasses four basic activities:

  - Quality planning
  - Quality assurance
  - Quality control
  - Continuous quality improvement

- Several different quality management programs use a total quality approach; however, the name of the program may vary depending on the philosophy, quality tools, and the pioneer credited with creating the program.

- If a specific quality tool has proved beneficial when working with continuous process improvement activities, then it should be used regardless of which quality management program has been adopted.

Management Terms

Balance scorecard A management tool that focuses on aligning key business practices and processes with the vision, mission, and strategy of the organization.

Benchmarking The process of comparing one's business processes, practices, and metrics to those of industry leaders.

Continuous quality improvement (CQI) A management process activity to make immediate or ongoing improvements to organizational processes or systems. The improvements are made by applying quality improvement tools. Also called *continuous process improvement*.

Control limit chart A chart with upper and lower limit specifications for a process or system.

Histogram A group of vertical bar graphs illustrating data points and the frequency of each data point.

Lean A quality program focused on eliminating waste.

Mean The sum of a set of values divided by the number of values; the average.

Median The midpoint in a series of values.

Mode The value that occurs most often in a data set.

Pareto chart A graphical bar view, where bars are in descending order.

Pie chart A circular graph divided into sections, where specific data is assigned to each section.

Plan–do–check–act (PDCA) A quality management program used to control and manage continuous improvement.

Process flow chart A diagram or algorithm that displays each step in a process.

Project charter A document, commonly prepared by a senior leadership team member or the project manager, that contains information about how a project will be managed.

Quality Meeting or exceeding customer expectations by delivering goods or services consistently with minimal to no variation from the expected outcome.

Quality assurance (QA) A quality management process established to monitor (audit) organizational standards and detect any variations from the organization's goods or services delivery desired outcomes.

Quality control (QC) A quality management process intended to ensure that necessary procedures are in place to support a quality outcome.

Quality management program A program that consists of methods used to achieve quality outcomes. Such programs include management activities and methodologies to support continuous quality improvement. Also called *quality methodology program*.

Quality planning A component of quality management that involves creating a plan to improve organizational performance outcomes.

Range The difference between the highest and lowest numbers in a set of values.

Scatter plot A graph in which individual data points are plotted in two dimensions to show their relationship.

Six Sigma A quality management program focused on achieving near-perfect outcomes.

Standard deviation The amount of variation or distance from the mean.

Total quality A commitment to creating a culture of quality across all levels of the organization, ensuring that the goods and service meet or exceed customer expectations and that continuous improvement is at the center of every quality initiative.

Trend A movement of a series of data points in a specific direction over time.

Value stream mapping (VSM) A methodical process, pertaining to the flow of organizational activities, that identifies the analysis and elements included in each of the activities that make up the process.

Variation A value or data point that differs from the mean.

Case Review: Improving Dispatch Times

The Boyed EMS director assigned the administrative team to review the organization's 911 system process flow and to identify areas where improvements were needed. Fortunately, the team had recently completed a 2-day introduction to quality management. The session had covered not only the role of the leadership team when working with quality programs, but also some of the differences among common quality management programs and tools used for continuous improvement. The assignment had perfect timing, because the group was eager to apply some of the tools they learned during the training session.

The leadership team members assigned to the project first created a quality plan that would include the appropriate approach in achieving the desired outcome. The plan included a process flow chart identifying each process within the 911 system:

- Request for service received by the dispatcher
- EMS crews notified of the request for service
- Unit response to the scene
- Arrival on scene
- Transport patient to the hospital
- Crew arrives at the hospital
- EMS crew transfers patient care to hospital staff
- Crew prepares the unit for the next response
- Crew is back in service

After each process was labeled in the process flow chart, the team defined the expected outcomes for that process, then measured each current process outcome against the organization's goal for each of the steps. The team analyzed the data and observed that all of the processes were meeting the organizational benchmarks except for the time it took to process a 911 call when first received at the dispatch center. Currently, it was taking dispatchers an average of 124 seconds to dispatch a call to the crews; the department's benchmark was 90 seconds.

During the improvement phase, the team was able to apply the tools introduced during the quality management training session—for example, the cause and effect (fishbone) diagram and the critical to quality tree—to improve the current underperforming process. It was determined that the dispatchers were taking too much time gathering information and providing medical care instructions, ultimately delaying dispatch of the units. It was also noted that there were not enough personnel during the afternoon and evening shifts to meet the call load demand. After informing the EMS director and communications center manager, the personnel schedule for those shifts was adjusted until additional personnel could be hired. After hiring the necessary personnel (two per shift), the dispatch team started meeting and exceeding the target threshold of 90 seconds or less.

The project team continued to monitor the activities, during the control phase and beyond, to ensure that the dispatch times continued to meet the organization's benchmark. After confirming that the improvements had been successful, the EMS director and the communication manager standardized the process by including the staffing level in the organization's SOPs.

The EMS director was impressed with the team's methodical approach to process improvement. After observing the results and the continuous improvement process, she made total quality part of the organization's culture and made continuous improvement training a requirement for all leadership personnel, who would then promote the quality activities throughout the organization. The director also requested value stream mapping for many of the systems in place within the organization (e.g., logistics, fleet services, purchasing, billing for service, 911 service delivery). The goal was to improve efficiency and eliminate those activities that did not add value.

Case Discussion

This was a relatively small project, but it allowed organizational members to work together on a process improvement project, use quality tools, and develop a quality management program approach that worked for the organization.

Case Review: Working with the Team for Quality

The Gold EMS Department was considered an industry leader for many years, and its employees were proud to be part of the organization. Mr. Miller, an assistant director of the Gold EMS Department, was promoted to EMS director after the former EMS director retired. Shortly after taking the post, Mr. Miller began to micro-manage his employees and implement new processes without sharing his vision with any of his leadership team. In addition, he requested information and assigned tasks to employees without including the employees' supervisors in the loop. Mr. Miller began requesting data to be collected that had already been collected, resulting in wasted time and effort. He refused to listen when employees attempted to share the data they had collected and were tracking on a regular basis. Mr. Miller's actions created a duplication of effort, implementation of processes that did not add value, and increased costs. His actions did not promote a culture of quality, and it did not take long before Mr. Miller met with resistance when implementing new processes. Employees grew increasingly frustrated and eventually the organization became stagnant.

Mr. Miller may not have had a clear plan, but if he did indeed have one, not sharing it prevented the organization from moving forward. Mr. Miller was eventually replaced. The Gold EMS Department then slowly regained a culture of quality, began delivering positive performance outcomes, and created an environment of inclusion for its employees. The new EMS director's vision was shared with all employees. It will take a while before the Gold EMS Department successfully meets its standard of delivering quality service; nevertheless, there is no doubt that with the introduction of the new culture, the organization will be back as an industry leader in the near future.

Case Discussion

Quality initiatives are about changing the status quo, and it takes real leadership and the flexibility to change if the data show a change is indicated. So where did Mr. Miller go wrong? This case has multiple issues, but the root cause of many of them is the lack of communication between Mr. Miller and his employees. Every individual in a leadership role must make every effort to communicate his or her vision and business expectations with the members of the organization.

Mr. Miller also attempted to micro-manage his employees, which not only led to employee frustration and disengagement, but also produced a failure in performance outcomes. For the EMS officer with numerous direct reports, it is important to ensure that employees are successful in their roles, to support their work initiatives, to guide them when necessary, and to encourage continuous learning.

Mr. Miller did not inquire about which division of the organization had a quality system in place. Therefore, he had no idea which processes and systems were being tracked, how the data were being collected, why the team members were collecting those data, what the data had shown in the past, and which performance improvements had been made as a result of the data collected. In his ignorance, he overlooked the systematic and organized quality assurance, quality control, and quality improvement management initiatives already in place. This issue goes back to one of the key responsibilities of an EMS officer hired to a new position: Evaluate the existing processes and systems before implementing new ones.

6

Customer Service

Learning Objectives

After studying this chapter, you should be able to:

- Explain the importance of quality customer service.

- Describe how to create a customer service plan.

- Describe the importance of, and methods for, following up on customer issues.

- Describe how to evaluate a customer service plan once it is implemented.

Introduction

The most important factor in an organization's success is satisfied customers. Without customers, a business organization would fail. Regardless of whether the organization is a for-profit or non-profit enterprise, customer service must be at the very core of the organization's culture of quality (one of the five business priorities [5 BPs]). The goal must be to exceed customer expectations in the hope that customers will reward you with their loyalty. *Good* customer service is no longer enough; your organization must *exceed* customer expectations.

There are two types of customers: external customers and internal customers. **External customers** are the traditional customers to whom your organization provides goods and services; they are outside of the organization, meaning that they do not work for your organization. **Internal customers**, in contrast, work for your organization and depend on your support to ensure that they have the necessary tools to better serve the external customers.

In emergency medical services (EMS), it can be difficult to think of patients as customers, or even clients. Although this text refers to them primarily as customers, they do not cease to be patients. Patients are one kind of customer with whom EMS professionals interact; the use of the term *customer* allows us to look at the patient from another perspective, from a wider angle.

The Importance of Quality Customer Service

There is nothing more frustrating to customers than poor customer service. Have you ever walked into a division within your own organization and heard the words, "We're busy right now. Come back later?" Consider the customer who arrives at a hotel with a confirmed reservation, only to find that no rooms are available, or the customer who receives different answers from different employees within the same organization. If the employees all work for the same organization, they should provide the same answers to questions on policies and procedures. These examples reveal a lack of communication among employees and management. Inefficient processes, poor employee attitudes, poor-quality products and services, and a failure to exceed customer expectations will certainly affect customer satisfaction.

Employees must embrace the organization's core commitment to customers if the organization is to succeed. As the EMS officer, you must create, implement, and evaluate a plan within your organization that embodies the attitude of exceeding customer expectations for your internal and external customers. People—whether internal or external to the organization—represent the first of the 5 BPs, and keeping them not just satisfied, but pleasantly surprised with the organization's services, must continue to be a priority.

Before you tackle the challenge of creating a customer service plan, ask yourself why having a customer service plan is important and what you are trying to accomplish by developing one. Having a customer service plan is critical because it helps differentiate your organization from its competitors. In addition, when customers have an opportunity to know an organization and understand what they can expect in terms of its services, then as long as their experiences are positive, the customers will be supportive of the organization. As the EMS officer, you will need to ensure that quality customer service goals, objectives, strategy, and tactics are included within the organization's (or functional workgroup's) strategic planning process.

A customer service plan is commonly created either by an employee project team with customer service experience or by the leadership team. Regardless of who creates the plan, upon its completion it must be shared with the organization's members, supported by the organization's leadership team, and routinely evaluated. Taking care of customers with the goal of meeting and exceeding their expectations must be part of the organization's culture. Although the delivery of customer service may vary depending on demographics, the service being requested by the customer and the resources available to meet and exceed those expectations must be considered as part of every customer service plan.

Creating a Customer Service Plan

The first step in creating a customer service plan is to determine who will be responsible for overseeing the process and ensuring that a customer service plan is created. The organization's leadership team must also determine who will be responsible for managing the customer service initiative once it becomes part of the organization's strategic plan.

The next matter to consider when creating a customer-centric plan is who your customers are and what they expect from your organization. This understanding is instrumental both in creating a customer service plan and in continually reevaluating that plan. After identifying the organization's internal and external customers, it may be beneficial to categorize customers further into primary, secondary, and tertiary rankings. For example, a patient would be considered an external primary customer, the patient's husband or wife would be considered an external secondary customer, and a neighbor may be considered an external tertiary customer. When working with internal organizational customers, any individual with whom you interact on a regular basis (e.g., finance manager, fleet manager, supply manager) would be an internal primary customer, and members within those functional units would be the internal secondary and tertiary customers. Identifying organizational customers helps the organization's leadership team and all members obtain and align the necessary resources to meet and exceed specific customer expectations.

Each customer will have slightly different requirements from the organization. Consequently, the plan developed should be specific enough to ensure quality customer service is delivered and flexible enough to address nontraditional customer requests, if at all possible. The customer service strategic plan must identify the organization's various types of customers and include what those customers expect from the organization and the organizational resources available to meet their requirements. The plan must also be routinely evaluated to ensure adjustments are made when necessary.

Managerial Leadership **BRIEFCASE**

Strategic Planning for Customer Service

During the strategic planning process, the strategic team members must address the planning of a customer service initiative. The approach to formulating a customer service strategic plan is similar to the approach for developing other operational or administrative strategic plan initiatives. Consider how the organization's vision applies to internal and external customer service and conduct a SWOT (strengths, weaknesses, opportunities, and threats) analysis. Consider the goals and objectives that must be achieved. Which tactics will the organization use to achieve the customer service strategy and thereby meet its objectives? The strategic planning team must examine what other successful customer-centric organizations are doing to meet and exceed customer expectations. Setting customer-centric benchmarks is beneficial when establishing the foundation for a strong customer service plan. (See the "Strategic Planning" chapter for more information on creating a strategic plan.)

Understanding Your Customers

External Customers

Understanding the different customer groups your organization serves is an essential part of the organization's strategic plan (**Figure 6-1**). Although it is critical to know how best to treat your patients from a medical emergency standpoint, it is also important to know what customers expect from your organization during nonmedical situations. In the healthcare industry, a provider's focus must reach beyond a single segment of the customer base; that is, the organization must have a customer segmentation plan to ensure that as many customer demands are met as possible. Customer segments might include geriatric customers, pediatric customers, young adults, customers of different cultures, and customers speaking different languages. Accommodating the needs of these various groups helps establish effective community partnerships between the customers and the organization.

Organizations identify customer segments as part of their quest to discover what customers want and/or need, and they then use this information to direct their delivery of key products or services. Within the EMS field, organizations must target all segments because their core service is safety—taking care of all persons who are in need of medical attention as well as providing

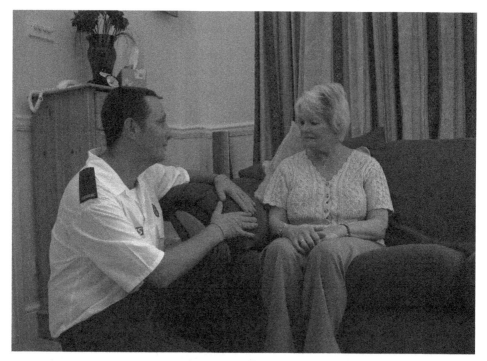

Figure 6-1 The customers in your jurisdiction will have differing needs and expectations.
© Jones and Bartlett Publishers. Photographed by Kimberly Potvin.

assistance to individuals with nonemergent health-related issues. Segmenting customers in EMS establishes a baseline in understanding the customers' expectations; it establishes a partnership between the organization and each of the customer segments and helps the organization adjust its strategic planning regarding its customer service goals. For EMS, establishing customer segmentation is not focused on selecting a customer segment and selling a product or service to just that group; rather, it considers how the EMS organization can best serve each customer segment and meet and exceed the customer expectations during a customer's request for service.

When attempting to define customer segments, the EMS officer must gather data to determine the customers' characteristics. These data can help the organizational leaders determine goals for serving the various customer segments and strategies for interacting with them. You must be creative and use tools that can capture accurate information that will contribute to the organization's customer-centric strategic plan. For example, the organization can conduct surveys; interview customers during nursing home facility visits; gather information during town hall meetings; review the area census to capture accurate demographics; and check with local building departments to find out which new subdivisions, nursing facilities, and daycare programs are coming to town. This information, although it may take some time to gather, will prove to be invaluable as the organization attempts to more closely align its services with its customers' needs.

Understanding customer needs prior to receiving a request for service is beneficial. For example, when attending to nursing home customers, some common needs may depend on whether the home is a skilled nursing facility, a long-term nursing facility, or an assisted living facility. The EMS organization servicing a nursing home should know whether the customers residing there require specific interventions, need to be transported to a specialty facility, and are able to communicate effectively. Beyond the expectations of facility personnel, what do the customer or family members expect from your organization during the service delivery experience? Properly assessing the demographic characteristics of the jurisdiction allows organizational leaders to determine the relative value of the service and what needs improvement. For example, having teddy bears available can help comfort a child in distress but will not have the same effect on an adult.

After identifying those individuals who would most likely use the organization's services, you must determine what they expect from the organization. Is their top priority fast response times, or is it that qualified and well-trained personnel are on-board each EMS unit? Is it important to the customer that he or she receives courteous service from EMS personnel, or that he or she is transported to his or her hospital of choice? Does the customer expect a ride home from the hospital once the services provided there are finished? The organization must make a concentrated effort to understand its customers' expectations. This can be done by conducting customer surveys, meeting with homeowners' organizations, having town hall meetings hosted by the department, participating in community events, and using social media to get feedback. Regardless of the activities used, it is imperative to get out into the community and to listen to customers. Once you know what your customers expect from the organization, then the organization can begin to align the customers' requirements with the organization's resources. It will be difficult to meet or exceed the customers' requirements when the organization does not have the necessary resources to achieve the customer service objectives.

An additional consideration, however, is that customers' expectations may not always be reasonable. For example, a patient's spouse may request that the patient be transported to a particular hospital, but you know that the requested hospital does not have the resources to treat the patient's medical issue and is also much farther away. In such cases, personnel must continue to do the best they can to care for the patient with the resources they have available, but if possible, personnel should explain to the customer why certain decisions are being made.

Internal Customers

Internal customers—those individuals and groups within your organization to whom you provide services—also require consideration when developing a customer service plan for the organization. A key strategy in working with internal customers is earning their trust and demonstrating that they can rely on you in your position, regardless of whether their position is above or below yours. Consider how you will earn that trust and motivate your employees. Which needs do your employees have that the organization can fulfill? Many elements in the work environment serve to support all members of the organization, including compensation, training, and appreciation. Some individual employees, however, may have additional needs—for example, a particular schedule because of a family scheduling conflict, or refresher training in a skill that has not been used recently. When you understand what your employees need to keep them active and effective members of the organization, employee relations will run much more smoothly and it becomes easier to retain employees. (Team building and employee relations are discussed further in the "Building the Team" chapter.)

Success in the BUSINESS WORLD

Exceeding Expectations

Organizations must make every effort to meet and exceed customer expectations and leave the customer with a positive lasting impression. The key is determining what the customer considers "meeting and exceeding expectations."

Zappos, an online shoe store, is committed to providing the greatest customer experience possible for its online customers. Customers want quality, variety, and availability in their shoes, but providing just these three elements is not enough to push a shoe retailer ahead of others. What has made Zappos a leader is its commitment to customer service. After assessing how the company was doing business and what needed to be done to gain market share, the Zappos leadership team made a move that turned their organization into a true customer service leader: They instituted free delivery and returns—a move that set Zappos apart from its competitors and exceeded customer expectations.

Interaction with the officers and managers above you, or officers of other divisions with whom you interact, must also be considered. Open, clear communication among these individuals and departments facilitates interactions and cooperation. Ask these officers what they need, share your own and your department's needs, and work together to ensure these needs are met. When an organization's internal customers work well together to meet needs, it becomes easier for them to also meet the needs of external customers.

Creating a Customer-Centric Culture

In the book *Creating Magic*, author Lee Cockerell, a former executive with the Walt Disney World Resort, speaks about the importance of creating magic for all of that organization's guests. Imagine customer service as embodying this philosophy. Fire protection and EMS are businesses, and patients are their customers. The goal for all organizational leaders is to ensure that they promote and support a customer-centric culture throughout the organization, as part of a general culture of quality. Some EMS professionals believe customers have no choice among EMS organizations, because they call for assistance and the one provider for that jurisdiction is dispatched to assist them. Not only is this the wrong attitude to have, but it is also an erroneous assumption: Just because an EMS organization is the only provider in town today, it does not mean the organization cannot be replaced by another EMS department in the future.

Adopting a customer-centric attitude within any public safety organization is critical not only from the standpoint of maintaining the organization, but also for building trust in the customers/patients whom you are there to assist during their emergencies. While many community members will never use your department's services, they may know someone who has, and word of mouth is a powerful advertising medium. Although these citizens may not use the town's EMS system themselves, they will get involved when it comes time to vote on keeping the current EMS provider or replacing it; raising taxes to support city, township, or county public service initiatives (including EMS); approving the purchase of a new ambulance unit or equipment; and providing raises for your personnel.

If your organization is providing an unacceptable level of service, rest assured that one or several citizens will express their displeasure about the service being provided to the town's leadership. This may lead to a change in department leadership or to the city, town, or county commissioner replacing the current organization with a new vendor. Your customers will take care of you if you do your very best to take care of them and provide them with a service that exceeds their expectations.

If a patient requests to be transported to a hospital that is a bit farther away than the closest hospital, what should the paramedic do? If the patient is stable, consider taking the patient to his or her hospital of choice if the system allows it. It may not be possible to meet every request made by a patient, because EMS personnel must follow their medical protocols and current organizational policies. However, certain requests will occur on a more frequent basis, and the leadership team must empower its employees to do what it takes to exceed customer expectations. This can be done by including common customer request scenarios in protocols or by creating a standard operating guideline (SOG) that describes how to address these situations.

Asking the patient, family members, and friends if there is anything that you can do for them or any questions that you can answer will go a long way toward building trust between customers and your organization. It is the responsibility of your organization and its members to create a positive impression in the patient's mind about your services.

The mindset of serving customers and exceeding their expectations needs to be part of the organization's core mission. Every member of the organization must understand that exceeding a customer's expectations is a priority within the organization and must become part of the organization's culture.

Leadership Buy-In

Exceeding customer expectations must be a company-wide initiative supported by all members of the organization. However, you as the EMS officer, as well as the rest of the leadership team, must make it a priority and let all members of the organization know that you fully support this initiative. This priority must be a core value that is both deeply rooted within the organization and continuously promoted.

Customer Service Training and Development

Your team members must understand what the organization expects from them in every aspect of their jobs, especially when serving customers. Customer service problems tend to arise when members of the organization who interact with customers do not clearly understand what is expected of them. Many organizations have an internal training and development program specifically designed to address customer service. If your organization does not have such a program for employees at all levels of the organization, now is the time to consider creating one.

Empowering Employees

To better serve customers, employees must be fully empowered to do their jobs. That is, they must be able to respond to customers' needs, follow up on customer requests or organizational promises, and deliver a quality product or service that will exceed customer expectations. They must also be empowered to admit that the organization has made a mistake when it has and to correct the problem.

A culture of customer service is deeply rooted in a culture of quality (see the "Creating a Culture of Quality" chapter) and depends on all members of the organization, not just the leadership. Empowering employees to resolve customer issues is a critical link in the process of addressing those issues quickly. This empowerment must include everyone within the organization—not just a handful of employees. If there is something a member of the organization can do to address a customer request and exceed the customer's expectations, the employee must be authorized to do it.

Managerial Leadership **BRIEFCASE**

Ensure Quality Customer Service by Hiring the Right People

When you are seeking a new team member for your division, you should recognize that this individual can become an internal customer and, if hired, would have an impact on both internal and external customers. The reputation of the organization depends on how employment candidates are treated as well as how qualified the candidate chosen is for the position. Consider the following questions:

1. Is the candidate qualified for the position? Ask the candidate to explain how he or she works with others and resolves issues. These skills are needed for both internal and external customers.

2. Could this candidate grow within the organization? Do not hire for just the present; hire for the long term. Ask the candidate what he or she can bring to the organization to help it become more customer-centric.

3. Does the candidate have the required customer service experience for the position? If the candidate does not have this experience, consider whether these skills would be needed immediately or whether it would be easy enough to train the right individual in these skills once hired.

4. When interviewing the candidate, be sure to listen well. Focus on the answers to your questions, but also listen to any questions or concerns the candidate may have.

5. When you have chosen a candidate for the position, notify the candidate by telephone, rather than by letter or e-mail. After the interview, this interaction offers the new hire the first glimpse of how the organization treats its employees, and you need to send a positive message to the new team member.

6. Attempt to get at least three references and determine which duties the candidate performs in his or her current job, whether he or she works well with others, how much direction the candidate needs to get a job done, which positive initiatives the candidate has led or facilitated, and whether the current employer would hire the candidate again.

7. Does the candidate want the job or just the title? Hire someone who is passionate about doing the work, rather than an individual who is just looking for a new title.

8. Ask the candidate what he or she expects from the immediate supervisor.

9. Make sure you have answered the candidate's questions before he or she leaves, and encourage the candidate to call you if he or she has any more questions. In addition, ask the candidate if it is acceptable for you to call him or her if you have any more questions.

Be organized and prepared so you can get as much as possible out of the time allotted with the candidate. Do everything you can to make the experience pleasant for both the candidate and yourself. After all, you are not just evaluating the candidate for hire—the candidate is also evaluating you and your organization.

If employees are not empowered to resolve customer issues, and the leadership team has not embraced a culture of exceeding customer expectations, the customer will not get the results he or she is seeking and the organization will fall short of its goal. As an EMS officer, you must clearly state your expectations of empowerment to those reporting to you. They must understand what empowerment means to them and what they can do with it. (See the "Building the Team" chapter for more discussion on empowering employees.)

Organizational Branding

The commitment to exceed both internal and external customers' expectations must be woven into the organization's culture of quality and embraced by all team members. In addition, the commitment to exceed customer expectations will serve as the foundation for creating a positive organizational brand. A **brand** is built on the value, perception, and feel of a product or service after a customer experience. The organization's brand image can be either positive or negative and will determine how the community perceives your organization.

A customer, whether by personal experience or by word of mouth, may immediately form an opinion of the organization. Thus the leadership team must establish a branding strategy. Everyone in the organization must be part of this initiative. Besides exceeding customer expectations and delivering quality service with the day-to-day emergency response service, the organization should take other steps to create a positive brand. For example, it may take a global approach and consider all of its services to the community. Providing additional services may strengthen the organization's brand and could include conducting home health visits, holding fall prevention seminars and home inspections, providing outreach programs, and aligning customer needs with the appropriate resources. The organizational leaders, when attempting to establish the organization's brand, must keep in mind that this brand will represent the organization as a whole and will serve as a means to set the organization apart from its competitors.

A brand requires at least two key factors: a product or service and an evaluator. As it pertains to this text, the brand represents the services provided by the EMS organization and the organization's overall manner of conducting business. The brand evaluation is conducted by customers who have used those services or have had some interaction with the organization.

In establishing a brand image, the organization must be consistent in its service delivery. The customers need to know what to expect when they request emergency medical services. Through this consistent service delivery, the organization begins to establish its brand. The goal is to ensure positive brand recognition and to have a community that values your organization above the rest. Other EMS agencies may be able to provide services to your customers, but your organization's positive brand will distinguish the organization from its competitors.

The members of the organization must determine which organizational brand they desire to project. If they make no effort to establish a brand, the customer will not know what to expect from the organization. For example, many citizens do not know how training differs for emergency medical technicians (EMTs) versus paramedics; they do not know that prehospital providers have standing orders and do not need to consult with a physician before every intervention; they do not know that they may be transported to a more-distant hospital that is equipped to manage the medical emergency; and they may wonder why an ambulance does not respond with lights and siren activated. Following are some important steps that an organization can take to establish its brand:

- Introduce your organization to the customer. This can be done before, during, or after an event. Regardless of whether the occasion is a town hall meeting, an EMS Week event, an open house, transport of a patient to the hospital, or a follow-up visit to see how well the patient is recovering, the organization must not stop promoting itself as the EMS brand of choice to its customers. It is during these exchanges between customers and the organization that the organizational members will have an opportunity to send a clear message about the organization and its mission, vision, attributes, and core values.

- Make sure the customer can distinguish your organization from the competition. Create a differentiating appearance (e.g., a logo, tagline, ambulances of a different color, different uniforms).

- Let customers know how well you will take care of them and what they can expect when they call on the organization. Engage customers and make them part of the system. Promote the organization's brand on a continuous basis. If customers have not used the service, they will not know what to expect until you tell them.

- Deliver quality service.

- Make sure you are doing everything possible to achieve a positive outcome for the customer. Exceed customer expectations.

The organization's brand will serve as the organization's public face regardless of whether customers have actually used its services. When external customers speak about the service provided

Management Leadership BRIEFCASE

Promote Your Organization

If your organization is performing at a high level, but customers do not know you exist, then they will probably go somewhere else. Get your service noticed, establish a brand, and promote it. Identify the things your organization does better than its competitors, and then let your customers know about it.

When given an opportunity to represent the organization during a speaking engagement, a town hall meeting, or an interaction with a single customer, it is important to stress that the organization is committed to delivering consistent service, is focused on meeting or exceeding customer expectations, works hard to establish long-term relationships with its customers, and, above all, cares about all of its customers.

by your organization, read about it, or see a department ambulance unit driving down the road, the organization's brand image should speak for the organization. When internal customers have a positive experience working for the organization, with members of different departments, or with other stakeholders on the organization's behalf, they will be more confident in their position and their work and will be more apt to promote quality customer service both internally and externally. In this way, ensuring quality service delivery and focusing on being a customer-centric organization will pave the way for establishing a positive brand image.

Outlining a Process for Quality Customer Service

Regardless of the industry, customers can become very frustrated when their concerns are not resolved, when they face a long wait before they are helped, or when they are passed from one department to another without being helped. Every organization must implement and maintain a customer-friendly process to meet the customers' needs. This process should not end at the point of service delivery, but rather must flow into all areas of the organization. A customer-friendly process will ensure that you deal with customer issues when they arise, and will also show customers that you are well prepared to address their concerns. A customer service plan will consist of several components that differ among organizations. Examples of such components include a central location where customer questions or concerns are managed and tracked for resolution, a customer survey distribution protocol, review of customer surveys, and follow-up with customers to ensure that their questions or concerns have been addressed. During the strategic planning process, therefore, it is critical to identify what works best for your organization to ensure the desired customer service outcomes.

Outlining a process for quality internal customer service is often accomplished simply through internal protocols, training, and effective communication. The steps described in the following subsections focus on how to serve external customers.

Establish a Central Location for Customer Issues

When a customer calls your organization to inquire about a particular service, to ask questions, or to speak with a member of the organization, that individual does not want to wait a long time on the telephone or in a lobby. To meet this expectation, the organization needs a central customer receiving site where customer questions or issues can be resolved thoroughly and quickly. Often, a receptionist will be able to address the customer's request. If the receptionist cannot answer the question or provide the requested information, the organization must be prepared to handle the issue through a set process.

The customer information center must be clearly identified. The medium for information exchange may take the form of the organization's website or a social media site, a transport billing statement, town hall meetings, or customer service cards. The goal is to establish a system that addresses customer questions and concerns immediately. This is one of the organization's many opportunities to exceed the customer's expectations.

Specify a Functional Unit to Address Customer Issues

Although every member of the organization must be prepared to address and remedy customer issues, the organization must have a single answering point for all customer requests to ensure that questions are answered and problems are resolved quickly. This may be a receptionist or a designated team. Having a central intake site allows the customer a contact point and keeps him or her from having to contact multiple departments in search of answers. The individual(s) assigned to this function must be well versed in the organization's overall processes and systems and be empowered to remedy any customer issue.

If the organization's customer service representative is not able to answer the customer's question or resolve the customer's issue, he or she must be knowledgeable enough to forward the query to the correct individual or functional workgroup in the organization. The key is to ensure that whichever functional workgroup is responsible for working with a customer, the members are well informed as to how best to assist the customer. A process flow chart will help ensure that the customer's issues are being addressed (**Figure 6-2**).

When a customer calls the organization inquiring about a bill received for a recent transport, that individual should be forwarded to the appropriate functional workgroup, which must be able to provide an immediate response to the customer. If a customer calls the organization inquiring about the treatment received while the customer was being transported to the hospital, the call must be forwarded to the administrative EMS office and the team must be ready to address the customer's questions.

Organizations will differ in terms of which functional unit is responsible for receiving and addressing customer complaints, questions, or requests. Regardless of which functional unit is responsible for addressing the initial customer service exchange, the customer's call must be logged, the incident must be tracked to ensure that it has been addressed, and if it is determined that a current organizational process is adversely affecting customer service, that process must be examined immediately. Having a central location where complaints, concerns, questions, and requests are received from customers is extremely important. However, knowing what to do once the call is received is just as important.

Having all members understand how to address customer service issues, questions, and requests is important not only for the customer, but also for the organization as it strives to ensure continuity with its customer service initiative. When a customer calls an organization to report a complaint, the last thing that person wants is to be transferred to functional workgroups who are unable to address the customer's specific concern.

Put the Plan in Writing

After the customer service strategic planning team or the organization's leadership team have determined the goals, objectives, strategies, and tactics for exceeding customer expectations and addressing customer concerns, the plan must be shared with the entire organization. The plan can be rolled out in a variety of ways:

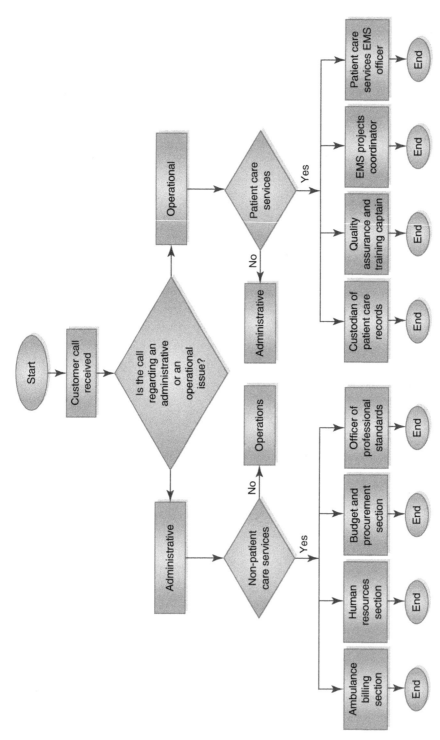

Figure 6-2 A process flow chart can help ensure customers are receiving quality and consistent service.

- It can be added to an employee handbook that is provided to every new and current employee.
- The plan can be reviewed during new-hire orientation and regular team meetings.
- It can be included in the organization's SOGs.
- A process flow chart can be created to help employees remember the customer service protocol.

The written guidelines and protocols regarding customer service should cover most, if not all, of the general customer concerns the organization expects to face. For example:

- If a customer is reporting a complaint about a crew being disrespectful, who within the organization will be assigned to address the complaint?
- If a patient asks the crew assisting her to notify her daughter that she is being transported to the hospital, how should the crew handle that request? Should they call from the scene, have a hospital staff member call, or not call at all because calling may be a Health Insurance Portability and Accountability Act (HIPAA) violation?

With all employees on the same page, the customer will receive consistent service and any issues with the plan will be easier to fix.

Following Up on Customer Issues
External Customers

Every organization must have a customer follow-up system. For external customers, after a service has been provided, the organization should attempt to ascertain the customer's level of satisfaction with the service rendered, especially in the case of negative experiences. Even if the organization has remedied the issue, a follow-up call or visit will demonstrate that your organization cares about resolving all customer issues and making sure that the customer has no further issues.

Internal Customers

Although much of this chapter has focused on external customers, you must not overlook your internal customers. Just as you seek feedback from your external customers, so you must do the same with your internal customers. Understanding what your internal customers want and need will assist you in being an effective managerial leader. If you want your team to exceed the customer's expectations, then you as the EMS officer must exceed the team's expectations. For example, determine what the team members need to stay engaged at work. Ask the team members; do not assume you know the answer. As the EMS officer, it is up to you to ensure that team members have everything they need to perform their jobs. This responsibility can include making sure they have the necessary equipment, training, and opportunities to perform their duties; listening to their concerns or ideas; encouraging them to grow within the organization; and supporting them professionally and personally.

Evaluating the Customer Service Plan

As an EMS officer and part of the organization's leadership team, evaluating a customer service plan is no different than reviewing the organization's or a functional-level workgroup's strategic plan. Both plans must be evaluated routinely and adjustments made as needed. Having a set time frame for when the leadership team or the customer service strategic planning team should meet to evaluate the plan is a must.

One helpful step in evaluating the current plan is to place yourself in the customer's shoes and go through the organization's customer service system. This will allow you to see firsthand whether the organization is falling short in resolving customer requests.

Compare your system's performance to that of other organizations. This can be done by conducting customer surveys and asking customers to rate your organization's services as compared to those offered by your competitors or other organizations they have used in the past. The goal is to get as much information as possible and to identify opportunities to make improvements. Also, this effort will help you gather information about services your competitors are offering that you are not. Get feedback from those who have used both services and listen to what they have to say.

As an organizational leader, it is as important to gather information from your internal customers as it is to gather information from external customers. Both customer groups deserve attention to ensure they continue to support the organization. All too often, though, organizations tend to spend much of their time and effort seeking ways to improve external customer service while neglecting internal customers. It is important not to wait for annual reviews to determine what an internal customer needs to do his or her job, how that person feels about the organization, and what input or feedback he or she has. As the first of the 5 BPs, people must be a priority for every organizational leader; therefore, the organizational leader must spend time in the trenches with the employees and continuously seek their feedback. An organization may also develop functional workgroup surveys, giving everyone in the organization an opportunity to evaluate the internal service provided by each functional group to internal customers. This allows functional workgroup leaders to learn not only how their section is perceived by other internal functional workgroups, but also what they need to do to improve internal customer service. An incentive can be awarded to the functional group that scores the highest.

Never stop asking for feedback. You will never know what the customer is thinking or wants until you ask. Customer loyalty depends on how well customers are treated throughout their entire experience with the organization.

Surveys

Surveys are good tools for capturing customer feedback and measuring your organization's ability to meet patient expectations. Surveying your customers demonstrates that the organization cares about them. To obtain this type of feedback, a survey card can be left with the patient or family member to be completed and mailed back at a later date. Surveys can also be mailed to each customer several days after the service was delivered.

The downside of this type of survey is that the customer has no obligation to complete the survey and return it. Several variables can impact whether a customer responds to such a questionnaire. It may be that the customer never received the survey, the customer is now deceased, in the aftermath of the emergency the customer forgets to return the survey, or the customer does not speak English. If the survey is web-based, some customers may find the process too complicated, and others may not have Internet access. Additionally, customers who were highly satisfied or highly dissatisfied would be the most likely to complete a survey, leaving it unclear where the organization stands with the majority of its customers.

The organization must make it easy for its customers to complete the surveys and return them. For example, mail surveys should be easy to read, with plenty of space for responses, and should be accompanied by a prepaid return envelope (**Figure 6-3**). Surveys that can be completed electronically should have step-by-step instructions. To reach customers who do not have Internet access, the organization must have a system in which the customer can provide feedback to a human representative.

Before submitting any survey to customers, answer the following questions:

- What will the organization gain by investing in surveys?
- Will the data be accurate?
- Will the sample of all the collected surveys be large enough to ensure statistical significance?
- Which survey medium will be used to gather the data?
- What will the organization do once it has analyzed the data?

Surveys can be used to elicit suggestions for service improvements and to ensure that current or proposed services are relevant to your customers and exceed their expectations. When creating a survey, it is important to determine the purpose for conducting the survey. Consider those aspects of the service for which you are most interested in obtaining feedback. For example, if your organization has recently increased its efforts to shorten time on scene, is a side effect of rushed EMS personnel that the patient/customer feels rushed or stressed?

To collect as much feedback from the customers as possible, select a survey medium that works best for the customer. Gathering information from a large sample is paramount because it increases the likelihood that the feedback received will be truly reflective of most of the customers' experiences, even for the customers who were not surveyed.

A variety of media can be utilized, but each medium comes with its own benefits and drawbacks. Surveys can be conducted through face-to-face interviews, telephone (live or automated) contacts, written (in-person) surveys, mailed questionnaires, or online media. When using a customer survey

Brevard County Fire Rescue Patient Satisfaction Survey

1. What was the location of your incident (city)?

_____

2. Name (optional)

_____

3. What is your age?
   18 to 24
   25 to 34
   35 to 44
   45 to 54
   55 to 64
   65 to 74
   75 or older

4. What language do you mainly speak at home?
   English
   Spanish
   Chinese
   Russian
   Vietnamese
   Other (please specify) _____

5. What is the account number and date of service listed on your statement (optional)?

_____

6. May we contact you with questions regarding your service?
   Yes, via telephone
   Yes, via e-mail
   No
   Telephone number and/or e-mail address

_____

Figure 6-3 Sample survey. *(continues)*

7. Please indicate whether you agree or disagree with the following statements:

	Strongly Agree	Agree	Somewhat Agree	Disagree	Strongly Disagree	N/A
A. The Brevard County Fire Rescue Team encouraged me to be transported to the hospital.						
B. The Brevard County Fire Rescue Team treated me with courtesy and respect.						
C. The Brevard County Fire Rescue team showed concern for my safety and comfort during transport.						
D. Brevard County Fire Rescue responded to my emergency in a prompt, timely fashion.						
E. Based on my experience, I would recommend Brevard County Fire Rescue to my friends and family.						

Comments (optional):

_____

_____

_____

8. Please read the following statements regarding your recent experience with Brevard County Fire Rescue. Choose the answer that best describes your experience.

	Excellent	Very Good	Good	Fair	Poor	N/A
A. Please rate your overall level of satisfaction with Brevard County Fire Rescue.						
B. Please rate your opinion of the emergency medical care provided by Brevard County Fire Rescue.						
C. Please rate the appearance of the Brevard County Fire Rescue team.						

Comments (optional):

_____

_____

_____

Figure 6-3 Sample survey. *(continued)*

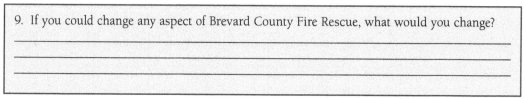

9. If you could change any aspect of Brevard County Fire Rescue, what would you change?

Figure 6-3 Sample survey. *(continued)*

to capture information about a service or product, it is important to take into consideration the medium being used. For example, face-to-face or in-person written surveys may be effective in getting information from the customer because it is more difficult to ignore the interviewer's request to complete the survey. However, the customer may be reserved or feel pressured when providing a response because the interviewer is watching. With telephone, mail, or online surveys, there is always the risk that the customer may not want to spend time completing the survey. These surveys may pose a greater challenge if there is no incentive, the survey takes a long time to complete, or the tools to complete the survey are not available (e.g., a customer without Internet access is asked to complete an online survey). Therefore, when creating a survey you must keep the customer in mind and create a survey that will not discourage customers from completing it.

Knowing what to do with survey information once it is obtained is just as important as gathering the data. It is not uncommon to review surveys, analyze the information, determine areas that need improving, and then neglect to create initiatives to make the necessary adjustments.

Guidelines for Creating a Survey

When creating a survey, keep it simple, ask pertinent questions, avoid long surveys, and explain why completing the survey is important and how the participant's feedback will help improve the EMS organization and service delivery.

First, every effort must be made to prevent the survey from becoming too complicated. Asking the customer to answer questions that use technical terms, that require essay answers, that have nothing to do with the service provided, or that require references to information not provided in the survey will simply cause customer frustration and discourage participation in completing the survey. The ideal survey is short and to the point. If possible, use a Likert scale for responses, where the customer is asked if he or she strongly agrees, agrees, is neutral, disagrees, or strongly disagrees. A number range of 1–5 is associated with these responses and can be used to generate an overall score. For example, Question 7 in Figure 6-3 uses a Likert scale to gauge customer satisfaction with the interactions with EMS personnel.

Second, the questions must center on the service provided to the customer and must consider demographics. For example, was the EMS crew courteous and respectful? Was service provided in a timely fashion? Were the customer's expectations met? Did the crew encourage transport to the hospital? Consider capturing the customer's gender, age, ethnicity, and primary language on the survey as well, because this information can help identify any customer segments that are not as satisfied with the service as others. Be sure that the information collected is kept private, and treat the information as you would any other HIPAA-protected data.

When determining which questions to include in the survey, consider those questions that will provide information about the organization's core services and key performance indicators.

Managerial Leadership **BRIEFCASE**

Customer Privacy

Privacy is always a concern, especially for members of the medical profession. The EMS officer must ensure that a system is in place to keep protected health information (PHI) secure and to release such information only to those who are authorized to receive it. Often, after an EMS request for service is made and care is subsequently delivered, a patient, family member, or friend requests information about the patient's condition. In addition, an attorney, an insurance company representative, and even law enforcement personnel (who were not on the scene) may request protected health information about a patient treated by your organization.

Every EMS organization must have a system in place to ensure that the release of protected health information is closely supervised and in compliance with the rules under HIPAA and any additional state privacy laws. Check with your organization's HIPAA compliance officer for guidance to ensure that the organization is following the appropriate guidelines when releasing such information. If the organization does not have a HIPAA compliance officer, consider the following steps:

- Attend a HIPAA training session.
- Assign someone to serve as the HIPAA compliance officer for the organization.
- Request proof of identity and any necessary authorization forms from anyone requesting information about a patient.
- If you are unsure whether to release PHI, *don't* do it!

Protection of PHI also comes into play when customers submit surveys or contact the organization through the organization's website. Customers should be reminded that any information submitted to the organization through these formats is not protected and may be viewed by a number of people within the organization, and that customers should therefore refrain from including sensitive information through these media.

Including questions that have nothing to do with the service provided may lead to confusion and discourage the patient from completing the survey. Also, avoid questions that are similar to other questions being asked; such questions are redundant and overcrowd the survey.

Third, avoid creating surveys that are too long. Surveys should not take longer than 5 minutes to complete. Long surveys will take time to complete and may discourage a customer from completing the survey.

Fourth, customers may choose not to complete a survey because it adds no value to them personally. As the survey provider, you must inform the survey participants how their feedback will impact the EMS organization and the services it provides. If the budget allows, and with appropriate approval, consider offering an incentive for completing the survey. Keep in mind, however, that many government organizations are prohibited from offering any gifts to customers for services rendered by the organization.

Do not conduct a one-time patient survey and then stop your data-gathering efforts. Rather, continuously measure the organization's customer service performance by attempting to expand the survey sample size, reevaluating the survey medium being used, and taking the necessary action once the data (information) have been collected. This ongoing process to improve customer service represents a key part of the organization's culture of quality.

As an EMS officer, creating customer surveys may not be your forte, but you should make every effort to gather customer feedback and thereby improve the organization. When asked to create a survey for the first time, confer with others who have created similar surveys in the past and do your own research into how to write an effective survey. Check with your organization's leadership team as well, in case there are specific requirements you must follow or certain questions you should avoid. If you have an opportunity to be part of a survey committee or a focus group or to participate in surveys, take advantage of it; this participation will better prepare you in the event you are asked to create a customer survey for your division.

Website

A website can be a powerful tool for conveying information about the organization. Moreover, the website can be used to acquire information from customers (**Figure 6-4**). For example, the organization's information technology (IT) team can create mechanisms on the website that allow customers to complete online surveys, but also can allow customers to make suggestions independent of surveys and to submit formal complaints.

The EMS organization's website also can include a mechanism that allows community members to join a focus group for the organization. The members of the focus group may then be given access to a page that contains questions of particular interest to the organization.

An organization may provide customer service cards that include the unit number and the name of the crew members who treated the patient or that can be used during a customer–organization business exchange. Such business cards typically include the department's website

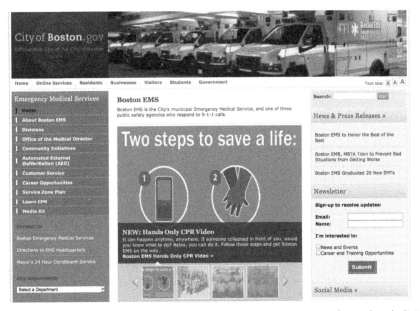

Figure 6-4 EMS organizations can use their websites to keep customers informed and elicit their feedback.

Reproduced from Boston EMS

address and may also have a quick response (QR) code that will link the customer to the website. The customer can then be guided to find the desired information on the website.

The website must be monitored and updated regularly to ensure that customer requests, suggestions, and concerns are addressed promptly. Obtaining input from customers is not enough; customers must know that the organization received the message, and they must be assured of how the organization plans to address the customer's message. Using every resource to gather information from customers while also promoting the organization contributes to a customer-centric organization.

The organization must ensure that no personal (protected) information is posted on the organization's website or on social media. If the website will be used to obtain customer feedback, the organization must include a statement on the website identifying the kind of information that can be included. A website that is not secured for privacy should not be used to convey sensitive and protected patient information.

Social Media

Social media can be a powerful tool for communication between an organization and its customers. To maximize its effectiveness in reaching customers through social media, the organization must identify the social media that are being used by its customers. For example, citizens who follow your organization might be sent Twitter messages publicizing a new piece of EMS equipment, notifying citizens of an EMS open house, or requesting feedback about a specific customer service topic. The goal is not only to communicate with these citizens via Twitter, but also to attract more Twitter followers—the more followers an organization has, the more people it is reaching when it tweets.

If the organization is holding an open house for community members, plans to purchase a new piece of equipment, wants to warn customers of potentially hazardous conditions, or needs to provide shelter information during a disaster, social media can prove a valuable tool in disseminating the necessary information. Adept use of social media tools, such as Twitter, Facebook, YouTube, Flickr, Instagram, and Google+, can increase the organization's exposure, promote the organization's brand, keep customers informed, and collect customer feedback. Social media are just one means through which to engage with customers, however, and should be used in conjunction with other informational tools such as media releases and media interviews.

Improving the Process

As part of effective customer service, it is critical to find ways to improve your organization's process for addressing and resolving customer issues. To start, the organization must make every attempt to capture the voice of the customer before and after service delivery. Knowing what the customer expects before he or she requests the organization's services will help reduce future customer concerns. As an EMS officer, you must routinely review the service being delivered by your business unit, identify what is working and what is not, listen to customer experiences, and make adjustments as needed to meet customer expectations.

After compiling data on customer experience, consider creating a process flow chart to create a visual map of the ideal customer service delivery process. You may consider creating process flow charts for individual scenarios, such as how to manage a customer's concern, when to move ambulance units into certain response areas for coverage, what to do when the patient care report will not upload, and what to do when your patient requires no medical intervention yet is in need of personal assistance. Focus on the areas in which your organization or department may be struggling. Not every customer-related process will require a chart, but this representation can be helpful, especially for new employees and for getting all employees on the same page, following the same process. Set processes like these are especially helpful if the process is related to a sensitive topic or if the situation requiring the process does not crop up often but consistency in process is still required. Each step in the customer service process should be evaluated to determine whether it adds value to the overall process. (See the "Creating a Culture of Quality" chapter for a discussion on how to create a process flow chart.)

Managerial Leadership **BRIEFCASE**

Providing Feedback to Team Members

Keeping team members informed about your organization's activities is essential. As an example, sharing information and receiving feedback made a significant difference for Brevard County Fire Rescue in Florida. This EMS organization was experiencing the following issues:

- Patient care reports were not being completed within the specified time frame.
- Complaints from a hospital about the organization's performance were at an all-time high.
- Some operational targets were not being met.

The leadership team looked carefully at how they were communicating with their internal and external stakeholders and realized that their expectations were not being thoroughly communicated to the team members. To address these shortcomings, the leadership team established a strategic communication plan consisting of five critical targets:

1. Clearly illustrate and explain the organization's expectations and the reasons they are important to the organization.
2. Ensure that employees understand the leadership team's expectations and make sure that all team member questions have been addressed.
3. Give feedback to the crews regarding patient care outcomes and seek feedback from employees.
4. Make every effort to ensure that good and bad news is delivered by the leadership team, and not by someone else, to prevent rumors and misinformation.
5. Monitor performance improvement after implementing the communication plan.

Brevard County Fire Rescue had a positive return from this commitment to communicating with all team members and promoting strategic communication across the organization. The leadership team was convinced that they could turn their low-performing organization into an industry leader. The leadership team began this journey by becoming more inclusive and opening its strategic communication to its internal and external customers. The plan yielded the following results in a year:

- 72 percent improvement by field personnel in thoroughly and accurately completing patient care reports
- 75 percent increase in letters of appreciation from the community
- 60 percent increase in the number of EMS charts processed during quality assurance review
- 40 percent improvement in accuracy in patient triage
- 10 percent improvement in acquiring a 12-lead electrocardiogram (ECG) on cardiac patients within 8 minutes of arrival on scene; average time was 6 minutes
- 4.71 patient satisfaction score out of a maximum of 5.0 on the Likert scale

WRAP-UP

Concept Review

- The most important factor in an organization's success is satisfied customers.

- You must create, implement, and evaluate a plan within your organization that embodies the attitude of exceeding customer expectations for your internal and external customers. Keeping people in their primary position—that is, as the first of the 5 BPs—must continue to be a priority.

- The first step in creating a customer service plan is to determine who will be responsible for overseeing the process and ensuring that a customer service plan is created.

- Understanding the different customer groups that your organization serves must be an essential part of the organization's strategic plan.

- When you understand what your employees need to keep them active and effective members of the organization, employee relations will run much more smoothly and it will be easier to retain employees.

- The goal for every organizational leader is to ensure that he or she promotes and supports a customer-centric culture throughout the organization, as part of a general culture of quality.

- Regardless of the industry, customers can become very frustrated when their concerns are not resolved, when they face long waits before they are helped, and when they are passed from one department to another without being helped.

- Every organization must have a customer follow-up system. For external customers, after a service has been provided, the organization should attempt to ascertain the customer's level of satisfaction with the service rendered.

- Understanding what your internal customers want and need will assist you in being an effective managerial leader. If you want your team to exceed the customers' expectations, then you as the EMS officer must exceed the team's expectations.

- As an EMS officer and part of the organization's leadership team, evaluating a customer service plan is no different than reviewing the organization's or a functional-level workgroup's strategic plan.

- Surveys are good tools for capturing customer feedback and measuring the organization's ability to meet patient expectations.

- A website can be a powerful tool for conveying information about the organization and for acquiring information from customers.

- To have the greatest effect in reaching customers through social media, the organization must identify those social media that are currently being used by its customers.

■ For the EMS leader, it is critical to find ways to improve the organization's process for addressing and resolving customer issues.

Managerial Terms

Brand An organization's reputation among actual and potential customers as determined by the organization's quality of goods and services and the market's perceptions of the organization.

External customers Individuals to whom an organization provides goods and services, and who do not work for the organization.

Internal customers Individuals who work for an organization and depend on the organization's support to serve the external customer properly.

Case Review: Exceeding Customer Expectations

Medical Team 2 was dispatched to the same address for a wellness check several days in a row around dinner time. When the crews arrived, they would interview the patient and conduct a patient assessment, but on all occasions the outcome was the same: There was no medical issue. After they assessed the patient, however, the crews would be offered milk and cookies prior to them leaving the scene.

Realizing that the caller just wanted some company, the crew began visiting the patient before dinner time on every shift. The crew, while still in service, spent some time with the caller and had a bite of a cookie and some milk. The team would then make sure that the patient was safe and ready for bed after dinner. The requests for emergency service stopped, and the crew made the visits part of their daily shift routine when they were on duty. It was clear that the patient was lonely and wanted someone to spend some time with her.

The patient was satisfied because the crew demonstrated a simple act of kindness and it was an exemplary display of customer service. The customer no longer requested a service call on a daily basis; however, the crews continued to visit the patient until her final days. This act of kindness and exceptional customer service benefited not only the patient, but the organization as a whole. For example, when visiting the customer the crews were not responding to the scene with lights and siren to a nonmedical request for service, the system was able to operate more effectively because the crews were not committed to a call that did not require medical attention, the crew remained in service and available if needed to respond to a true emergency, and resources were appropriately aligned to better serve other customers.

Case Discussion

Meeting and exceeding customer expectations must be a priority for every organization. Whether stopping to check on a customer, bringing in the garbage cans from the roadside as you approach the house, or even getting the mail or newspaper, even the smallest efforts go a long way. As the EMS officer, it is important to promote a culture of quality customer service when providing patient care or just assisting someone in making that individual's life a little easier. EMS professionals focus on attending to those who are sick and injured, but—just as important—they realize that they are community ambassadors. The community will turn to EMS professionals not only during a medical emergency, but also during other events in which the customers seek personal assistance.

The assumption that EMS is only in the emergency delivery business is no longer valid. Service delivery in this industry goes beyond managing and transporting critically ill and injured patients. The EMS profession is in the "people" business, which includes emergent care, nonemergent care, and even assistance with nonmedical situations. EMS customer service goes beyond the day-to-day medical operations and is about helping people in a time of need.

Case Review: Expanding the Components of Service Delivery

During the department's quality assurance process, the Jones EMS agency noticed an increase in requests for service for nonmedical complaints and committed to identifying the reasons for the calls and determining what the organization could do to assist the customers. Jones EMS was committed to aligning the appropriate resources to meet or exceed its customers' requests for service. Establishing a plan to meet the requests for service was important for the organization from financial, operational, and customer service standpoints. The organization's EMS staff established a plan that proved to be beneficial to the organization and the customers whom they were called upon to serve. The plan was divided into five parts:

1. The organization reviewed all EMS requests for service for the previous month and identified which customers requested services more than three times in that month. The EMS team then reviewed these customers' charts to determine the reasons for requesting services on a frequent basis (and whether the reasons were medical). The team separated out those patients who were requesting EMS because they were experiencing a medical emergency and required transport to the hospital from those who had no medical complaints. The customers who were not experiencing medical emergencies but required some personal assistance were classified as "Superusers." Some of these customers were requesting transportation to their doctor appointments; others needed a ride to the grocery store, needed their prescriptions filled at the local pharmacy, were homeless and needed a place to sleep, or were just lonely and wanted company.

2. After identifying the Superusers from the previous month, the team conducted a home visit with each of these customers to establish a rapport and determine which services the customer actually needed.

3. Once the team members determined the reason for requesting EMS, they were able to assist with obtaining the appropriate resources to meet each customer's needs. For example, the team might connect the customer with a local community network that would provide meals, transportation to scheduled doctor appointments, family counseling, information pertaining to shelters, and even phone calls to those customers who needed someone to speak with them on a daily basis. In addition, the services were free.

4. After the home visit was conducted and the customer had been informed of the numerous services that were in place to meet his or her specific needs, the team followed up with a phone call twice a week with each customer. The phone calls added value to the program because they demonstrated to the customer that the agency's commitment did not end with the home visit. After tracking the Superusers for 3 months, it was found that their phone calls had tapered off. If the calls diminished to once a month and eventually ended, the customer was no longer considered a Superuser.

5. For the program to be successful and to ensure that the resources needed were available, routine quality assurance of the program was required. In addition, the crews were supported by the organization's leadership team to continue to assist those customers who did not require medical assistance but still needed an occasional helping hand. The Jones EMS organization established strong community partnerships not only with its customers, but also with the organizations that would be making the resources available to those customers. This was important because patients were being referred to a third party and, as the referring agent, the Jones EMS organization needed to make sure that specific resources were available.

The program was new to the organization's members and was a different service than providing care to a critically ill or injured patient. Nevertheless, it was understood and now part of the organization's culture that the Jones EMS Department was in the business of more than just managing those patients who required medical attention.

Case Discussion

After the first month of working with known Superusers, the Jones EMS organization was able to reduce the number of repeat callers by 85 percent. EMS delivery is a business where many customers seek medical attention on a regular basis. As an EMS officer, it is important to understand the EMS response activity taking place within your organization. This will allow for better planning and a better ability to serve all your customers. In today's ever-changing landscape of medical care, some organizations have partnered with local healthcare organizations to provide mobile integrated healthcare services (community paramedicine) within their community. Such a service adds value to any community but requires additional skills in patient care and must be supported by local healthcare organizations. Funding and training are, therefore, at the very core of this program.

Mobile integrated healthcare comprises a variety of programs that help patients, for example post-admission follow-up, social services, and home health care. These programs can help ensure that the patient is doing everything that the doctor has recommended while the patient is at home to reduce the possibility of being readmitted to the hospital. For example, when conducting home visits with patients with congestive heart failure, the mobile integrated healthcare paramedic will work with those patients to ensure they do not forget or refuse to take their diuretic medication. Similarly, this type of paramedic will visit patients with diabetes and discuss the importance of maintaining a good diet and taking their insulin. The Superuser program falls under the umbrella of mobile integrated healthcare as a community paramedicine initiative. It focuses on those patients who have no medical complaint yet need some day-to-day assistance with personal nonmedical needs. The approach taken by the Jones EMS Department was simple: fill in the gaps that were preventing customers from getting the assistance they needed, while aligning the organization's resources to meet the customers' requests.

7

Strategic Planning

Learning Objectives

After studying this chapter, you should be able to:

- Discuss the purpose of strategic planning.
- Identify and describe the two types of strategic plans.
- Identify and describe the steps of the strategic planning process.

Introduction

This chapter introduces the EMS officer to organizational and functional-level strategic planning processes. The strategy planning process must be thorough and systematic, and it must have leadership support and employee buy-in if it is to succeed. Establishing a mission and vision statement for the organization will be one of the first priorities for the strategy planning team. In addition to analyzing the organization's performance outcome data, the organization's operational strengths and weaknesses must be addressed. The strategy planning team must also determine any opportunities for improvement and evaluate the current market conditions and the organization's competitors. Creating a strategy will be the first step in establishing administrative or operational goals that maximize performance and align business resources to achieve improved service delivery outcomes.

Purpose of Strategic Planning

Strategy may be defined as the art of devising or employing plans or stratagems to reach a goal. You use strategy every day. For example, when you get up in the morning, your goal may be to get to work on time. You then formulate a strategy that will help you achieve that goal. When you are at the grocery store, your goal may be to keep your spending to a minimum; once you confront the many choices for food purchases, you strategize how to make that happen.

As an EMS leader, when you are assigned the responsibility of providing direction to the organization or a functional-level unit (section or division), having a strategic plan must be a priority.

A **strategic plan** is an organizational plan designed to clearly and concisely communicate how the organization will achieve its desired future organizational goals. It is essentially an organizational roadmap that provides direction between the current administrative and operational state of the organization and where the organization's leadership team would like it to be in the future. Although every organization may have a different framework that it uses for creating, implementing, and evaluating a strategic plan, the intent in creating such a plan will be the same.

A strategic plan is developed through multiple brainstorming sessions; conducting a strengths, weaknesses, opportunities, and threats (SWOT) analysis; and assessing internal and external business activities. Using the five business priorities (5 BPs) of the organization as reference points, establish goals, objectives, strategies, and tactics to move the organization in the desired direction. Once implemented, this plan must be routinely monitored to ensure that all team members stay on course. Attempting to create organizational goals without first considering multiple ideas, conducting a SWOT analysis, seeking input from internal and external stakeholders, referencing the organization's core priorities (5 BPs), and clearly having a mission and vision statement will result in ineffective organizational goals. Therefore, before creating a strategic plan, organizational leaders must first determine the purpose for creating the plan, understand which steps must be part of the strategic planning process, and have a clearly defined vision for the organization.

Creating a strategy must be part of every organization's plan when determining its short- and long-term business goals. As market conditions change, that strategy may need to be revised to avoid becoming obsolete. As an EMS officer, you may be asked to assist with the organization's strategic planning process, or you may take it upon yourself to do so for your department. Achieving the strategic plan's overarching goal—to get the organization from where it currently is as a business (mission) to where it wants to be (vision)—requires aligning organizational resources and making organizational improvements to service delivery. However, it is up to the leadership team to establish the importance of the organization's strategic plan. The purpose for creating a strategic plan should be one that everyone on the team supports.

Success in the BUSINESS WORLD

Bags Fly Free

One organization that has been very effective with its strategic planning is Southwest Airlines. Southwest Airlines, as part of its strategic plan, does not charge for customer baggage, whereas most other airlines do charge a fee when passengers check their bags. Southwest Airlines has differentiated itself from its competitors by not adding an additional expense for its passengers. This has helped establish its reputation as an airline where "bags fly free."

Determining what to include in the plan, implementing the plan, and then routinely evaluating the plan will almost certainly require some trial and error. In any industry, organizational leaders must understand the business they are in and create a strategic plan specific to that market. EMS crews may not be offering snacks or beverages throughout transport like airline crews (at least, like cabin stewards in the past), but every EMS organization must have its own strategic plan geared toward leading it to improved outcomes and differentiating it from competitors. After the organizational leaders have determined the organization's purpose and identified why the implementation of a strategic plan is critical for the organization, they will need to define the organization's mission, because the strategic planning process must always begin with a clear and concise organizational mission statement. Put simply, organizational leaders must first understand why the business exists before determining which improvements will be made.

Types of Strategic Plans

As part of the strategic planning process, if the EMS officer is assigned to lead a strategic planning initiative, he or she will need to determine whether the plan will be created for the organization as a whole or will be specific to a division within the organization. If the strategic plan is to include performance improvement initiatives across all levels of the organization, then it is referred to as an **organizational (or corporate) strategic plan**. If the EMS officer is assigned to create a strategy for a single functional-level group or division, then a **functional-level strategic plan** should be the plan of choice. Creating either type of plan will require many of the same activities, but the goals for completing the plans will be different.

Organizational or Corporate Strategy

Organizational (or corporate) strategy focuses on evaluating current organizational activities, then establishing organization-wide administrative and operational goals. The activities that must be evaluated as part of the strategic planning process include finance, internal and external customers,

Managerial Leadership BRIEFCASE

Corporate Versus Functional-Level Strategy

A corporate strategic plan includes all areas of the organization; a functional-level strategic plan focuses on the services, processes, and systems of a specific area or division. A functional-level strategic plan should also support the corporate strategic plan so that all divisions within an organization, regardless of their own goals and objectives, ultimately contribute to the success of the entire organization's goals and objectives. In addition, a functional-level strategic plan helps team members assigned to a specific functional unit remain focused on the goals of their section. Be sure to include your team members when developing such a plan, because their input and support will be critical to the plan's survival.

service delivery resources, market competition, and scope of business provided. Then, by working through the strategic planning process, administrative and operational activities can be improved or adjusted to match or exceed the competitors' service delivery outcomes. To achieve this aim, the strategic plan must focus on improving not only the organization's internal activities, but also the organization's reaction to external market conditions. As the EMS officer, this is when understanding the organization's "big picture" will prove beneficial.

The creation of a strategic plan must be a collaborative process between the organization's leadership team and the front-line members of the organization. The leadership team must ensure that input is encouraged from all levels of the organization and must attempt to gather input from customers as well. The ultimate goal when creating an organizational strategic plan is to improve organization-wide performance and effectively align business resources. Having an organizational strategic plan will allow for necessary business and resource adjustments as the market environment continues to change.

Functional-Level Strategy

Functional-level strategy involves creating a plan within a functional-level workgroup that will contribute to attaining the organization's vision. Such a strategy differs from an organizational strategy in that it focuses on a functional level, rather than on the organization as a whole; however, it still must support the overall plan for the organization. A functional-level strategic planning team will use many of the same strategic planning tools employed to create an organizational strategic plan, except that the planning process centers on the administrative and operational business activities within a functional-level unit.

Before creating a functional-level strategic plan, the leadership team must assign a strategic planning team to this process, each member must have the opportunity to provide input, and the following areas must be evaluated:

- Functional-level unit administrative and operational activities
- Functional-level unit market competitors or drivers
- Areas where the functional-level unit is performing well and where it is not

The Strategic Planning Process

Once the organization's leadership team has agreed on a purpose for creating a strategic plan, it is time to create that plan. The organization will benefit not only from having a strategic plan, but also from the many activities that take place during the course of the strategic planning process, including the following:

- Creation of a mission and vision statement
- Improved communication among team members as they work through the strategic planning process

- Identification of organizational strengths and weaknesses through SWOT analysis
- Identification of opportunities, through SWOT analysis, that will help the organization improve its service delivery
- Identification of threats, through SWOT analysis, that are currently found in the marketplace and may impact the organization's service delivery system
- Compilation and analysis of data pertaining to different areas of the organization
- Setting of organizational goals
- Familiarity with duties conducted by other functional-level groups within the organization

Regardless of the type of strategy (organizational or functional level) under development, the strategic planning process activities must be thoroughly evaluated and systematically completed throughout the process. Every EMS organization must have an up-to-date strategic plan that is supported by the organization's leadership team and employees across the organization.

It is important to break down strategic planning into manageable parts so each of the required activities will be easier to analyze and manage and the team members will not become overwhelmed (**Figure 7-1**). The strategic planning process should be broken down into five steps:

1. Create a mission and vision statement.
2. Conduct a SWOT analysis.
3. Establish goals, objectives, strategy, and tactics.
4. Implement the plan.
5. Routinely evaluate the plan.

Creating Mission and Vision Statements

The first step when creating a strategic plan is to formulate a **mission statement**. If the organization already has a mission statement in place, ensure that it clearly states the purpose of the organization. When creating a mission statement, the strategy team must ask the following questions:

- Why does the organization exist?
- Which service is the business providing today?
- How is the organization going to improve?

The mission statement should not be lengthy. If it becomes too long, the message may not be easy to follow and may cause the reader to lose interest. Ideally, the message will make a lasting impression and leave the reader wanting to know more about the organization. Moreover, the mission statement will clearly identify the service currently being provided by the organization.

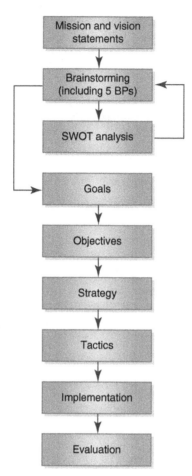

Figure 7-1 The strategic planning process.

When creating a mission statement for the first time or rewriting the organization's current mission statement, the process should not be rushed. Rather, input from all members of the organization should be diligently gathered. Creation of a mission statement offers a golden opportunity to evaluate the current processes and systems that are part of the organization. It is also an opportunity to bring employees together where they can work with each other, get to know each other, learn from each other, and gather information about all areas of the organization. The goal is to create a statement that all members support and are proud to promote throughout the community. Examples of EMS organization mission statements are listed in **Figure 7-2**.

Once a clear and concise mission statement has been created, then the organization's strategy planning group can begin to create a **vision statement**. If the vision will encompass

---

Miami Dade Fire Rescue
We protect people, property and the environment by providing responsive professional and humanitarian fire rescue services essential to public health, safety and well-being.
Reproduced from Miami Dade Fire Rescue.

MedStar Mobile Healthcare
To provide high quality patient care in an effective and cost efficient manner with accountability to system performance standards.
Reproduced from MedStar Mobile Healthcare.

King County Medic One
King County Medic One is a public service organization, a critical link in our regional emergency medical service system, providing high quality, advanced patient care.
Reproduced from King County Medic One.

New York City Fire Department
As first responders to fires, public safety and medical emergencies, disasters and terrorist acts, FDNY protects the lives and property of New York City residents and visitors. The Department advances public safety through its fire prevention, investigation and education programs. The timely delivery of these services enables the FDNY to make significant contributions to the safety of New York City and homeland security efforts.
Reproduced from New York City Fire Department.

Figure 7-2 Examples of mission statements.

the entire organization, then it will be a corporate (or organizational) vision statement. Alternatively, a vision statement can be specific to a functional-level work group. The creation of a vision statement requires a thorough analysis of data and input from organizational or functional-level workgroup members. As with creating the mission statement, this process will take some time to complete and must have senior leadership support. The vision statement must be clear, concise, and descriptive as to how the organization sees itself in the future. Words like *creating, establishing, achieving,* and *implementing* to discuss future activities are helpful additions. The vision statement must be simple enough that it is easy to follow and short enough to paint a clear picture of where the organization is headed. Examples of EMS organization vision statements are listed in **Figure 7-3**.

The main reason for creating a strategic plan is to guide the organization from its current mission statement (organizational or functional-level mission) to a future vision statement (organizational or functional-level vision). The organization's mission and vision statements serve as a guide for the strategy team as they create the rest of the strategic plan.

Boston EMS

Boston EMS' vision is to expand upon our role as a critical public safety agency that delivers exceptional pre-hospital emergency medicine in an urban environment. The department will remain at the forefront of EMS advancements, driving progress in clinical care, operations, research and training. As a leader in all-hazard emergency preparedness, we will enhance our workforce and community's ability to be resilient when confronted by man-made and natural disasters. Boston EMS will continue to be viewed as a challenging, diverse and rewarding place to work as well as a model for other EMS agencies.

Reproduced from Boston EMS.

District of Columbia Fire and Emergency Medical Services

The vision of the DC Fire and Emergency Medical Services Department is to be a performance based organization in which a well-trained, multi-disciplined skilled workforce utilizes state-of-the-art equipment, technology and apparatus to provide the highest quality of fire and emergency medical services. To our residents and visitors the DC Fire and EMS Department strives for excellence in emergency preparedness, education and response, to enhance our customer focused innovative initiatives as industry leaders, while overcoming expanding risks.

Reproduced from District of Columbia Fire and Emergency Medical Services.

Allegheny County Emergency Medical Services

Our vision is committed to responding to the changing needs of EMS agencies throughout Allegheny County by providing educational programs and initiatives that will train our current and future EMS leaders in becoming recognized innovators and providers of comprehensive, cost-effective, and clinically sophisticated emergency medical services.

Reproduced from Allegheny County Emergency Medical Services.

Toronto Paramedic Services

Toronto Paramedic Services meets the changing needs of the community for pre-hospital and out-of-hospital care and believes that by the timely application of the advances of both the art and science of medicine to the practice of emergency medical services, we can decrease suffering, improve the health of the community and save lives.

Reproduced from Toronto Paramedic Services, www.torontoparamedicservices.ca.

Figure 7-3 Examples of vision statements.

Conducting a SWOT Analysis

Performing a SWOT analysis is the second step of the strategic planning process and must be completed once the organization's mission and vision statements have been clearly presented. A SWOT analysis is a brainstorming tool that is used to analyze information about an organization's current and potential future state by evaluating internal and external business activities. The strategy team follows these steps when working with the SWOT tool:

- Separate each section: strengths, weaknesses, opportunities, and threats.
- Know which sections of the SWOT tool will be used to evaluate internal versus external business activities.
- Brainstorm the organization's or functional-level workgroup's strengths, weaknesses, opportunities, and threats.
- Capture and analyze the data in each section of the SWOT tool.
- Encourage the submission of ideas from all internal and external organizational stakeholders to formulate goals.

Once the four components have been separated, the strategy team needs to identify the organization's or functional-level workgroup's strengths and weaknesses. Because the strengths and weaknesses directly pertain to internal activities, these two components are included in the internal analysis area of the SWOT tool (**Table 7-1**).

Next, the strategy team needs to determine which opportunities and threats may play a role in the organization's or functional-level workgroup's future. These two components are considered external business activities, originating outside the organization.

Once the SWOT tool has been established, you can begin gathering data and filling each quadrant for analysis. To gather the data, the strategy team must consider the 5 BPs (people, financial management objectives, learning objectives, strategic objectives, and a culture of quality) as core priorities when brainstorming and generating ideas. Then, as ideas are collected, the strategy team must determine whether the ideas being presented are internal or external and where they fall within the four quadrants of the SWOT tool.

Internal business activities that can be used to determine what the organization or functional-level workgroup is doing well (strengths) and where it needs improvement (weaknesses) include the following:

Table 7-1 Internal and External Components of SWOT	
Internal	**External**
Strengths	Opportunities
Weaknesses	Threats

- Employee feedback
- Performance outcomes
- Evaluation of processes and systems
- Customer surveys
- Equipment and resources

The strategy team must then gather secondary data (data captured by someone else) pertaining to external activities that may have an impact on the organization or the functional-level workgroup. Examples of secondary data sources include the following:

- Market environment: Increase or decrease in business taxes, increase or decrease in real estate costs, recession
- Industry standards: The implementation of laws or rules that govern emergency medical services delivery
- Technology: New software, new equipment
- Competition: Competitors that are providing the same or similar services and pose a threat to taking market share

A sample SWOT analysis appears in **Table 7-2**.

Once the information is gathered and all four quadrants of the SWOT tool have been filled in, the strategy team must review the activities placed within each section. It is important to continue the brainstorming session to create new ideas from the SWOT list. Keep the 5 BPs at the core of the decision-making process, and determine which goals will need to be established to move the organization from its current state toward the organization's vision. The leadership and strategy team must continue to encourage organization-wide feedback and input during the brainstorming sessions.

Establishing Goals, Objectives, Strategy, and Tactics

Establishing goals, objectives, strategy, and tactics is the third step of the strategic planning process. These four elements function together, but differ in their structure and purpose.

Goals and **objectives** answer the question of *what* you are trying to accomplish. Goals are broader, more general statements, whereas objectives are more specific and measurable.

The strategy team uses the activities included in the SWOT analysis when brainstorming for specific goals. For example, once the SWOT tool has been completed and all four sections have been addressed, then the strategy team analyzes the information in each of the sections, taking each bullet point within each section, and, with input from all members of the organization or group, establishes specific goals using the SWOT information as a guide. Some sample goals include the following:

Table 7-2 Sample SWOT Analysis	
Internal	**External**
Strengths (Build upon) ■ Well-trained paramedics and EMTs ■ Modern and reliable equipment ■ Healthy partnership with the medical community ■ Low employee turnover ■ Community support ■ Cardiac and stroke care outcomes above national average ■ Positive and consistent revenue stream from transports	**Opportunities (Capitalize)** ■ EMS grants ■ Sharing station lease agreement with another agency ■ Increasing revenue by dispatching for other organizations in the area ■ Vendors reducing purchase prices for bulk orders ■ Emergency department physicians hosting lectures and hands-on training for EMS personnel ■ Support to expand services to meet mobile integrated healthcare demand ■ Invitation from homeowners' group to have an EMS representative participate during town hall meetings

Weaknesses (Improve)
■ EMT and paramedic pay less than national average
■ No educational incentive program
■ Minimal staff to complete assignments
■ Inconsistent quality management system
■ Lengthy response times
■ Minimal backup units
■ Lack of organizational or functional-level workgroup strategic planning
	Threats (Identify root cause and adjust)
	■ Change in technology
	■ Change in market conditions
	  - Increase in gasoline prices
	  - Decrease in property tax, creating a decrease in general government funds
	  - Increasing cost of employee healthcare benefits
	  - National recession
	■ Changing industry standards
	  - Required EMS personnel credentialing
	  - Required equipment
	  - Increase in mandated training requirements
	■ Outsourcing of EMS
	■ Dissatisfied customers
	■ First-responding agencies seeking to take over transport services

■ Goal: We must meet or exceed the EMS contractual response time agreement.

■ Goal: Ensure up-to-date medical protocols.

■ Goal: Provide a quality assurance analysis of performance outcomes pertaining to EMS service delivery.

During brainstorming, the strategy team must refer to the SWOT analysis and the 5 BPs to ensure that the goals introduced support the core organizational priorities. Many goals may be suggested, but the final list of goals should include between five and seven. Included with each goal should be a time frame for accomplishing that goal. Goals are usually set for completion within a 12-, 18-, or 36-month period.

The strategy team must make it a point to meet regularly (e.g., on a monthly or quarterly basis) to ensure that the organization is still moving toward the set goals. During such reviews, the strategy team can determine whether the process of achieving the goal is on target, whether the plan needs to be adjusted, or whether the goal is outdated and no longer worth pursuing.

Regardless of the target date for completing a goal, the strategy team must routinely evaluate the progress to ensure that the organization or the functional-level workgroup remains on target to meet the deadline. It is paramount that not just the members of the strategy team, but all individuals directly involved with the goal, remain highly engaged and committed to achieving the goal.

Once a set number of goals have been established by the leadership team and/or strategy team, then it is time to create specific objectives. Objectives provide detailed information about what, specifically, is to be accomplished to support the goal. They should be measurable so that progress can be evaluated and the strategy team can determine if the organization or functional-level workgroup is close to achieving the goal or if the goal has already been met.

The following are examples of strategic objectives from the goals stated above:

- Objective: An ambulance will be on-scene within 6 minutes or less (travel time) 95 percent of the time.
- Objective: Every 6 months (June and December) the department's medical protocols will be reviewed. The first 6-month review will consist of adult care and the second 6-month review will consist of pediatric care.
- Objective: Patient transfer of care to emergency department staff upon arrival at the hospital must not exceed 15 minutes.

When creating a strategic objective, consider using **key performance indicators (KPIs)**. A KPI is a specific performance measure, used to measure strategic objective outcomes, that is essential for the sustainability of the organization's strategic goals. For example, the following KPIs may be used:

- EMS response times
- On-scene times
- Hospital turnaround times
- Customer survey results

Consider using the mnemonic SMART when creating goals and objectives to ensure that the goals and objectives message is clear:

- *Specific:* The goal must be specific for everyone to understand it.
- *Measurable:* The strategy team must be able to measure the progress of achieving the goal and determine whether the organization is on target to accomplish the goal.
- *Achievable:* Although it is important to challenge the organization as it moves from its current state toward the idealized vision, the goal must not be set so high that it is impossible to attain.
- *Realistic:* The goal must be realistic and pertinent to the organization's mission.
- *Time-bound:* The strategy team must clearly establish deadlines, which then must be shared with all participating members of the organization.

Strategy and tactics answer the question of *how* something will be accomplished. The strategy is the approach you will take to accomplish the goal, and the **tactics** are the tools used to accomplish the goal. For example:

- *Strategy:* Make sure that all EMS units are equipped with the necessary tools that will assist in reducing response times.
- *Tactics:* Place global positioning system (GPS) modules in every unit, ensure that all area map books are up-to-date, ensure that all mobile data terminals clearly display the address of the incident location, and routinely evaluate crews' knowledge of their response area.

A strategy clearly defines, within a narrow scope, how the organizational team members plan to achieve a goal. Having a clear strategy then allows the strategy team and organizational

Managerial Leadership **BRIEFCASE**

Strategic Plan Questions

When creating your organization's strategic plan, ask the following questions:

- Are there organizational mission and vision statements?
- Is the organization monitoring its competitors?
- Have the organizational leaders committed time to complete a SWOT analysis?
- Has the strategy team created SMART goals and objectives?
- Do the objectives, strategy, and tactics support the goal?
- Are the 5 BPs clearly stated, and do the goals support the priorities?
- What is the organization doing right and what needs improving?
- What input, if any, is being sought from internal and external stakeholders?

Answering these simple questions will get your organization moving in the right direction.

members to begin planning which tactics to use to achieve the goal. Tactics can include any activity, resource, equipment, or people necessary to get the job done. Once you reach the point of identifying the tools necessary to achieve each goal, the plan is almost complete.

Implementing the Plan

Strategic planning is not complete once the plan has been created. The fourth step in the strategic planning process is implementing the plan. Once the goals are set, objectives have been specifically defined, a strategy has been crafted to achieve the goal, and tactics are in place to achieve the goals, then the leadership team must articulate the plan to internal and external stakeholders. If the organization's internal and external stakeholders do not understand the strategy, it will be difficult for them to follow it. Communicating the strategic plan clearly so that all parties thoroughly understand it is essential, so the medium used to share the plan is important. Depending on the size of the plan, the organizational or functional-level unit leaders may choose to share the plan during a meeting, disseminate the plan via e-mail, post it on a website, or mail the plan to stakeholders.

Disseminating a strategic plan, especially within a large organization, may be a bit challenging. Therefore, it is recommended not to wait for the final product to introduce the organization to a strategic plan. Make it a point to share the progress and outcomes along the way. This ensures feedback from the team members, but also allows for an easy introduction to the plan. Introducing the plan incrementally or in phases may allow for better understanding of what end goal the organization is attempting to achieve. Once the final plan is shared, it should not take the organizational members by surprise.

Although the strategy team leader will ultimately be responsible for managing the strategic plan, each of the goals created during the strategic planning process needs to be assigned to an organizational team member. This person may be a member of the strategy team or a functional-level team member. Depending on the complexity of the goal, more than one team member may be assigned to routinely measure the progress of each goal and to ensure that the organization continues moving toward its target. When creating a strategic plan, the strategy team may specify a number of goals that should be accomplished at the 1-, 3-, or 5-year mark. In turn, before the strategic plan is rolled out, the strategy team leader must determine how often the strategy team will meet to evaluate the progress of the plan and its goals: Routine follow-up meetings are considered part of the strategic planning process.

Although a strategic plan can have an actionable time span anywhere from 1 to 3 to 5 years, goals must be set for completion at 6-, 12-, 18-, or 36-month increments. Identifying these interim milestones allows for adjustments and quicker results in a constantly changing business environment. Their existence also emphasizes the importance of following through on the implementation process. It is tempting to think the hard work of strategic planning is complete once the plan has been written, but, in fact, implementation of the plan is an essential component. Without implementation, the plan is not serving its purpose.

Evaluating the Plan

The fifth and final step of the strategic planning process is evaluating the plan after it has been implemented. Many strategic plans fail because the plan is not routinely evaluated. As noted earlier, regular follow-up meetings are needed to ensure that the plan is still on target to achieve the strategic goals, the goals are still appropriate, and there are no changes in the organization's or functional-level workgroup's priorities. To ensure that the strategic plan is still up-to-date and to evaluate the progress made in accomplishing the plan, the strategy team must meet on an ongoing basis.

Because market environments and industry requirements can change, the organization's leadership and strategy team must be able to adjust rapidly to their dynamic environment. What was once considered a strength may become a weakness over time, and what was once a weakness may no longer be a weakness—but it may also be an even greater weakness than when the strategic plan was first devised. An opportunity may no longer be available, or perhaps there are more opportunities to seize. A threat may have dissipated, in which case you will want to avoid wasting time and energy on it. More ominously, a threat may intensify, and without regular evaluations of the plan, it may be too late to make any adjustments to ameliorate the growing threat.

Evaluate the strategic objectives to ensure that they are specific enough and that the strategy team is able to measure the progress in achieving the goal. Evaluation will also reveal if there is minimal progress in achieving the desired goals due to ineffective tactics.

It is paramount that the strategy team routinely evaluates the plan not only to ensure that the plan is still on target to reach the set goals, but also to assess the internal and external priorities of the organization. The leadership and strategy team must continue to refer to updated SWOT analysis, performance outcome data, and the 5 BPs during any such reevaluations.

As the EMS officer assigned to lead a strategy team, you should consider the following points when evaluating a strategic plan:

- Meet with your strategy team and key members of the organization after implementation of the plan to ensure everyone understands his or her role.
- The evaluation of a strategic plan must be a collaborative process among the leadership team, strategy team, and members of the organization. Internal and external stakeholder buy-in and input are extremely important. Ask what is working and what is not, what you can do better as an organization, what you should change, and what you should keep.
- The leadership and strategy team must be ready to make necessary adjustments regarding goals, objectives, strategy, and tactics.
- The strategy team must ensure that the goals, once set in place to move the organization forward, continue to have a direct link to the information obtained through the SWOT analysis, performance outcomes, and 5 BPs. This is part of the organization's commitment to total quality management.

Success in the BUSINESS WORLD

The Importance of Reevaluation

Southwest Airlines, Walmart, and Toyota have survived turbulent economic times. One key factor in their survival is that these companies all had strategic plans for operating in a very difficult economy. These organizations reduced spending and found ways to deliver their products and services more efficiently than their competitors. They were successful because they prepared for downturns and were able to adjust as necessary to ensure that they met the current market demands. It is critical that after a strategic plan is implemented, the leadership and strategy team meet regularly to determine whether the organization is still on target to meet the organizational or functional-level unit goals set within the strategic plan. Goals may need to be adjusted if internal and/or external conditions have changed.

WRAP-UP

Concept Review

- The strategy planning process must be thorough and systematic, and it must have leadership support and employee buy-in if it is to succeed.

- The strategic plan is an organizational plan designed to clearly and concisely communicate how the organization will achieve its desired future organizational goals.

- The purpose of a strategic plan is to get the organization from where it is as a business (mission) to where it wants to be (vision), which requires aligning organizational resources appropriately and making organizational improvements to service delivery.

- An organizational (or corporate) strategic plan includes performance improvement initiatives across all levels of the

organization. A functional-level strategic plan is appropriate if the EMS officer is assigned to create a strategy for a single functional-level group or division.

- Organizational (or corporate) strategy focuses on evaluating current organizational activities, then establishing organization-wide administrative and operational goals.

- A functional-level strategic planning team will use many of the same strategic planning tools used to create an organizational strategic plan, except the resulting plan centers on the administrative and operational business activities within a functional-level unit.

- Regardless of the strategy selected, the strategic planning process activities must be thoroughly evaluated and systematically completed throughout the process.

- The mission statement should clearly identify the service currently being provided by the organization.
- The creation of a vision statement must include a thorough analysis of data and input from organizational or functional-level workgroup members.
- SWOT analysis is a brainstorming tool used to analyze information about an organization's current and potential future state by evaluating internal and external business activities.
- Goals and objectives answer the question of *what* you are trying to accomplish, whereas strategy and tactics answer the question of *how* something will be accomplished.
- Communicating the strategic plan is essential to ensure its effectiveness, so the medium used to share the plan is important.
- To ensure that the strategic plan is still up-to-date and to evaluate the progress made in accomplishing the plan, the strategy team must meet on a regular basis.

Managerial Terms

Functional-level strategic plan A plan created by and for members working in a division of an organization.

Key performance indicators (KPIs) Specific performance measures essential to the sustainability of an organization's strategic goals.

Mission statement A statement that identifies what you are doing now as an organization—that is, the purpose of the organization.

Objectives Instructions used to support a goal. Objectives must be specific and measurable.

Organizational (or corporate) strategic plan The overall strategy that is created to meet and exceed an organization's overall mission.

Strategic plan An organizational plan designed to clearly and concisely communicate how an organization will achieve its desired future organizational goals.

Strategy The approach taken to achieve a goal.

SWOT analysis A brainstorming tool used to analyze information about an organization's current and potential future state by evaluating internal and external business activities; its components are strengths, weaknesses, opportunities, and threats.

Tactics A set of actions or processes used to achieve the organization's strategic plan.

Vision statement A statement that identifies where the organization should be in the future, and that serves as the compass of the organization.

Case Review: Getting the Organization Moving Again

Captain Wayne had been promoted to oversee a functional-level unit (division) within his organization. The division had been one of the most productive divisions within the organization; however, over the past 2 years, it had become unproductive and had failed to meet service delivery standards. Over that time span, the division had ceased to offer new products and services to the community, the employees seemed directionless, unhappy customers were at an all-time high, there had been missed opportunities to improve service delivery, and the services were routinely threatened by the organization's competitors. The division was at a standstill.

Captain Wayne identified the primary reason the division was at a standstill: It did not have a formal strategic plan in place, so the functional-level workgroup had no direction and no idea as to how to chart its course. One of the first actions taken by Captain Wayne was to bring all of the members of the team together and take the time to explain why creating a strategic plan was the first order of business. The team supported this initiative and was encouraged to provide input during the continuous strategic planning process. After the formal implementation of a functional-level unit strategic plan, the plan became part of the division's culture, and the division began to see positive results. The group needed a leader with a clearly defined vision, a plan, and the wherewithal to get all members involved in the planning process.

After the implementation of the functional unit's strategic plan, the team members understood the mission and vision set by Captain Wayne. The team, using the SWOT analysis, identified the unit's strengths, weaknesses, opportunities, and threats. The team became informed of the service their competitors were offering to the citizens and were able to make the appropriate adjustments and remain competitive. By evaluating the unit's strengths and weaknesses, they noted that their service delivery and well-trained EMTs and paramedics were among the organization's key strengths. However, the organization's salaries were not comparable to those in other EMS organizations; therefore, the morale and employee retention suffered. By implementing a strategic plan and incorporating the plan as part of the organization's quality management program, the functional-level unit (division) began identifying areas of waste and was able to make adjustments that resulted in cost savings for the organization. These savings resulted in improved financial health and ultimately an increase in wages and the purchase of much needed equipment.

Case Discussion

Like Captain Wayne, you cannot afford to wait until your organization or functional-level unit fails to meet its desired performance outcomes before you undertake strategic planning. When you create a strategic plan, that plan must be supported by the leadership team; however, it will be the team members who will execute the plan on a daily basis. Given this fact, input and active participation from all members of the organization must be encouraged. Having a formal strategic plan will serve as a roadmap for the direction in which the organization is heading. Its development is paramount if the organization plans to remain competitive and to adjust to changing market environments.

All members of the organization must be given an opportunity to be part of the strategy team and be encouraged to submit input. Either the strategy team or the leadership team must visit the front-line team members and get their input. It is important that all members understand not just the importance of having a strategic plan, but even more so the importance of thoroughly committing time and analysis to each of the strategic planning sections. When creating a strategic plan, it must be routinely emphasized that the plan is intended to support internal and external organizational and functional-level unit business activities. When no strategic plan exists, the organization and its members will continue to carry out their daily work routines, but will have no idea what the organization's or functional-level unit's vision is and will not know when or how to adjust to changing business conditions. Over time, the organization will most likely become stagnant because there is no plan to move the organization in a specific direction. Finally, the strategic plan should always be evolving, so it must be reevaluated regularly and internal and external stakeholders included as part of the strategic planning process.

Case Review: Strategic Planning

The fire chief calls the EMS division chief into the office and asks her to share her division's strategic plan with the other functional-unit managers (e.g., Budget Office Manager, Division Chief of Fire Suppression, Fleet Manger, Logistics Manager, and Communication Center Manager). He is having a team meeting next month with the command staff (functional-unit managers) and would like the EMS division chief to give a presentation of the EMS division's strategic plan at that meeting. The chief would also like her to describe each step of the strategic planning process and to share the final plan with the team. She will have 3 weeks to complete the plan. Will she be ready?

As it turns out, the EMS officer involved in this case was ahead of the curve because she had taken the initiative to create a strategic plan for her functional-level unit before she was asked to do so.

This EMS officer took advantage of the 3 weeks' notice prior to the presentation to evaluate the current plan, highlight which goals had been either accomplished or were on target to meet the set deadline, describe which adjustments had been made to the plan due to changes in market or industry conditions, and describe which method of communicating the plan was used upon rolling out the plan. When initially creating the strategic plan, it took the EMS officer and members of a strategy team approximately 2 months to complete the plan.

During her presentation to the command staff, the EMS division chief was able to describe both her functional-level unit's strategic plan and the process involved in creating such a plan. The chief was appreciative of her and the team's hard work and efforts in providing such a thorough presentation. After the meeting, the chief asked the EMS division chief to be part of the organization's strategy team and asked for her assistance in creating a strategic plan for the organization.

Case Discussion

As an EMS officer, you will be counted on to bring fresh ideas to the table, discuss your vision and goals for the organization or your functional-level unit, and be prepared to manage changes to internal and external business activities. The ultimate goal is to move the organization in the right direction to achieve the desired business outcomes. You are now in a managerial-leadership role, and you must be available to the chief of the department, the senior leadership team, and the front-line team members for guidance and assistance. Those around you will expect accurate information and will seek your advice. Always try to go above and beyond when working on projects and with your day-to-day responsibilities.

Provide the chief what he or she is asking for and then some. If the chief does not need the additional information, there is no harm done: It is always better to under-promise and over-deliver. As an EMS officer or someone in another type of leadership position, you must not wait to create a strategic plan for your functional-level unit or your organization.

The time frame for creating a strategic plan may vary depending on the team's meeting schedule, the number of participants assisting throughout the strategic planning process, the amount of information that needs to be analyzed, and the scope of the strategic plan (i.e., for a functional-level unit versus the entire organization). The strategic planning process offers an opportunity to get to know the organization or functional-level unit, and that opportunity should not be squandered in the haste to meet a deadline. Organizational and functional-level unit leaders should be less concerned with how quickly a strategic plan can be completed, and more focused on getting the strategic plan done right the first time.

8

Managing a Crisis

Learning Objectives

After studying this chapter, you should be able to:

- Explain the relationship between risk and crisis.

- Discuss the components and implementation of an injury prevention program.

- Describe how to anticipate a crisis.

- Discuss how to create a crisis management plan.

- Identify and describe the steps in managing a crisis.

- Discuss the effects that crisis events have on an organization.

Introduction

Crisis management is part of every EMS officer's responsibilities and affects four of the five business priorities (5 BPs): people, strategic objectives, financial management objectives, and culture of quality. A crisis can be caused by numerous situations—for example, a natural disaster, a medical emergency, not meeting a deadline, an event that is negatively affecting your organization, or economic difficulty. The EMS officer may not see a crisis looming on the horizon, but if there is a crisis plan in place and the organization or division adopts an anticipatory (and not reactionary) stance, the organization will be better prepared to address and manage the crisis. Establishing a crisis management action plan that includes key steps in dealing with a crisis will help the organization manage the crisis, keep it from growing, look for internal and external organizational ramifications from the crisis, prevent tunnel vision, and identify how to bring closure to the crisis. A crisis is one situation in which having the right team members assigned to the right roles and doing the jobs they do best can make a great impact on the outcome.

Every organization will have differences in its organizational structure, the roles and responsibilities assigned to each EMS officer, and the elements included in a crisis management action plan. A managing (rather than a supervising) EMS officer would likely be called upon either to manage or to assist with the resolution of internal or external crises. This chapter focuses primarily on managing administrative crises, as the primary duties of the managing EMS officer are administrative. It highlights the importance of having a crisis management action plan and identifies some key points when confronting a crisis. Understanding the importance of managing risks and crises is critical to the EMS officer.

Understanding Risk and Crisis

As an EMS officer, you must be prepared to manage internal and external risks and crises. **Risks** are processes, systems, stakeholder activities, and other business activities that may turn into crises if not monitored or managed appropriately. They are natural side effects of doing business and can develop from both actions and natural occurrences.

An internal risk is one that originates within the organization, whereas an external risk is one that originates outside the organization. If not managed appropriately, either type of risk has the potential to become a **crisis**, a situation that poses a serious threat to a single customer, a community, or the organization and its **stakeholders**. Examples of internal risks include the following:

- Doing business with a vendor that does not have a good reputation
- Opting not to purchase the extended warranty when purchasing ambulance units
- Implementing priority dispatching for all 911 requests for service
- Purchasing nonessential equipment with budget reserve dollars
- Reducing staffing by closing an EMS station during nonpeak hours

External risks, too, have the potential to turn into crises if not managed or prepared for appropriately. Examples include the following:

- Market competition
- Crews being exposed to communicable diseases
- Events that pose safety challenges for the rescuers (e.g., natural disasters and terrorist events)

Having a plan to monitor and manage risks before they become crises must be a priority for the EMS officer, and every effort must be made to anticipate a crisis before it occurs. Avoidance of a crisis situation benefits the community, the organization, and stakeholders. As an EMS officer, you should actively look for those operational and administrative risks—do not wait for a crisis to occur to begin preparing a **crisis management plan**.

A crisis poses a challenge to those being affected by it as well as those attempting to mitigate the crisis. Such an event can be caused by internal or external stakeholders, and can be triggered by natural, human-made, market, or technological forces that pose a direct threat to customers, community, the organization, or the organization's stakeholders. Examples of internal crises include line-of-duty deaths or injuries, internal stakeholder layoffs, budget cuts resulting in a reduction of service, and an audit finding of noncompliance with legislative mandates. Examples of external crises include mass-casualty incidents, vehicle accidents involving an ambulance, a protected health information (PHI) security breach, and natural disasters.

Regardless of its size and origin, each crisis requires immediate attention. The first priority must be providing for the safety of all involved in the incident, ensuring that customers are being appropriately supported, rapidly obtaining the necessary resources, resolving the crisis as soon as possible, and preventing any negative publicity directed toward the organization as a result of the incident.

Anticipating a Crisis

You may not be able to stop a crisis from happening. Nevertheless, if you thoroughly understand the internal and external business activities within your area of responsibility and remain alert to anticipating a crisis before it happens, the better prepared you, your team, and the organization will be in managing the crisis.

Crises Without Warning

You may not know when a crisis is on the horizon and how it will affect your customers, community, organization, and stakeholders. Events that occur without warning may include multiple-casualty crashes involving a mass transit bus or a commercial airliner, an active shooter event, or an unfunded mandate placed on the organization. For both internal and external crises, instilling a culture of preparedness and ensuring that all team members understand their role before a crisis happens will be critical. It is not a question of *if* a crisis will occur under your watch, but rather *when*.

Having a basic systematic approach that can be used to manage internal and external crises when they erupt without warning signs is critical so an effective response can be implemented immediately. The organization's members must know their fundamental duties when a crisis occurs within the organization as well as during a large and complex emergency.

As an EMS officer, you must expect that crisis situations will surround you, and you may have no time to prepare for them. Therefore, how you have prepared in advance and how you manage the incident will play a major role in determining the outcome.

Crises with Warning

Some situations allow organizational leaders enough time to prepare for making a specific response. For example, the threat of an impending hurricane, a winter storm, a volcanic eruption, heavy rain with the potential for severe flooding, a mass gathering, and a pandemic are all situations that may lead to a crisis, but there is typically enough time to prepare for the specific event and plan accordingly. Many crisis situations that emerge with warning create cyclical threats on a regular basis—for example, hurricanes in Florida, winter storms in the Northeast, and a heightened alert of terrorist activities in areas of public gathering such as tourist events or during specific holidays. Because these situations are more likely to yield a crisis, EMS, fire, and police organizations will be well versed in the management protocol for them and will have a crisis management plan already in place. Ideally, an initial crisis management plan will be in place well before a threat arises, and that plan should be flexible enough to realign the response to meet the needs of the specific crisis. No organization should wait for a crisis to occur before beginning its management preparations.

Organizational leaders must make it a priority to anticipate organizational crisis situations before a crisis strikes by assessing the immediate organizational risks and determining the potential hazards that might turn a risk into a crisis. Sometimes risks will be readily evident. For example, a hurricane may be quickly approaching the east coast, with city officials turning to you for direction: Should they implement a mandatory evacuation or allow citizens to remain on the barrier island during the storm? The hazards in such a case are storm surge, high winds, power outages, and poor accessibility to victims during and after the storm. In this situation, organizational leaders have time to assess the external risks and hazards and to make the appropriate decisions to avoid a crisis situation.

An example of an anticipated internal crisis is a situation in which most of the organization's revenue is obtained through user insurance payments and county-wide taxes, but the current economy is unstable and healthcare reform is being introduced. Both of these changes are considered serious hazards with the potential to directly affect the organization's service delivery if a drop in revenue occurs.

These examples outline risks that, if not effectively managed and routinely monitored, can potentially turn into crises. Focusing on those key risk areas and understanding which hazards create the potential for a crisis event must be a priority to avoid a crisis. The EMS officer must make every attempt to routinely evaluate internal and external risks and hazards, monitor organizational processes and systems, analyze customer feedback, determine areas of potential risk, review data and performance outcomes regarding impending crises, ask organizational employees where they see potential risks and hazards, and research what other organizations are doing to prepare for crises. In addition, the EMS officer must make a point to review organizational spokes that have the greatest risk of becoming a crisis (e.g., operations, logistics, dispatch, budget support, fleet, and customers). (See the "Dynamics of EMS Leadership and Organizational Structure" chapter for more discussion of organizational spokes.)

Limiting Risk to Personnel

Injury prevention and personnel safety are key components in preparing for—and potentially preventing—a crisis. Therefore, organizational leaders must conduct risk assessments to ensure the safety of their personnel and those they serve. In addition to the impact to life and property, there is also the financial impact associated with employee injury. This can range from medical care for the employee, workers' compensation, paying overtime to fill the position while the injured individual is out of work, repairing damaged equipment, and any investigation to ensure compliance with state and federal occupational safety regulations. Creating and implementing an injury prevention and safety program within your organization must be a priority and it must start with the leadership team.

To create an injury prevention and safety program, organizational leaders must first conduct a workplace risk assessment. The following steps will help with this assessment:

- Review any preexisting injury prevention and safety plan.
- Review specific injury prevention policies, procedures, and forms and any risk assessment documents.
- Collect data such as:
  - Recent inspections
  - Recent injuries
  - Workers' compensation
  - How often training was conducted and which training topics were covered
- Visit office workstations and remote sites to get input from employees regarding their preparedness to deal with unsafe situations.
- Review any documentation pertaining to injury prevention or safety inspections at work stations, department vehicles, employee and visitor common areas, lunch rooms and cafeterias, conference centers, and other areas that are considered high traffic areas or where employees congregate.

Injury prevention must be part of the organization's culture and must be driven by the organization's leadership team. The organizational leaders must show a commitment to injury prevention and safety by participating in injury prevention drills, attending injury prevention classes, visiting workstations, and asking employees for feedback about injury prevention. Leaders must demonstrate this commitment across the different functional workgroups, not just those at the highest risk of injury.

An injury prevention and safety program consists of numerous key activities that must be ongoing; for example, the plan must include a communication mechanism (regular meetings, bulletins, e-mails, posters, one-on-one interviews) of how employees will be informed of regular safety updates, employees must know what to do when faced with an unsafe situation, clear state and federal compliance regulations pertinent to the work environment must be posted, there must be routine safety worksite inspections and continuous injury prevention training, and the leadership must maintain records of all injury and safety activities, including accident investigations.

For an injury prevention plan to be successful, it must be clearly written in an accessible format and must be supported by policies and procedures. The following components must be part of an injury prevention and safety plan:

- Perform any safety activities mandated by state or federal occupational safety and health officials.
- Conduct safety meetings with new and senior employees on a regular basis.
- Conduct routine drills (at least twice a year) and have employees assume their assigned roles while working through hazardous scenarios.
- Create and implement an Organizational Hazard Assessment Form specific to worksite, office, and pre-hospital environments; for example, the forms may ask the following questions:
  - Do outlets have surge protectors?
  - Is the furniture sturdy and safe for use?
  - Are there trip hazards in the office and throughout the station?
  - Are stairwells lighted appropriately and do they have non-skid lining?
  - Are work stations ergonomically friendly for employees who spend a lot of time at their desks?
  - Are EMS crews using the necessary personal protective equipment when working with patients?
- Ensure non-public safety employees know how to detect unsafe situations such as electrical hazards; fire safety hazards, such as blocking exits with storage equipment; and inappropriate storage and use of flammable material.
- Ensure all non-EMS employees are trained in basic first aid and how to use a fire extinguisher.
- Establish a building evacuation map.
- Provide the necessary equipment to protect the rescuer and render assistance to other employees.
- Designate an on-scene and administrative safety officer.
- Determine how and when to conduct a post-accident or near-miss analysis, document all findings, and report the findings to the appropriate officials.
- Practice proper lifting techniques.
- Provide continuous injury prevention and safety training and resources across the organization.
- Create a safety committee.

Employees must be provided with the necessary tools and training to support an injury prevention environment. If a hazard is observed, it must be reported and corrected immediately. Waiting to correct a hazard or a potential risk may not only result in fines and additional work, but may also severely impact life and property and contribute to an internal crisis.

Injury prevention and safety practices must be an ongoing event. Therefore, incentives should be provided to those individuals who actively participate and follow the injury prevention and safety policies and procedures. The best approach to an injury prevention and safety program is to promote the importance of using safe practices before an injury occurs.

Creating a Crisis Management Plan

Having a crisis management plan in place before a crisis occurs is critical because it provides the necessary framework to manage the incident and allows for a rapid deployment of activities necessary to mitigate the crisis. The content of the plan must be simple and straightforward enough for everyone to understand during a crisis and must be easily accessible for any team member's use. Remember, however, that any plan must be tailored to the organization's specific operational capabilities. Public safety organizations typically have crisis response plans already established for external large-scale incidents, but EMS officers and organizational leaders must also be prepared for those internal crises that affect the organization directly and that impact its stakeholders.

The plan may be created and published in a booklet form or as a standard operating guideline (SOG). The organization's leaders may also choose to make quick-reference crisis management materials readily available at every employee's workstation (**Figure 8-1**). These quick-reference materials can provide instructions regarding what to do in the event of a specific crisis. Regardless of the format of the plan, the approach to crisis management must be shared with all personnel and agencies that will assist during a crisis management event.

Crisis management does not end with the development of the plan, however. The organization must practice, on a regular basis, how to use that plan, and every team member must be familiar with his or her role during a crisis so less uncertainty will occur when an actual crisis occurs. No plan can include all the answers necessary to manage every specific crisis, but such a document can certainly set the direction to begin mitigating the crisis effectively.

The organization's leadership must be prepared to manage both administrative and operational crises. They may choose to have separate plans for internal and external crises, or they may create a single plan that addresses both. Regardless of which approach is chosen, some key activities should always be considered when creating a crisis management plan:

- Include a well-coordinated and comprehensive approach to prevent duplication of work and resources and to promote safety throughout the incident.
- Establish an incident command system (ICS) either upon arrival at the scene (external crisis) or upon being notified of an impending crisis event (internal crisis).

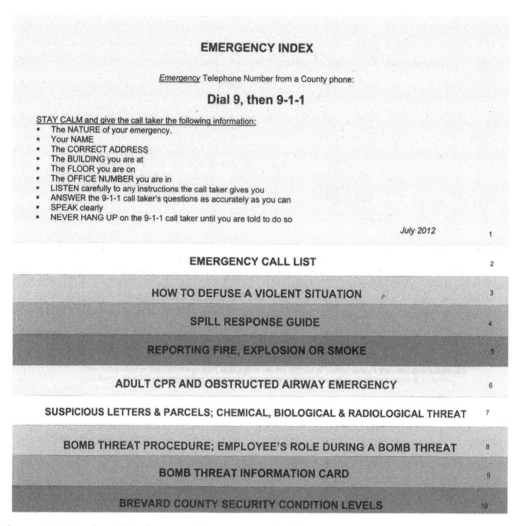

EMERGENCY INDEX

Emergency Telephone Number from a County phone:

Dial 9, then 9-1-1

STAY CALM and give the call taker the following information:
- The NATURE of your emergency.
- Your NAME
- The CORRECT ADDRESS
- The BUILDING you are at
- The FLOOR you are on
- The OFFICE NUMBER you are in
- LISTEN carefully to any instructions the call taker gives you
- ANSWER the 9-1-1 call taker's questions as accurately as you can
- SPEAK clearly
- NEVER HANG UP on the 9-1-1 call taker until you are told to do so

July 2012   1

EMERGENCY CALL LIST   2

HOW TO DEFUSE A VIOLENT SITUATION   3

SPILL RESPONSE GUIDE   4

REPORTING FIRE, EXPLOSION OR SMOKE   5

ADULT CPR AND OBSTRUCTED AIRWAY EMERGENCY   6

SUSPICIOUS LETTERS & PARCELS; CHEMICAL, BIOLOGICAL & RADIOLOGICAL THREAT   7

BOMB THREAT PROCEDURE; EMPLOYEE'S ROLE DURING A BOMB THREAT   8

BOMB THREAT INFORMATION CARD   9

BREVARD COUNTY SECURITY CONDITION LEVELS   10

Figure 8-1 Sample quick-reference crisis management guide.
Courtesy of Brevard County Board of County Commissioners.

- Share the crisis plan (objectives, strategy, and tactics) with internal and/or external stakeholders as soon as possible.
- Ensure that the necessary resources are available.
- Ensure that the plan is easy to use and includes simple process flow charts.
- Include the big picture of the organization and the root cause of the crisis (e.g., whether the crisis is the result of one or more specific hazards).

- Assign a spokesperson to disseminate information pertaining to the crisis (ideally in place before the crisis occurs; see the "Communications" chapter).
- Include the organization's expected outcomes when dealing with internal and external crises.
- Include protocols for postincident analysis and critical incident stress debriefing (CISD).
- Specify how the leadership team and those involved in mitigating the crisis will communicate with each other: face-to-face, phone, e-mail, social media, texting.
- Prepare for a crisis before it occurs. Practice often. Conduct table-top exercises.
- Determine which team members will be involved in managing the crisis, and define those team members' responsibilities.
- Routinely evaluate the plan. Determine who will be responsible for updating the plan, and include the management of specific crisis situations within the current crisis management plan.
- Consider internal posting of an emergency index at each team member's workstation. Such an emergency index can provide specific instructions for what to do when employees encounter a potential crisis. For example, which essential information must be reported when requesting help from 911 or from the leadership team regarding the incident? Which initial activities should employees perform when they encounter a specific crisis (e.g., hazardous chemical spill, explosion, bomb threat, medical emergency)? What are the instructions for administrative staff on how to perform certain life-saving activities (e.g., cardiopulmonary resuscitation [CPR] and use of a fire extinguisher)? An emergency index can serve as a valuable tool when a potential crisis emerges, and can help employees take immediate action to begin addressing the incident.
- Stress the importance of ensuring and working in a safe environment by promoting situational awareness, injury prevention, containing the crisis, isolating the crisis, and mitigating the hazard before it spreads.
- Include input from the team members. The plan must be executed by all team members. There must be no freelancing.

Effective written and verbal communication is essential among all members of the organization, especially during a crisis. Although EMS and other public safety personnel routinely train and may have actively participated in crisis situations, administrative staff members may not have the same experience. Consequently, the plan must be comprehensive, clear to understand, concise in its instructions, and easy to follow. If it is not, the members of the organization may find it difficult to execute the plan. Including technical jargon may create challenges for some team members in understanding what is required during a crisis.

Conversely, including diagrams, such as process flow charts, in addition to text should make the plan easier to follow.

For the crisis action plan to be effective, obtaining input from the management crisis team, practicing how to manage a crisis situation with all staff members, and ensuring that all members understand their roles during an emergency are essential. It is not enough to put the plan down on paper and store it on a shelf. Instead, every member assigned to the crisis management team must participate in preparing for crises and discuss his or her role during a crisis. Table-top exercises allow employees to make mistakes while practicing and to identify any secondary crises that could occur during the management of the crisis.

It often takes a real crisis for an organization to realize that it is not adequately prepared to manage a crisis. In any case, it is beneficial for the organization to be proactive and anticipatory rather than reactionary.

There will certainly be differences when managing different crises, as no two crises are the same and the demands will be different. The leadership team will need to adjust the response accordingly to mitigate the crisis. Nevertheless, effective crisis management all starts with a plan and the assurance that every organizational member understands his or her responsibilities before a crisis occurs.

Planning for an Internal Crisis

Internal crisis events may not require the same resources or multijurisdictional personnel support as large and complex external crisis situations do. Therefore, organizational leaders may opt to develop a crisis management plan intended exclusively for internal crisis management. **Figure 8-2** shows an example of an internal crisis management preparedness plan.

When attempting to manage an internal organizational crisis, it is beneficial to use principles similar to those applied when managing an external crisis. Such principles clearly emphasize an organized approach to crisis management and delineate a central point of command, roles and responsibilities of those participating in the event, necessary resources to mitigate the crisis,

Managerial Leadership BRIEFCASE

Planning for a Crisis

When a crisis erupts, it typically comes without warning and can range from a small event to a large incident. Any crisis has the potential to pack a catastrophic punch. The key to managing such an incident is to have a crisis plan ready before a crisis occurs. You cannot possibly prepare to manage every crisis that comes your way, but by having a plan you will be ahead of the curve. The plan in the briefcase must include the flexibility to adjust before and during a crisis, and include guidelines for bringing the crisis to a close.

Jones EMS Department
CRISIS MANAGEMENT PREPAREDNESS PLAN

DIVISION: Operations	**SUBJECT:** CRISIS MANAGEMENT PREPAREDNESS PLAN (INTERNAL)	**SOP#** TBD

Purpose: To ensure a consistent approach to **internal** organization crisis management by establishing a crisis action preparedness plan.

Types of Crises: Examples of internal crisis situations that may be encountered by the Jones EMS Department or specific to one of the department's functional workgroups:

— Disruption of EMS service delivery

— Disruption of office resources (IT, power outage, damage to office building)

— Workplace violence

— Legal action taken toward the agency

— Media reports of poor EMS service delivery by Jones EMS

— Sexual harassment by department employee

— Being investigated for billing fraud

Priorities: To gather as much information as possible pertaining to the incident, determine the risk or crisis, prevent or resolve the risk or crisis to stakeholders and organization quickly.

— What happened?

— Which activity is causing the crisis?

— Are there any injuries or fatalities?

— Is the crisis still active?

— If there is an immediate threat to life and property, has 911 been notified?

— If there is no immediate threat to life and property, has the leadership or crisis management coordinator been notified?

1. **Response Checklist:** To establish a thorough and systematic approach to managing internal crisis situations. *External crises such as disasters or large-scale emergency incidents will be managed as dictated by the organization's standard operating procedures specific to the incident and direction of the on-scene incident commander.*

If Internal Risk or Crisis Poses a Life Threat

A. Get to safety

B. Report the incident to 911

C. Assist victims

D. Conduct an accountability check for employees

Figure 8-2 Example of an internal crisis management preparedness plan. *(continues)*

If Internal Risk or Crisis Poses No Life Threat

    A. Perform a risk-crisis assessment

        a. What is the probability of the risk becoming a crisis within 24–72 hours?

                    Low—Moderate—High

        b. What is the probability that the crisis will cause life threats to internal and/or external stakeholders?

                    Low—Moderate—High

        c. What is the probability that the crisis will affect the organization and prevent it from doing business?

                    Low—Moderate—High

2. **Roles and Responsibilities**

    A. Incident Officer (managing to executive officer level)

        a. Establish a member of the leadership team as the incident officer.

        b. Determine the goal, objective, strategy, and tactical approach to mitigate the crisis.

        c. Ensure that the risk or crisis is being addressed.

        d. Ensure support team members are involved with mitigating the crisis.

        e. Be transparent and honest when discussing the situation with stakeholders.

        f. Be available to meet with the community and discuss the crisis once it is no longer a threat to the organization or the community.

        g. Request feedback from stakeholders once the crisis has been resolved.

    B. Crisis Management Coordinator (entry level to managing officer level)

        a. Support the crisis incident officer.

        b. Coordinate the strategic and tactical response to mitigate the crisis by the crisis management team.

        c. Coordinate logistical support.

        d. Coordinate duties between functional workgroups when mitigating the crisis.

    C. Crisis Management Team (organization team members)

        a. Provide the tactical response to mitigate the internal crisis.

        b. Assist staff members in resuming business operations.

        c. Communicate with and assist stakeholders by answering questions.

        d. Notify and work with family members of injured employees.

    D. Public Information Officer

        a. Coordinate the release of information with senior leadership.

        b. Determine who is affected by the crisis and who the target audience is.

        c. Keep the message clear and simple to follow.

        d. Organize press conferences.

        e. Disseminate press releases.

        f. Be available for media interviews.

        g. Document the event and record all activities used to mitigate the crisis.

Figure 8-2 Example of an internal crisis management preparedness plan. *(continued)*

CHAPTER 8:** Managing a Crisis **233**

3. **Communication:** Ensure a consistent and effective medium of communication during a crisis situation.
   A. Face-to-face
   B. E-mail
   C. Text
   D. Social media
   E. Portable, mobile, or base station radio

4. **Stakeholders:** Provide the necessary information and direction to key stakeholders and those who are affected by the crisis situation.
   A. Internal
      a. Agency functional workgroups
      b. Field crews
      c. City or county elected officials
   B. External
      a. Community members
      b. Vendors
      c. Customers
      d. State EMS office
      e. Local hospitals

5. **Resources:** Ensure that resources are available and aligned to appropriately manage and mitigate the crisis.
   A. Have a predetermined operation center that can be accessible during crisis situations and provides access to:
      a. Telephone
      b. Computers/Internet
      c. Fax and copy machine
      d. Overhead projector
      e. Conference call capabilities
      f. Erase boards
      g. Office supplies
   B. Identify the necessary equipment or actions needed to resolve the crisis.
   C. Determine how to get the equipment and crisis team to the location of the crisis.

6. **Definitions:** Provide consistent terminology and definitions when mitigating a crisis situation.
   A. Crisis: A situation that poses a serious threat to a single customer, a community, or the organization and its stakeholders.
   B. Crisis review audit: An inspection of the organization's current operational risks, processes, systems, weaknesses, and threats.
   C. Risk: A process, system, stakeholder activity, and other business activity that may turn into a crisis if not monitored or managed appropriately.
   D. Stakeholder: A person or a group that has a professional or financial investment in something such as an organization or business. There can be both internal and external stakeholders.

Figure 8-2 Example of an internal crisis management preparedness plan. *(continued)*

    E. After-action report: A document that is created after an incident occurs and often includes a snapshot summary of the incident, the goals and objectives in managing the incident, performance outcomes, lessons learned, and actions taken to better prepare for future crisis situations.

7. **Postincident Review:** A postincident review shall be conducted after every response to a crisis.

8. **Update Plan:** Ensure that the plan is updated and risk assessments are ongoing.
    A. Risk assessments must be performed
        a. When updating the plan
        b. Post crisis
        c. When a risk has been identified
    B. The plan must be reviewed annually and after an incident.
    C. Update forms used during a crisis situation
        a. Emergency employee contact list
        b. List of functional workgroup resources
        c. Lessons Learned form
        d. Risk or Crisis Assessment form
        e. Mitigation Activity form
        f. Press Release form
        g. Operational Activity and Incident Action Plan form (primarily used during external crisis situations)

9. **Training:** Ensure that all members of the organization are well informed as to the appropriate procedures and actions to be taken when encountering a crisis situation by participating in:
    A. Functional exercises: Scenario based; teams have an opportunity for decision making and activity by participating in hands-on evolutions with local functional workgroups.
    B. Full-scale exercises: Scenario based; teams have an opportunity for decision making and activity by participating in hands-on evolutions involving state or federal agencies.
    C. Table-top exercises: A facilitated training exercise where activities take place without hands-on evolutions. Table-top exercises are designed to evaluate the organization's approach to decision making and policies pertinent to the scenario. The exercise is usually held in a classroom setting.
    D. All office staff personnel should receive crisis response training annually to include overview of the plan and new updates.

10. **References:** Provide direction in seeking additional information to remedy and support the actions to mitigate the crisis.
    A. Standard operating guidelines and procedures
    B. Policies
    C. Bulletins
    D. Protocols
    E. Emergency management plan
    F. Mission statement
    G. Strategic plan
    H. Finance

Figure 8-2 Example of an internal crisis management preparedness plan. *(continued)*

communication terminology that all team members understand, identification of personnel who will address the media regarding the incident, and the importance of safety for all involved.

Planning for an External Crisis

EMS and other public safety personnel are proficient in working with and managing external crises. EMS personnel are taught to execute the organization's adopted mass-casualty incident (MCI) plan, active shooter plan, and other crisis management plans, and they understand their role before such a crisis occurs. **Figure 8-3** shows an example of an external crisis management plan.

National Incident Management System

As an EMS officer, there is a high probability that you will be involved with managing crisis situations of varying sizes and complexity. When dealing with public safety and nonpublic safety crisis situations, organizations may choose to use the **National Incident Management System (NIMS)** as part of their crisis management plan. NIMS provides a standardized framework for managing an incident. The use of NIMS, which is integrated with the National Response Plan (NRP), assists responders in preparing for and managing crisis situations occurring at the local, state, and national levels. Although NIMS is not a response plan, it can be used as the foundation for developing a coordinated and organized approach to a crisis. The primary goal in using NIMS is to ensure that EMS and other public safety organizations implement a standard **incident command system (ICS)** to achieve a positive outcome. An ICS is a basic command structure for the organization and specifies coordination of tasks between the incident commander (IC) and the section chiefs or functional workgroups and personnel on scene. It also promotes effective communication regarding how the scene will be managed.

ICS existed well before NIMS was created, having originated after a series of California wildfires occurred in the 1970s. NIMS was introduced by the federal government after the terrorist attacks on September 11, 2001, with the goal of creating a standardized ICS, thereby achieving effective coordination, collaboration, communication, and interoperability among organizations on the scene of multijurisdictional crisis events. As an incident grows and additional responders and resources are dispatched to assist with operations there, a coordinated approach is needed to align the necessary personnel and equipment resources and manage the scene. It is imperative to consolidate all agencies involved in the response of a crisis situation under one organized, unified command structure. During a moderate- to large-scale incident, multiple agencies will respond to the scene. Rather than each of these agencies working independently, the ICS calls for the senior commanding officer for each agency to unify and establish a single command center. When there are at least two commanding officers from different organizations working together and sharing command authority as one command center, the situation is referred to as **unified command**.

Jones EMS Department
MASS-CASUALTY INCIDENT PLAN

DIVISION: Operations	SUBJECT: Mass-Casualty Incidents	SOG# 123

Purpose: To provide procedures for the identification and handling of mass-casualty incidents.

Guideline: This mass-casualty incident (MCI) procedure is to be used for any incident when the number of injured exceeds the capabilities of the first-arriving units to efficiently triage, treat, and transport the victims. For Jones EMS Department, this MCI procedure will be initiated on all incidents involving five or more victims.

A. **Responsibilities of Command**

1. Remove endangered persons and treat the injured.
2. Stabilize the incident and provide for life safety.
3. Ensure that the functions of extrication, triage, treatment, and transportation are established as needed and carried out.
4. Conserve property and preserve evidence.
5. Provide for the ongoing safety, accountability, and welfare of all emergency service personnel throughout the entire incident.

B. **Response:** When an MCI is determined, the incident commander should request the necessary resources needed to mitigate the situation. The following response levels should be considered the minimum resources required to manage a specific number of victims. The *Florida Incident Field Operations Guide* (FOG) was a reference for this SOG.

1. The MCI alarm assignment will be:
   a. One district chief
   b. Division chief of EMS or designee
   c. A safety officer
   d. Two engine or truck companies (whichever is closest)
   e. Two transport-capable rescues or closest ambulance units
2. Level 1 MCI (5–10 victims, minor MCI)
   a. Minimum response of one MCI alarm.
   b. Dispatch will notify the assistant chief of operations or designee.
   c. Dispatch will notify the EMS division chief.
   d. One safety officer will be assigned to the scene.
   e. Dispatch will issue a staff page.
   f. Jones EMS Communication Center will notify the closest hospitals in the general area of the MCI and the regional trauma center.
   g. Jones EMS Communication Center will notify the on-duty PIO.

Figure 8-3 Example of an external small- to large-scale incident response crisis plan, specific to a mass-casualty incident response. *(continues)*

3. Level 2 MCI (11–20 victims, minor MCI)
   a. Minimum response of two MCI alarms.
   b. Dispatch will notify the assistant chief of operations.
   c. Dispatch will notify the EMS division chief.
   d. One district chief will be assigned to the scene.
   e. Dispatch will issue a staff page.
   f. One safety officer will be assigned to the scene.
   g. Jones EMS Communication Center will notify all hospitals in the general area and the regional trauma center.
   h. Jones EMS Communication Center will page the EMS medical directors.
   i. Jones EMS Communication Center will notify SCATS.
   j. Jones EMS Communication Center will notify the on-duty PIO.
4. Level 3 MCI (21–99 victims, major MCI) = FOG Level 3
   a. Minimum response of three MCI alarms.
   b. Additional alarms or units should be requested as the situation dictates. Contact Jones EMS Office of Emergency Management (OEM) for special resources. Consider two to three climate-controlled buses to hold, treat, and transport Green-level victims.
   c. Dispatch will notify the assistant chief of operations or designee.
   d. Dispatch will notify the EMS division chief.
   e. Dispatch will issue a staff page.
   f. Two or more safety officers will be assigned to the scene.
   g. Jones EMS Communication Center will notify all area hospitals, regional trauma center, and any additional facilities in the region if indicated.
   h. Jones EMS Communication Center will notify the EMS medical directors for possible response and assistance.
   i. Jones EMS Communication Center will notify SCATS.
   j. Jones EMS Communication Center will notify the on-duty PIO.
5. Level 4 MCI (100–999 victims or more, major MCI)
   a. Minimum response of three MCI alarms.
   b. Additional alarms or units should be requested as the situation dictates. Contact Jones EMS Office of Emergency Management (OEM) for special resources. Consider two to three climate-controlled buses to hold, treat, and transport Green-level victims.
   c. Dispatch will notify the assistant chief of operations or designee.
   d. Dispatch will notify the EMS division chief.
   e. Dispatch will issue a staff page.
   f. Two or more safety officers will be assigned to the scene.
   g. Jones EMS Communication Center will notify all area hospitals, regional trauma center, and any additional facilities in the region if indicated.
   h. Jones EMS Communication Center will notify the EMS medical directors for possible response and assistance.

Figure 8-3 Example of an external small- to large-scale incident response crisis plan, specific to a mass-casualty incident response. *(continued)*

i. Jones EMS Communication Center will notify SCATS.

j. Jones EMS Communication Center will notify the on-duty PIO.

k. Notify the OEM for the purpose of requesting local, regional, and possibly state resources up to and including USAR teams, the Metropolitan Medical Response System (MMRS), and other special teams or resources if indicated.

6. Level 5 MCI (1000 victims or more, major MCI)

a. Minimum response of three MCI alarms.

b. Additional alarms or units should be requested as the situation dictates. Contact Jones EMS Office of Emergency Management (OEM) for special resources. Consider two to three climate-controlled buses to hold, treat, and transport Green-level victims.

c. Dispatch will notify the assistant chief of operations or designee.

d. Dispatch will notify the EMS division chief.

e. Dispatch will issue a staff page.

f. Two or more safety officers will be assigned to the scene.

g. Jones EMS Communication Center will notify all area hospitals, regional trauma center, and any additional facilities in the region if indicated.

h. Jones EMS Communication Center will notify the EMS medical directors for possible response and assistance.

i. Jones EMS Communication Center will notify SCATS.

j. Jones EMS Communication Center will notify the on-duty PIO.

k. Notify the OEM for the purpose of requesting local, regional, and possibly state resources up to and including USAR teams, the Metropolitan Medical Response System (MMRS), and other special teams or resources if indicated.

C. **First-Arriving Officer:** Assumes command and implements those sections of EOP 1.0 through 5.0 appropriate to the incident, including announcing the location of the command post.

1. Perform a size-up to include:

a. The number of victims involved in the incident.

b. Safety concerns (e.g., hazardous materials, fires, collapse hazards).

2. If the numbers of sick or injured exceed the capabilities of the first-arriving units to efficiently manage the scene, command should declare an MCI, designate the "Level MCI," and request additional resources early.

3. Designate a triage, treatment, and transport group.

4. Designate a Level II staging area for:

a. Engines, trucks, and rescues (not for transport), or other resources.

b. A separate staging area for transport vehicles (for patient transport only) where they can enter and depart the scene readily and safely.

c. As additional units arrive, command will establish divisions/groups and assign personnel to the following areas if necessary:

i. EMS branch

ii. Triage group

Figure 8-3 Example of an external small- to large-scale incident response crisis plan, specific to a mass-casualty incident response. *(continued)*

      iii. Treatment group

      iv. Transport group

  5. Additional assignments should be made or divisions/groups established based on the complexity of the incident. These may include, but are not limited to:

      a Staging group

      b. Landing zone (LZ)

      c. Extrication group

      d. Hazardous materials group

      e. Safety officer

      f. Rehabilitation (rehab) group

      g. Critical incident stress debriefing (CISD)

      h. New medical designations

  6. Treatment capability (T-Cap), ambulance capability (A-Cap)

      a. Command, EMS, and transport groups must know the area hospital's ability to accept and treat victims (T-Cap).

      b. During any MCI, Jones EMS Communication Center will contact all hospitals in the area to obtain their T-Cap information.

      c. In the case of a large incident that may require many transport vehicles, Jones EMS Communication Center will poll other agencies for their ambulance capability. The A-Cap will provide Jones EMS Communication Center with the number of vehicles that each agency has available to respond.

D. Divisions and Groups

  1. Triage group:

      a. Use the radio designation "triage group."

      b. Organize the triage team to begin the initial triaging of victims using triage tags. Consider a team of two personnel per 10 victims.

      c. Jones EMS will use triage tags for any incident with five or more victims.

      d. During the initial triage phase, use the START (Simple Triage and Rapid Transport) system for adult victims and JumpStart triage system, if available, for children age 8 or younger.

      e. Some agencies may initially use colored ribbons to identify the severity of victims, not triage tags. The ribbon colors coincide with the colors on the triage tags used by Jones EMS.

      f. Affix a triage tag to each victim in a visible location (around the neck if possible); remove only enough of the lower portion of the colored tag necessary to identify the condition of the victim. Retain the torn-off portion of the tag, and deliver it to the triage group supervisor for tracking.

      g. Advise command as soon as possible of the total number and category of Red, Yellow, Green, and Black victims.

      h. Coordinate with the treatment group to ensure that victims are moved to the appropriate treatment area in the priority of their injuries and/or illness (i.e., Red category victims are moved before Green category victims).

Figure 8-3 Example of an external small- to large-scale incident response crisis plan, specific to a mass-casualty incident response. *(continued)*

    i. Ensure that all areas around the scene have been checked for potential victims, walking wounded, ejected victims, and other individuals, and that all victims have been triaged.

    j. Report to command upon completion of duties for further assignments when triage is completed.

2. Treatment group:

    a. Use the radio designation "treatment group."

    b. Assign a person to assist with the documentation.

    c. Establish a centralized treatment area or areas.

    d. Ensure that all victims are re-triaged upon arrival to the treatment area utilizing a secondary exam, and then document the assessment findings on the triage tag.

    e. Personnel assigned to treatment areas that assess or treat victims will document pertinent findings on the triage tag.

    f. All victims in treatment areas must be monitored and constantly re-triaged, as their conditions may change, creating the need to move them to another treatment area.

    g. Ensure that adequate equipment and personnel are available to effectively treat the victims.

    h. Considerations for a treatment area:

       i. Think big; make sure the treatment area selected will accommodate all the victims and personnel.

       ii. Consider weather, safety, and possible hazardous materials needs (e.g., decontamination, runoff, wind direction).

       iii. Designate an entrance and exit to each treatment area for good access and to aid in victim movement.

       iv. On large-scale incidents, divide the treatment area into three distinct and separate areas based on triage priorities: Red, Yellow, and Green. Colored flags or tarps will be used to mark each treatment area.

       v. The immediate care (Red) area must be closest to the transport area to facilitate rapid departure; the delayed care (Yellow) area will be the next closest area to the transport area; and the minor care (Green) area should be farthest away and well removed from the Yellow and Red areas to eliminate roaming Green victims from interfering with patient care.

       vi. Communicate with the transport groups to coordinate transport of the appropriate patients.

3. Transport group:

    a. Use the radio designation "transport group."

    b. Designate an area where transport units can enter and depart the scene safely. Also consider the need for an air transport area (LZ) with easy access if indicated.

    c. Maintain a "transport group log."

    d. Assign a documentation aide with a second radio to assist with the log and communications.

Figure 8-3 Example of an external small- to large-scale incident response crisis plan, specific to a mass-casualty incident response. *(continued)*

    e. Establish continuous contact with Jones EMS Communication Center to determine the
        T-Cap of area hospitals and the A-Cap of other transport agencies. Use an approved tacti-
        cal channel assigned by Jones EMS Communication Center.
    f. Coordinate transport of victims from the treatment areas.
    g. Communicate with the LZ regarding the number of patients to be transported by air.
    h. When vehicles are prepared to transport victims, the transport group or their aide will
        contact Jones EMS Communication Center and supply them with the following
        information:
        i.   The transporting radio ID number.
        ii. The number of patients going to a specific facility.
        iii. Their priority (Red, Yellow, or Green).
        iv. If any Green patients are immobilized on backboards, the receiving facility must be
             notified.
        v.   The transporting vehicle should not contact the receiving facility directly unless there
             is a change in patient condition or further medical control is required.

E. References
    1. State *Field Operations Guide* (FOG)

Figure 8-3 Example of an external small- to large-scale incident response crisis plan, specific to a
mass-casualty incident response. *(continued)*

The basic ICS structure can be expanded or collapsed as the incident requires, but certain
basic personnel are always likely be included (**Figure 8-4**):

- **Incident commander (IC):** The IC is the one position that must be implemented immediately
  and must not be terminated until the crisis is resolved. The IC is responsible for developing
  the incident objectives and for all aspects of implementing the crisis management plan, which
  includes working directly with the operations section chief, logistics section chief, planning
  section chief, and finance section chief.

- **Public information officer (PIO):** The PIO is responsible for disseminating information
  about the incident to the news media, to incident personnel, and to the community. This
  information is released during media interviews, press releases, and social media. (See the
  "Communications" chapter for more discussion about working with the media.)

- **Safety officer (SO):** The SO is responsible for the safety of on-scene personnel. He or she
  monitors scene safety and ensures that operational activities are being conducted safely.

- **Operations section chief (OSC):** The OSC is responsible for the operational management of
  the crisis and the development of the strategy and tactics used to mitigate the crisis.

- **Logistics section chief (LSC):** The LSC is responsible for providing necessary resources to
  assist in mitigating the crisis.

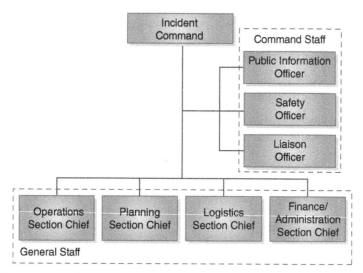

Figure 8-4 Incident command system structure.

- **Planning section chief (PSC):** The PSC is responsible for capturing and analyzing scene data, which are then used to plan the response to the crisis event. The PSC also prepares and writes the incident action plan (IAP) for adoption by the IC.

- **Finance/administrative section chief (FSC):** If financial and/or administrative duties must be handled during the incident, the IC may appoint a finance/administrative section chief, who is responsible for addressing and managing administrative and financial requests during the incident (e.g., employee record keeping for hours worked, vendor contracts, documentation for reimbursement after the crisis ends). The finance/administration section is used primarily during large incidents, but may also be activated during small incidents.

In addition to the necessary personnel, certain elements will be required in managing an incident with the ICS. The first is an incident command post (ICP) or emergency operations center (EOC), where the leadership team can confer and determine how best to execute the organization's crisis management plan and address the current crisis. Here the OSC can update other key organizational leaders on the planned strategy and tactics during the crisis management planning meeting. Once the plan is approved by the IC, it is formalized into an **incident action plan (IAP)** and shared with personnel involved in the incident. The IAP may be updated every 8, 12, or 24 hours, or as needed to meet the needs of the operation. It contains information necessary to the management of the scene, including the following items:

- Incident name
- Date
- Time

- Weather
- Participating units
- Operational sections
- Operational objectives
- Strategy and tactics
- Situational awareness updates
- Logistical plans
- Medical plans
- Temperature
- Additional information as dictated by the incident

It is within the ICS where detailed objectives and IAPs are created to appropriately manage the crisis. As an EMS officer, you can incorporate incident command and other crisis management courses into the organization's educational plan so that personnel will be better prepared when asked to use these skills. Every member of the organization, but especially those in leadership roles, must attend NIMS training to learn how to manage risks and crises should they occur.

Managing the Crisis

When determining how best to manage an internal or external crisis, it all starts with having a well-designed and thorough crisis management plan in place. Being able to anticipate, identify, manage, and monitor organizational risks and hazards is as important as managing a crisis.

Management of a crisis should follow these basic steps:

1. Avoid the crisis.
2. Confirm the crisis.
3. Implement the crisis management plan.
4. Contain the crisis.
5. Resolve the crisis.
6. Conduct a post-crisis analysis.

Avoid the Crisis

Although handling a crisis well is an important skill, it is much better to avoid the crisis in the first place, if at all possible. As an EMS officer, you will deal with small and large internal and external crises on a regular basis. This experience can assist you in identifying potential impending crisis situations before they occur, then managing and monitoring conditions in an effort to keep the situation from becoming a crisis.

When attempting to avoid a crisis, make it a point to conduct **crisis review audits**—inspections of the organization's current operational risks, processes, systems, weaknesses, and threats.

Success in the BUSINESS WORLD

Prioritizing the Customer

In 1982, Johnson & Johnson, the maker of Tylenol (a brand of acetaminophen), experienced an organizational crisis of epic proportions. The Chicago media reported that several Chicago residents had inexplicably died within a very short time period and authorities had no idea as to the cause. The events left Chicago-area communities and medical practitioners puzzled and concerned. Once the victims became ill, EMS was summoned and the victims were transported to the hospital, where they died shortly after.

After these deaths started, two fire fighters were discussing the sudden unexplained deaths of the victims and made a connection among them. One of the fire fighters checked with one of the paramedics who transported one of the victims, and this contact confirmed his suspicion: The victims had all taken a Tylenol capsule before becoming ill. Authorities were alerted, and the medical examiner confirmed that the Tylenol capsules taken by the victims had been laced with cyanide.

The information was released to the public, but Johnson & Johnson's leadership team heard about the confirmation only after a reporter contacted the organization for comment. Marketing experts at the time said Johnson & Johnson would never recover from this crisis. Although the company was not responsible for the poisoning, its leadership team immediately responded to the crisis and took some bold actions to resolve it.

Johnson & Johnson's chief executive officer, James Burke, had made it clear to all employees that the company's philosophy was that people came first and property was second. This culture was present before the crisis occurred, and it remained strong throughout the crisis. The leadership team remained extremely transparent and kept the public informed about what they were doing to remedy the situation. For example, Johnson & Johnson:

- Removed all 31 million Extra Strength Tylenol bottles from every store, which cost the company $100 million
- Introduced new triple-sealed, tamper-resistant bottles
- Provided coupons for $2.50 off any Tylenol purchase
- Sent sales representatives to provide ongoing presentations to the community and medical professionals, reinforcing the safety of the product
- Activated a crisis hotline (toll-free number) that was updated regularly to keep customers informed of the organization's actions
- Allowed consumers to return any previously purchased Extra Strength Tylenol capsules, which would be replaced with the new triple-sealed, tamper-resistant bottles at no charge

Johnson & Johnson managers had no idea that the Tylenol Extra Strength capsules would be laced with cyanide and that the company would be enveloped by a crisis few business organizations had experienced. The leadership team had no warning about what was about to happen—yet the organization was prepared for the crisis before it ever occurred. The organization would do what it took to place the consumer first. The internal stakeholders already knew what was expected of them. Once organizational members know their roles, it is much easier to adjust and realign resources as needed to manage a crisis.

Within a year of the crisis, Johnson & Johnson had nearly regained the market position it had held prior to the incident and had saved the reputation of both the organization and the Tylenol brand. CEO Burke was given the Presidential Medal of Freedom and was named one of the greatest CEOs of all time. More than 30 years later, many business experts commend Johnson & Johnson's handling of the crisis as one of the best ever in business. The individual(s) responsible for the terrorist act were never found.

Johnson & Johnson did acknowledge some things it could have done differently. For example, the company did not have a designated public affairs program and did not engage with the media on a regular basis before the crisis. The media did not let Johnson & Johnson off the hook quickly, but rather remained committed to airing and printing the story for several days after the discovery of the cyanide-laced capsules was made. However, the organizational leaders did acknowledge that the crisis could have been a lot worse.

By conducting routine (e.g., annual) crisis audits, the organization or the functional workgroup will be able to avoid some potential crises. In addition, the EMS officer may consider incorporating crisis management into the organization's or functional workgroup's strategic plan. Using SWOT (strengths, weaknesses, opportunities, threats) analysis to identify specific risks and potential crisis situations will be extremely valuable in attempting to avoid a crisis. During such an analysis, the EMS officer and the crisis management team can review the organization's weaknesses and threats to identify and manage any potential risks or a crisis brewing on the horizon. (SWOT is discussed in more detail in the "Strategic Planning" chapter.)

After completing the SWOT analysis and determining the areas of risk (weaknesses and threats) that are most likely to lead to crisis events, the EMS officer or other organizational leaders must prioritize the activities taken in response to the results from most severe to least severe. This will set a priority for which risks should be monitored, managed, or eliminated first. Furthermore, in an attempt to avoid a crisis, the EMS officer must make it a priority to receive input from organizational team members, the crisis team, and organizational leaders. This will allow for a "big picture" approach and will assist in identifying key areas that might otherwise be missed within a specific functional workgroup or the organization as a whole.

Confirm the Crisis

Confirming the crisis is important because it provides the "go/no go" decision-making point for implementation of the crisis management plan. There is a delicate balance between anticipating a crisis and jumping to conclusions before a crisis event is confirmed. You should not hold off on activating the crisis management plan if there will be a delay in confirming the crisis. You can always discontinue the activation of the crisis plan and immediate response. In an actual crisis, a delay in implementing the plan can prove detrimental and can set the organization behind—rather than in front of—the event.

Crisis confirmation hinges on the answer to the following question: Does the event threaten harm to one or more individuals, the community, the organization, and/or the organization's stakeholders? Once that question has been answered, you must determine the hazards that are the root cause of the crisis and begin mitigating the situation.

Implement a Crisis Management Plan

Crises can occur at every level of the organization, and the EMS officer must be able to rapidly assess the situation to determine the following:

- Whether the crisis is internal or external
- The root cause of the crisis
- The impact the crisis will have on external stakeholders, the community, the organization, and internal stakeholders
- The appropriate crisis plan to mitigate the situation

Management of each crisis event will be different. The goal of every crisis plan is the same, however: to provide easy-to-follow information for rapid deployment during a crisis. This format allows the crisis management team to begin mitigating the crisis as soon as possible.

For example, there is no need to deploy public safety units or to establish a command system for an internal computer network failure. Such a network failure will affect only internal stakeholders, who will not be able to get their jobs done. Although this situation can be extremely frustrating and may keep projects from being completed in time, it does not pose any immediate risk to life or property. As the EMS officer ensuring that all facets of the system under your responsibility are operating effectively and efficiently, you will need to address internal crises with urgency and have a specific plan to address them.

Now consider the example of an ambulance accidentally hitting a pedestrian on the way to an emergency. Although it is also an internal crisis, this event poses different challenges to the EMS organization. The organization will need to address its response policy, answer questions about the driver, attend to the victim and his or her family members, deal with negative publicity, conduct an investigation to determine any legal ramifications, and offer support to the ambulance crew. The network failure and the ambulance incident are two very different internal crisis events, but both can be managed from the same basic crisis management plan.

The EMS officer must consider using the same initial crisis management efforts when managing an external crisis. These basic crisis management activities serve as the fundamental framework of both internal and external crisis management:

- Ensure safety for all personnel.
- Account for all personnel.
- Determine the immediate impact zone and ramifications.
- Attempt to determine the root cause of the crisis and hazards.
- Ensure that resources are requested immediately.
- Prepare to deploy the crisis management goals, objectives, strategy, and tactics.
- Establish the ICS as needed.
- Brief the PIO. If the organization does not have a designated PIO, a member of the leadership team must assume that responsibility.
- Determine how the organization will communicate with internal and external stakeholders (e.g., face-to-face, e-mail, social media).
- If the crisis is the result of the organization's action and has impacted life or property, be upfront and transparent with those who are affected by the incident.
- Take control by demonstrating a command presence, working with team members, and collaborating with other organizations to achieve resolution of the crisis.
- Provide support for personnel (e.g., food, shelter, medical aid) if the crisis event has resulted in an extended operation.

These activities help determine the best approach for mitigating the crisis. For example, should they implement the organization's MCI plan, active shooter plan, hurricane plan, negative media plan, organizational negligence plan, or a plan that deals with internal administrative issues? Specific crisis management plan ideas must be introduced and discussed during SWOT analysis exercises, crisis management "lessons learned" events, and table-top exercises. The leadership team is responsible for making sure that these crisis management activities take place as part of the strategic planning process, training, and postincident review, thereby ensuring that the plan is up-to-date and organizational members are well informed.

In a crisis situation, time will be critical—and there will be no time to play catch-up if the crisis is not addressed promptly. Whatever initial activities the organizational leaders choose to pursue as the initial approach to crisis management, there will always need to be some adjustments to better meet the needs of the crisis.

Take care of all those involved in the crisis. Such assistance may take the form of rescuing victims, debriefing (discussing the event and how it affected the team member), professional counseling, or listening to a member's input.

As the EMS officer, you will be expected to provide answers, especially during a crisis situation. You need to be prepared for this responsibility, and keep your skills sharp in readiness for a crisis that occurs without warning. Because large and complex crisis events do not happen every day, leaders tend to become complacent and may forget some of the skills for managing a crisis over time.

Contain the Crisis

After initially implementing the crisis management plan, the EMS officer (or, in large events, the IC) must immediately work on containing the crisis and preventing it from causing more damage. Request resources immediately and as needed to contain the crisis, allow the team to do the work they have been trained to do, and do not be afraid to ask for help or input from other organizations (e.g., through a mutual aid agreement or a state or federal coordinated resources system) and from colleagues who have experienced similar incidents. The EMS officer should acknowledge that he or she will need to rely on the team. This does not remove any of the responsibility of being in charge, but as the managerial leader you have to trust your people, especially if you are unfamiliar with certain aspects of the operation. Managerial leaders often feel the need to provide their input, change operational plans, or assume the responsibility for completing a task even if they are completely unfamiliar with the process. This kind of tinkering can prove to be catastrophic, especially during a crisis, and demoralizing for the team members who are truly familiar with the process. Surround yourself with talented team members and let them do their jobs, especially during crisis situations.

Resolve the Crisis

Bringing closure to a crisis begins with taking a snapshot of the crisis; noting the events, actions, and outcomes; and ensuring that every detail has been addressed and resolution has been accomplished. As the situation evolves, the EMS officer must ask whether the crisis is still a crisis. If an unstable condition still exists and has the potential to harm individuals, the community, or the organization, it is still a crisis. When determining whether the crisis has been resolved and what to do during this phase, the organization's leadership team must consider the following questions:

- Does the crisis still pose a threat to the organization, internal and external customers, or the community? If the incident required the activation of operations, planning, logistics, and administrative/finance sections, the senior leadership member or IC must communicate with each section chief to ensure that no sections remain in crisis condition before determining that the crisis has been resolved.

- Is the crisis still active in one or more areas? If the crisis is occurring in more than one location, all areas must be thoroughly evaluated to ensure there is no longer a threat for the redevelopment of the current crisis.
- Are all team members accounted for? Ensure that they are and that no resources are removed until the crisis has been officially resolved.
- Is the leadership team available to answer questions? The leadership team must be available to meet with and answer questions from the media and internal and external customers. The organization must assign a spokesperson to provide ongoing information to the media and internal and external customers. The flow of communication must not stop once the crisis is over.
- Are there legal concerns? Involve legal counsel if the crisis has ongoing legal ramifications.

Conduct a Post-Crisis Analysis

Depending on the crisis, an investigation may follow the crisis resolution. For example, the National Traffic and Safety Board (NTSB) investigates airplane crashes, law enforcement officers investigate multiple-vehicle accidents, and fire investigators investigate fires. When an organization is responsible for a crisis, an internal investigation is required. Organizational leaders must ensure transparency in their investigation if the crisis negatively impacted customers and the community. This transparency can be facilitated by enlisting nonorganizational members to become part of the investigative team, so that the results will be impartial and unbiased. Organizational leaders must demonstrate a willingness to resolve the crisis expeditiously and to get the answers necessary to ensure that the crisis does not reoccur. Acknowledge when your organization makes a mistake; this willingness to admit fault demonstrates to customers and the community that the organization is doing its best to care for its customers.

After a large incident, an **after-action report** must be completed. It is typically created by the crisis management team or someone designated by the team who was involved in the overall

Managerial Leadership BRIEFCASE

Recognition Primed Decision Making

Among the many management activities included as part of the EMS officer's role, there will certainly be many requiring the need for quick decisions. Making a decision under stressful situations, as most EMS and other public safety professionals do on a regular basis, does not allow for much consideration time and could mean the difference between life and death, or a business decision that could negatively impact the organization. The ability to rapidly assess a situation or a patient's presentation is very important.

The **recognition primed decision making (RPD)** approach to decision making consists of being able to provide a solution or taking action to a problem during a stressful period by essentially using past experiences, identifiable patterns that were present in previous situations or intuition. For example, a crew is interviewing a patient who is complaining of bed sores on her back. The patient is alert, cooperative, and oriented, with several bed sores noted on her back. The patient informs the crew that she is fine and does not need to go to the hospital. However, the paramedic crew on scene observes the patient's body movement (pattern) and recognizes that the patient is presenting as a patient experiencing a dissecting abdominal aneurysm. The crew highly encourages the patient to be transported to the hospital and the patient finally agrees. Upon arrival at the hospital, the patient is diagnosed with having an aortic abdominal aneurysm and is immediately taken to surgery.

As another example, an EMS officer is responding to the scene of a commuter bus accident on the interstate. Upon being dispatched and listening to the description of the incident as described by the 911 callers, the EMS officer makes a decision to request aeromedical transport and additional ambulance units to the scene and to backfill the surrounding stations because all frontline units will be at the scene rendering care at a prolonged event. The EMS officer also requests a heavy-duty wrecker for stabilization and two additional mass transit buses—one for the walking wounded who would be transported to the hospital for evaluation, and the other for those who were not injured but needed to be transported to a specific location for further transport arrangements. The EMS officer did not wait until arrival at the scene to confirm that these assets were needed; rather, she requested the assets based on previous experience with similar events. As a result, the necessary equipment arrived quickly.

When using RPD, there is possibility that one's intuition will be incorrect, leading to under- or over-triaging of a situation; therefore, organizational leaders must ensure that safety is the first priority in any decision-making process. If a decision is made with safety in mind and it turns out that the actions were excessive, unneeded resources can be turned away.

There may be no time to use a classic decision-making process where the individual making the decision thoroughly assesses the situation by weighing the pros and cons of different strategies and discusses the approach with other leadership members prior to making a decision. This classical approach may be useful in many situations, but when used during an emergency situation may consume valuable time. EMS officers and other public safety personnel can strengthen the RPD model by learning about their profession, reviewing post-incident critiques to determine how best to manage specific situations, and identifying patterns during incidents that can later be used in similar situations. EMS officers will continue to be exposed to stressful situations where rapid decision making will be a priority; therefore, acknowledging and strengthening the RPD approach will serve public safety providers as an extremely valuable tool.

operation. This report must answer a series of key questions: What happened? What went right? What went wrong? What can be improved upon? An after-action report should be required by the crisis management plan. It provides an opportunity to learn and reflect on the strategies, tactics, and challenges that emerged during the crisis.

Learn from the experience of the crisis and how it was managed. Review the actions of the crisis management team and the content of any SOGs. Making adjustments in these areas is more easily done when a crisis is fresh in your mind.

Effects of Crisis on the Organization

It is not enough just to manage and contain the crisis at hand. There may be additional, related issues that can turn into crises if they are not handled quickly. For example, suppose one of your ambulance units is dispatched to the wrong address, and the delayed response to the real scene contributes to the unsuccessful resuscitation of the victim. You are notified of the crisis and begin working with the team members to understand how this problem happened and how to prevent it from happening in the future. But what do you do if the incident is leaked to the media and broadcast on the evening news? Now your organization is labeled not only as a contributor to the victim's death but also as an organization that has poor business performance. What else is looming, and how will you address this new crisis that morphed from the initial crisis?

Keep your eyes open during a crisis, and you will see that there is more going on beyond the original crisis that needs to be remedied. If negative allegations are made, you will need to deal with them immediately. In the era of social media, once a negative message begins to gain traction, it will be difficult to contain.

If a crisis situation is handled well, however, it can be a boon to the organization. An efficiently mitigated crisis can improve or reinforce an organization's reputation and brand. It can also improve confidence and teamwork in the organization's personnel who have brought a crisis situation to a successful resolution.

WRAP-UP

Concept Review

- Having a crisis management action plan that includes key steps in dealing with a crisis will help the organization manage the crisis, keep it from growing, look for internal and external organizational ramifications from the crisis, prevent tunnel vision, and identify how to bring closure to the crisis.

- Internal risks originate within the organization; external risks originate outside the organization. If not managed appropriately, either type of risk has the potential to become a crisis.

- The first priority in a crisis is ensuring the safety of all persons involved in the incident.

- Having a crisis management plan in place before a crisis occurs is critical because it provides the necessary framework to manage the incident and allows for a rapid deployment of activities necessary to mitigate an actual crisis.

- When attempting to manage an internal organizational crisis, it is beneficial to use principles similar to those used when managing an external crisis, because these principles clearly emphasize an organized approach to crisis management.

- You may not be able to stop a crisis from happening; however, if you thoroughly understand internal and external business activities and remain alert, you, your team, and the organization will be better prepared for managing the crisis.

- Identifying a basic systematic approach that can be used to manage internal and external crises prior to an actual event's occurrence is critical so a response can be implemented immediately.

- Being able to anticipate, identify, manage, and monitor organizational risks and hazards is as important as managing a crisis.

- Although handling a crisis well is an important skill, it is much better to avoid the crisis in the first place, if at all possible.

- Confirming the crisis is important because it provides the "go/no go" decision-making point for implementation of the crisis management plan.

- Management of each crisis event will be different. The goal of every crisis plan is the same, however: to provide easy-to-follow information for rapid deployment during a crisis.

- After initially implementing the crisis management plan, the EMS officer or incident commander must immediately work on containing the crisis and preventing it from causing more damage.

- Bringing closure to a crisis begins with taking a snapshot of the crisis; noting the events, actions, and outcomes; and ensuring that every detail has been addressed and resolution has been accomplished.

- Learn from the experience of the crisis and how it was managed.

- It is not enough just to manage and contain the crisis at hand. There may be additional, related issues that can turn into crises if not managed quickly.

Managerial Terms

After-action report A document created after an incident, often including a snapshot summary of the incident, the goals and objectives in managing the incident, performance outcomes, lessons learned, and actions taken to better prepare for future crisis situations.

Crisis A situation that poses a serious threat to a single customer, a community, or the organization and its stakeholders.

Crisis management plan A plan that includes key activities necessary for managing a current organizational threat or crisis, customers, and the community. An incident action plan may be included within a crisis management plan.

Crisis review audits Inspections of the organization's current operational risks, processes, systems, weaknesses, and threats.

Finance/administrative section chief (FSC) The individual responsible for addressing and managing administrative and financial requests during a crisis incident.

Incident action plan (IAP) The formal documentation of activities pertaining to incident goals, objectives, strategies, tactics, and other pertinent information specific to an incident.

Incident command system (ICS) A system implemented to manage disasters and crisis incidents in which section chiefs report to the incident commander.

Incident commander (IC) The individual responsible for developing the incident objectives and for all aspects of implementing the crisis management plan.

Logistics section chief (LSC) The individual responsible for providing necessary resources to assist in mitigating a crisis.

National Incident Management System (NIMS) A Department of Homeland Security system designed to enable federal, state, and local governments and private-sector and nongovernmental organizations to effectively and efficiently prepare for, prevent, respond to, and recover from domestic incidents, regardless of their cause, size, or complexity.

Operations section chief (OSC) The individual responsible for the operational management of a crisis and the development of the strategy and tactics used to mitigate the crisis.

Planning section chief (PSC) The individual responsible for capturing and analyzing scene data that are then used to plan the response to a crisis event, and for creating the incident action plan.

Public information officer (PIO) The individual responsible for disseminating information about a crisis incident to the news media, to incident personnel, and to the community.

Recognition primed decision making A method of rapidly solving problems by implementing a solution that has been previously used in similar situations.

Risks Processes, systems, stakeholder activities, and other business activities that may turn into crises if not monitored or managed appropriately.

Safety officer (SO) The individual responsible for the safety of on-scene personnel.

Stakeholders Individuals or groups that have a professional or financial investment in something, such as an organization or business. There can be both internal and external stakeholders.

Unified command Use of an incident command system in which each agency involved works together and shares command authority as one command center.

Case Review: Cruise Ship

The Jones Fire and EMS organization was faced with a potential crisis when a cruise ship with several thousand passengers was reported to have listed, meaning that it had inclined to one side, creating an unstable environment. The ship was several miles off shore when the incident occurred and immediately returned to port. More than 100 passengers were injured, experiencing minor to serious injuries.

When the report was received at the 911 communication center, multiple fire, EMS, aeromedical, mass transit, and law enforcement units responded from the surrounding areas. The number of units and agencies requested to assist was part of the response plan when dealing with an event of this magnitude. Because all agencies routinely worked and trained together, the incident command system was immediately established. The lead organization assumed command and assigned an operations section chief, who then took responsibility for the EMS operational activities at the scene. Triage, treatment, and transport groups were established, and the victims were rapidly offloaded and processed. In this situation, all the victims were evacuated from the ship and transported to local emergency departments for care without incident.

Case Discussion

In this example of an external crisis, although the incident commander, section chief, EMS crew members, and other support staff were challenged in managing more than 100 patients in a short period of time, preparation and coordination through a mutually accepted crisis plan proved beneficial to crisis mitigation. The management of the crisis was conducted flawlessly because all multijurisdictional agencies had routinely participated in functional full-scale and table-top exercises for numerous crisis situations. The key to their success in this incident was the commitment to training, coordination among agencies, and existence of a predeveloped crisis plan. The crisis plan included not only the actions required by the responders, but also a checklist of the necessary activities and resources that would be required as part of a large-scale incident.

Case Review: Use of Controlled Substance

The Bartlett EMS organization's chief of EMS operations was surprised when he received a phone call from a local reporter requesting an interview to discuss the tampering with controlled substances by one of the organization's paramedics while on duty. Allegedly, a paramedic, while on duty, was withdrawing Valium from a secured vial and replacing it with water. This medication was part of the controlled substance supply on board the ambulance unit and was used to treat patients as directed by the department's medical director. The reporter wanted to know who the individual was, which controlled substance was used, whether the paramedic placed patients in jeopardy during patient care, whether the paramedic was being placed on administrative leave pending the outcome of an internal investigation, whether the situation was being reported to local law enforcement and the state EMS office, and whether the organization was concerned about the public losing trust in its service delivery.

The organization's leadership team had already identified a public information officer (PIO), who had been designated as the official spokesperson for the organization prior to this incident and was responsible for working closely with the local media. In addition, the PIO was responsible for creating a crisis management team and working with them to establish a crisis management plan for the organization. The organization's leadership team, the PIO, and the organization's team members knew exactly what was expected of them prior to a crisis event. The plan required keeping the PIO and the leadership team front and center during all press conferences and media interviews. The organizational leaders were also expected to maintain transparency while being extremely sensitive to the situation and ensuring the privacy of the individual in question.

After the PIO and leadership team discussed with the reporter what had transpired, the event was not blown out of proportion and the organization was given the opportunity to explain the actions being taken to ensure that this situation would not occur again. During the preparation of the crisis management plan and a table-top exercise, a similar scenario had been presented and the crisis management team had been able to discuss what to do in case of tampering with any controlled substance. The preparation, the assignment of a PIO prior to a crisis, and the steps taken to ensure that all team members knew their roles during a crisis resulted in a seamless execution of the crisis management plan.

Case Discussion

Upon receiving the reporter's phone call, the division chief of EMS knew that he was facing two crises. First was the internal crisis—that is, the allegations of inappropriate use of controlled substance by an employee. Second was the threat to the reputation of the organization within the community. The division chief, using the organization's approved crisis management plan, was able to execute the required set of activities to address the situation at hand appropriately.

- Notification of the chief of the department and the medical director, informing them of the situation
- Suspension of the employee, with pay, per the organization's employee conduct policy
- Placement of the unit out of service and dispatch of an EMS supervisor to meet with the crew and conduct an inventory of all medications administered by all crew members assigned to the unit
- Removal of all controlled substance medication vials assigned to the unit, which were then sent to an independent laboratory for testing
- Notification of the state's Bureau of Emergency Medical Service, as requested per statute, local law enforcement, and the Drug Enforcement Administration

The division chief of EMS was able to conduct a thorough investigation because the EMS functional workgroup had already established a crisis management plan that included the steps required when facing the tampering of such medications by an employee.

Action also needed to be taken to protect the organization's reputation within the community. After the story appeared on television, radio, print media, and online, the organization began receiving phone calls from concerned citizens. The Bartlett EMS organization was committed to being as transparent as possible with the local media and community members without interfering with the investigation. This was achieved by displaying the current controlled substance medication policy, laying out each step of the investigation process and who was part of the investigation, and explaining what the organization was doing to ensure this situation did not happen again.

The outcome of the case resulted in the firing of the employee after it was determined that the evidence showed the medication had been removed from the vial. Although the organization's members did experience some challenges as they worked to remedy the crisis, having a crisis management plan proved to be beneficial, as it provided a map for ensuring that all essential steps necessary to work through the crisis were addressed.

CHAPTER

9

Budgeting

Learning Objectives

After studying this chapter, you should be able to:

- Describe the purpose and elements of a financial management plan.

- Describe the budgetary process for an EMS organization.

- Identify and describe the most common types of budgets.

- Identify and describe the most common expenses.

- Identify and describe the most common revenues.

- Describe the purchasing processes used by EMS organizations.

- Discuss the considerations involved in using a billing company.

Introduction

This chapter introduces the EMS officer to basic financial terminology and procedures that are used in the EMS industry. Every organization is different, of course; thus you must become familiar with your own organization's and own functional workgroup's **budget**. This chapter will not cover every detail of budgeting, but it does aim to give the new EMS officer the tools needed to work with basic organizational budgets.

If you are a seasoned EMS officer, you probably know how to create, implement, and evaluate budgets. Fortunately for EMS officers without this financial background, many EMS organizations have a budget office staffed with employees who are well versed in generally accepted accounting principles (GAAP), budgeting, billing, and collections. Some organizations hire certified public accountants (CPAs) as part of their staffs to ensure that all financial transactions have the appropriate oversight. As an EMS officer, you do not need to become a CPA or earn a financial or accounting degree. Nevertheless, as a leader within the organization, you must understand the financial and accounting activities that occur daily within your organization. Stated in terms of the five business priorities (5 BPs—people, strategic objectives, financial management objectives, learning objectives, and a culture of quality), you must focus on the **financial management objectives** to ensure that your organization or division stays on track and within its budget.

As a new EMS officer, you will most likely be assigned a budget for your division or at least be asked to provide input during the budgeting process. You can take several steps to ensure your success while participating in this process:

- Keep in constant communication with the individuals responsible for the final budget preparation. They will be able to answer questions, provide guidance, and help you after the budget has been adopted.

- Continue to monitor revenues and expenses within your area of responsibility.

- Do not wait until budget preparation time to begin formulating a financial management plan to meet your division's strategic objectives. Procrastination leads to poor planning and may result in essential items being left out of the budget.

- Develop strategic goals with detailed and comprehensive financial management objectives.

- Anticipate, plan for, and monitor unfunded mandates and unexpected expenses.

- Have a contingency plan for managing your budget.

If you know all of the services your organization provides to your customers, and if you stay engaged with the organization's budgeting process, you will be able to manage your area of responsibility more effectively and efficiently.

Financial Management Plan

Financial management, like other responsibilities assigned to an EMS officer, requires you to have a plan, execute the plan, and review the outcome regularly. Budget preparation requires you to forecast revenues and expenses, ensure that those revenues and expenses align with the budget, and monitor daily activities to ensure finances stay within the limits of that budget. By following these three basic steps, you can build a solid foundation in financial management.

A **financial management plan** conveys the "big picture" of the organization's strategic and financial goals and can be useful when deciding what to include in the organization's budget. Creating a financial management plan is similar to creating a strategic plan, except that the elements are focused on the financial aspects of the organization.

Managerial Leadership **BRIEFCASE**

Strategic and Financial Management Objectives

Strategic objectives may be specific, focusing on a single area, or they may cover many areas that directly affect your division or the organization. Financial management objectives are similar to strategic objectives but are specific to activities that involve monetary transactions.

Financial Goals and Objectives

The organization's financial goals must support the organization's strategic plan. In turn, the financial management plan should include financial management objectives; strategy; tactics; and budgetary activities such as revenue, capital expenses, and non-capital expenses. The intent of this plan is to show where set budgetary dollars will be allocated, what the justification for these allocations is, and which funds will be used for existing or new expenditures. The financial management plan should include financial benchmarks and a mechanism for monitoring revenues, expenses, and other financial activities; these elements will help the organization stay within the budgetary constraints.

Financial management objectives are financial benchmarks set by the organization's leadership, functional workgroup managers, or budget team, and are intended to support the organization's or unit's financial or strategic goals. (See the "Strategic Planning" chapter for information on using the SMART mnemonic to create goals and objectives.) The financial management plan ensures that the financial management objectives are being met, thereby ensuring that profit margins, key initiatives, and purchases are not overlooked. EMS officers cannot develop a budget for meeting financial management objectives if financial goals have not been developed. For example, the EMS officer may need to replace ambulance units, stretchers, cardiac monitors, or other equipment; to make sure funds are available for this purpose, the officer will need to budget for the particular items.

Forecasting and Demand Analysis

Along with organizational leaders and assigned budget team members, you will be asked for input on the budget. The organization's leaders will most likely be responsible for **forecasting** the organization's overall financial position based on the organization's current financial, operational, and economic conditions. In contrast, the EMS officer will likely be responsible for budgeting for key items that fall under his or her responsibility (e.g., capital improvement, replacement of major equipment, maintenance of regular equipment and supplies, employee training, introduction of new services, and payroll).

Determining how much it will cost the organization to execute each financial objective, and how much revenue the organization can expect to receive in the forthcoming fiscal year, can take some research and educated guesswork. How much will it cost to provide additional service to an unprotected response area? How should you factor the cost of an ambulance unit over the next 5 years? How much will tires, oil changes, and fuel cost for the year? How much should be set aside for salaries and benefits? These and many more questions are topics of discussion during budget preparation.

To represent expenses and revenues as accurately as possible, look first to those items that have been included in the organization's budget in the past. Trends in expenses can often be helpful indicators of future needs. For example, if expenses for general medical supplies have risen 5 percent per year over the last 5 years, you might forecast that next year the organization will need 5 percent more money available for general medical supplies than it did this year. When forecasting and obtaining a historical picture, it is best to use at least 3 to 5 years' worth of data in your evaluation.

Forecasting is not a foolproof method of determining budget needs, however. A consistent source of revenue may unexpectedly decline or disappear, new expenses may appear suddenly because of a natural disaster, and other unexpected events may change the organization's financial picture without warning. When preparing a budget, it is important to look at many variables beyond previous budgets, such as the economy, technology, changing demographics, and services that your competitors are providing to their customers. Analyze as much data as possible while reviewing potential obstacles.

Undertaking a **demand analysis** may also help when you are creating a budget, or even when you are just trying to strengthen the organization's financial position within the industry. A demand analysis involves researching the amounts that customers are willing to pay for a service, the number of units they are willing to purchase, and other factors that provide information regarding how customers perceive a product or service. The better understanding of customer demand provided by such an analysis gives a needed—and valuable—perspective on the budget. For example, the EMS officer might be considering an increase in the transport fees charged to customers. A demand analysis survey, however, might reveal that customers (patients) do not support these higher rates. If the proposed increase were presented in the budget and then reviewed by the public, community members would most likely express their concerns to local government officials or the private EMS department's governing board—that is, the people who are responsible for approving the increase. Perhaps the data from the demand analysis also indicate that customers are not happy that your organization does not transport patients to their hospital of choice, and that many customers are requesting a competitor provide nonemergency transports when needed. Having this information in hand allows you not only to make the necessary financial adjustments to your budget, but also to adjust your customer service to better meet customers' demands.

Pulling the Plan Together

When creating a financial management plan, consider the following guidelines:

- Plan for growth and ways to achieve the organization's short-term and long-term strategic goals.
- Align the organization's priorities with the organization's financial management plan.
- Direct the organization to remain true to its core mission and vision.
- Control spending to ensure that the organization remains fiscally viable.

- Communicate the progress of the organization's financial status to its leaders so adjustments may be made and the plan may be fulfilled.
- Gather budgetary data that enable you to make informed decisions about the organization's direction.
- Coordinate the appropriate resources to accomplish tasks.

Reviewing your organization's strategic plan will enable you to identify the financial management objectives needed to achieve the organization's (or functional unit's) strategic objectives (**Figure 9-1**). (See the "Strategic Planning" chapter for more information on creating a strategic plan.)

All the elements of the financial management plan, when pulled together, should present a focused plan for accomplishing the goal(s). For example, suppose the STAR EMS System is facing growth in terms of more requests for service. Its leadership team will need to support that growth if STAR is to effectively serve its customers. The strategic goal in this case might be to expand services to a specific area within the response jurisdiction that is experiencing a greater demand for service due to a rapid increase in the number of single-family homes built there. During the budget preparation process, key financial management objectives will need to be included in the budget to support the organization's strategic goal—for example, to place an additional

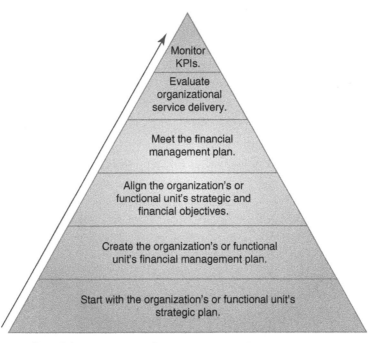

Figure 9-1 Using a financial management plan.

Success in the BUSINESS WORLD

Know Your Purpose

Being an organizational leader entails never losing sight of the organization's core mission and purpose. It is easy to stray from the organization's core mission during prosperous financial times, but doing so may result in operational and financial challenges for the organization.

Starbucks, known to many of us as a leading coffee provider, was once known for doing more than just selling coffee. In 2003, Starbucks ventured into music production; in 2006, it released its first movie. Other entertainment business projects followed. Soon after it jumped into these fields, however, Starbucks began experiencing some turbulent operational and financial times. In 2008, Howard Schultz, the company's former CEO, was brought back to replace current CEO Jim Donald and turn around the once-prosperous, but then-struggling company. At that point in its history, formerly loyal Starbucks customers were going elsewhere for coffee, Starbucks stock had plummeted, and store sales were down.

Schultz was committed to making some drastic changes to once again improve Starbucks customer loyalty and realign the company's service delivery. Starbucks needed to focus on its business priorities, mission, and purpose if it was going to remain in business. Schultz eliminated approximately 18,000 jobs, closed 977 stores, and ordered that all Starbucks stores be closed for a day so that employees (baristas) could be retrained. Closing stores for the one day cost the company $6 million—but the Starbucks team was determined to do what it took to get back to the company's core mission and return to what once had made it a coffee-selling giant. By 2014, Starbucks had turned itself around and was once again the coffee giant we all know. Starbucks acknowledged that it had lost focus on its mission and purpose for a time, and needed to return to its roots.

Within most EMS organizations, there are opportunities to provide services beyond treating the sick and injured and transporting them to the most appropriate facility—for example, providing home health evaluations, giving immunizations, holding community safety classes, transporting nonemergent ambulatory customers to doctor appointments, and so on. EMS organizations should certainly continue to expand their slate of offerings by seeking additional service delivery opportunities that will benefit the organization, the community, and its customers—but this expansion must be done cautiously and without losing sight of the organization's core mission and purpose: taking care of patients.

station with two new units in the response area during the next budget year. Before they can include the new station and ambulances in the budget, the budget team must know how those new resources will be funded. In this case, the goal is the expansion of service, the financial management objective is determining the financial needs associated with construction of a new station and implementation of two additional ambulance units, and the strategy and tactics focus on how the objectives will be funded.

As another example, suppose the Gill EMS Chief has determined that the department's ambulance units need to be replaced, and the goal is to replace all four units within the next three years. The financial management objectives will be to purchase two ambulance units this year, one ambulance unit next year, and one ambulance unit the following year. The strategy will be to purchase the units by finding a purchase price that is within the organization's forecasted budget assessment. The tactics used to keep the purchase price within the budgetary threshold may include contacting multiple ambulance vendors, obtaining a bulk price by ordering more than one ambulance at a time, and having the warranty work done by the department's fleet mechanics.

The Budgetary Process

Creating and working with a budget for any organization can be challenging, time consuming, and stressful. Nevertheless, helping to create a budget, attending budget workshops, and assuming the responsibility of staying within budget are the best ways to understand the operation and administration of the organization.

Managing an organization's budget is very similar to managing a personal or household budget. Your organization's budget is much larger and more complicated than your household budget, but the underlying concepts are much the same. The organization needs the funds to keep it functioning; that is, a steady flow of revenue is required if the organization is to remain viable. The organization often must reduce its spending, and it must not spend money on items that are not included in the budget. To ensure that it stays within its budget, the organization must regularly evaluate its budget activities; the financial management plan and financial management objectives can help with this monitoring.

The term **fiscal year** (or *budget year*) is used to describe the year for which a budget is meant to be used. The fiscal year is not required to match the calendar year. Each organization determines the dates of its fiscal year and then works within that schedule for accounting purposes. Preparations for a new fiscal year actually begin well before the first day of that fiscal year, with the requirement that a fiscal year's budget be completed and approved prior to the beginning of the fiscal year. Depending on the size of the organization, the budget preparation phase can range from 4 to 6 months or longer.

As the preparation of the budget approaches, directors, managers, and functional unit leaders typically will be summoned to a "budget kickoff" meeting. In larger organizations, a representative from the budget office, the chief executive officer, the chief financial officer, or another senior executive will discuss the upcoming year's financial management plan, including budget goals, budget reductions, financial management objectives for core services, deadlines for capital improvement/replacement plans, and budget targets for each unit and the organization overall. In smaller and/or volunteer organizations, the budget preparation process may be somewhat different, with either the chief or a city official being assigned to complete most of the department's budget. The size of the department and the number of personnel available to assist in completing the budget make a significant difference in how complex and how challenging the process will be.

Highly trained accounting professionals will often oversee the budget process. However, as an EMS officer, you will be involved because you will be overseeing a unit that is assigned a budget. If you are in a supervisory role, oversee the delivery of goods or services, have employees reporting to you, oversee projects, and/or are responsible for purchases, then you will likely have a budget assigned to your operations.

The basic steps in the budgetary process are as follows:

1. Identification of the organization's (unit's) needs and required resources
2. Budget request preparation
3. Review and approval of the budget request
4. Adoption of the approved budget
5. Administration of the approved budget

The first step—identifying the organization's (or unit's) needs and required resources—is done through the financial management plan. In a larger organization, aligning your section's specific strategic goals with the organization's larger strategic goals before the official budget process starts gives you time to determine how each financial objective will be achieved to meet the strategic goals set for your unit. Even in a small organization, the financial management objectives for the organization as a whole must agree with the strategic objectives for the organization. As you consider how you can meet these goals and objectives, it is important to allow some time for adjustments and follow-up from vendors. If you wait until the last minute to ask them for data and other input, you run the risk of not having all the necessary information ready for submission to the budget committee. By establishing a financial management plan, the EMS officer will know how each strategic goal will be supported by each financial objective and will be able to manage the budget effectively.

The second step of the budgeting process is to prepare the actual budget request. If the budget process is new to you, ask questions and learn from those who have been through this process before. Consider meeting with those staff who are responsible for overseeing the entire budgetary process and asking questions before the budget preparation meetings begin.

Your approach to creating the actual budget is determined by whether the organization chooses a top-down or a bottom-up approach. In a top-down budgeting process, the leadership team provides the financial management objectives and other budgetary parameters to the managers, giving managers a firm starting point, but also providing little room for adjustment based on the manager's own research. In contrast, in a bottom-up budgeting process, managers have more flexibility in pursuing the financial management objectives that will best meet their unit's strategic goals.

An organization's budget takes the form of a **budget worksheet**—an itemized list of expenses (e.g., employee salaries and benefits, billing services, fleet services, station maintenance and renovation, training, administrative supplies, medical supplies, and support services) and an itemized list of revenue sources (e.g., transport reimbursements; property taxes; response contracts with cities, townships, corporations, or government agencies; and grants). This information also helps identify the organization's fixed costs and variable costs. **Fixed costs** are expenses that must be paid independent of output changes—for example, building rental, leased equipment, and loan payments. In contrast, **variable costs** are dependent on output. That is, as the output increases, so will the costs—for example, gasoline, utilities, and office supplies. Total revenues, total expenses, and the difference between the two may be found at the bottom of the budget worksheet. This summary gives an overall picture of the organization's or unit's budget activities, including any net profit (i.e., the amount of revenue left over once all expenses and adjustments have been made) or net loss (i.e., revenues – expenses = profit or loss).

Ensuring that the organization's revenues and expenses meet the forecast requires thorough planning and constant monitoring of the organization's budget activities. There are several different types of budgets you may be required to create; more information on these types appears later in this chapter.

Once the budget has been prepared, it must be reviewed and approved by the individual(s) and/or department in charge of the organization's **master budget**. In smaller organizations, this may entail simply meeting with the chief or director, who can then approve or modify your budget, or send it back to you for adjustment. For EMS sections within larger public safety organizations or fire departments, the budget may be reviewed by the chief of your division; then, along with the other departments' budget requests, it may move to a team of leadership members, a budget director, and local officials for approval. Several rounds of review and adjustment of the budget may be necessary. In addition, the public may be allowed to review the full department's budget request via a town hall meeting or other forum, with ultimate approval coming from a local leader (e.g., mayor).

After all of the functional units' budgets are collected and consolidated into a master budget, it is recommended that each functional unit manager be prepared to present and discuss his or her budget with the department's senior leadership and finance team. Such a budget preparation presentation can serve as a "dry run" to answer any potential questions that might arise from the governing board or elected officials, identify any potential errors, and ensure that key budget items are included in the presentation prior to submission for final approval. Among the key items to include in this presentation are the following:

- Presentation structure
- Trends and issues
- Operating revenue summary

- Non-operating revenue summary
- Operating expenditure summary
- Non-operating expenditure summary
- Position summary
- Capital improvement plan
- Service level impacts
- Summary

The presentation must be easy to follow, cover all key points found within the proposed budget packet, and include a summary at the end of the presentation.

A budget preparation presentation is not the same as a budget workshop. A budget workshop is held to determine the expectations of senior leadership regarding the goals, expectations, and financial parameters for the following year's budget; clearly identify financial management objectives and the forms and justification required for purchases; and discuss any new changes to consider during the current budget preparation cycle and the expectations pertaining to capital equipment/improvement expenses. The workshop will also include allotted time to meet with senior organizational leaders to address budget questions during the budget preparation process. Ultimately, the goal of such a workshop is to ensure that the functional workgroup managers continue to work within the parameters set by the organization's leadership team and deliver an operational budget as outlined during the workshop. In addition, it is important to clearly set budget process benchmarks (**Table 9-1**). An approved budget must be

Table 9-1 Sample Budget Process Schedule	
Dates	**Activities**
January 5	Budget kickoff meeting with all division managers and senior leadership team
February 23–28	Division budgets due for initial review between division managers and chief executive officer
March 1–5	Final review of master budget between the chief executive officer and the department's budget representatives
March 15	Department's master budget is finalized and delivered to the organization's (private company) or city or county's (public company) budget office
April 2	Master budget is presented to the city council, county board, or board of directors for review
May–June	Budget is reviewed by the city council, county board, or board of directors
July	Requested adjustments to budget are made by the city council, county board, or board of directors
August	Budget approval by city council, county board, or board of directors

adopted prior to the beginning of the new fiscal year and is administered according to the details of the final budget.

Staying Within the Budget

Every organization prepares its budget differently, and budgets will have many more items than those mentioned in this chapter. To help managers track budget activities, some organizations provide monthly or quarterly budget activity reports. These reports help managers stay within the budget during each period. Many organizations use 1-year budgets, but some may use 3-year or 5-year budgets.

When a budget line item, whether a revenue or an expense, will have multiple entries during the budget period, the EMS officer must track actual amounts against budgeted amounts. For example, if repeated purchases are made for a specific line item (e.g., office supplies), the manager must track the amount of allocated money remaining in that line item. If the manager does not know the amount of money remaining for that line item and continues to approve purchases, that line item will most likely go over budget and may cause the organization to fail to meet a specific strategic goal. Such a difference between a budgeted amount and the actual amount is called a **budget variance**.

A budget variance can be either positive or negative. For example, if an organization budgeted $150,000 to purchase one ambulance, but the actual purchase price was $128,000, there is a positive budget variance because the actual price was less than the budgeted amount. Conversely, if $150,000 was budgeted for a new ambulance but the actual price was $160,000, then there is a negative variance and this item is over budget. Someone within the organization must monitor budget variances to ensure the organization remains within its overall budget limits. In addition to detecting a budget variance, it is as important to identify the root cause of the variance and take the necessary corrective actions to ensure that it does not keep occurring. Be aware that a

Managerial Leadership **BRIEFCASE**

Simplifying Budget Management

Developing and managing a budget can be overwhelming. To simplify this process, it is helpful to consider the EMS organization's (or unit's) budget to be no different from your home budget. At home, you likely use either a paper or software ledger to ensure that you have enough money to pay bills, buy groceries, buy clothes, and take vacations. At times, you must refrain from making purchases because there is not sufficient money in your account. You may be short on money because you did not budget appropriately, because you overspent on a nonbudgeted item, or because your revenue projections were inaccurate and you did not have as much money available as expected.

positive variance may also have potential negative ramifications. If you overestimate the amount of money needed for particular line items, that inaccuracy may negatively reflect on your planning and research skills. With any budget variance—positive or negative—you should document the factors that contributed to the variance.

Types of Budgets

The two main types of budgets you create as a manager will likely be an operational budget and a capital budget. An **operational budget** includes all the basic expenses an organization requires to remain operational, such as station utilities and rent, salaries, and benefits. It can be difficult to keep track of these expenses, so it is helpful when one staff member or a finance officer is assigned to routinely monitor such activities to ensure they stay within budget. The operational budget is presented as a **line-item budget**, which clearly separates each budget activity by description and funding account. It is commonly a static budget, meaning that it cannot be changed during the budget year, and typically has a life span of one year.

A sample operational budget appears in **Figure 9-2**. This example includes a limited number of line-item expenditures and revenues. Although each item in an operational budget appears on its own line, the budget worksheet should still be divided into sections based on the type of expense/revenue or the account from which expenses will be paid or in which revenues will be

XYZ EMS Department Operation Expense Budget			
Fiscal Year October 2014-December 2015			
	Commitment Items	Adopted Budget	Actuals
	Salaries and Benefits		
1351	Executive Salaries	41,452.00	39,027.70
1352	Regular Salaries	8,671,879.00	7,798,398.74
1353	Regular Wages-Salaries	370,694.00	392,300.35
1354	Labor Distribution	1,276,726.59	1,123,430.11
1355	Overtime	726,288.00	725,360.38
1356	Annual/Sick Pay	139,912.62	47,080.14
1357	FF Supplemental Co	50,094.00	53,917.61
1358	Innovation Awards	123,768.00	102,400.00
1359	FICA Taxes	840,809.00	769,244.50
1360	Retirement	1,789,525.00	1,951,463.21
1361	Health Ins Premium	2,160,179.00	1,948,981.78
1362	Life Ins Premium	10,891.00	18,167.23
1363	Workers' Comp	471,393.00	447,903.11

Figure 9-2 Sample operational budget. (*continues*)

	Utility Services		
3301	Heating Fuels	5,044.99	1,508.87
3302	Electricity	40,204.00	20,295.54
3303	Water & Sewage	4,799.18	3,723.70
	Station Rentals and Leases		
4102	Station Rentals and Leases	41,670.00	15,143.44
4103	General Liability	99,182.00	98,425.94
4104	Bldgs & Contents I	63.70	63.70
4105	Ins Outside Agency	22,257.00	22,257.00
	Other Current Charges & Obligations		
5501	ALS Vehicle Lic/Veh Permits (every 2 yr)	3,000.00	3,000.00
5502	Clinical Laboratory License	250.00	250.00
5503	DEA License for Controlled Substance	750.00	750.00
	Operating Supplies		
6601	Operating Supplies	32,032.94	11,749.42
6602	Fuel/Gas	870,912.23	866,333.47
6603	Medical Supplies	150,000.00	48,000.00
6604	Linen	1,225.00	1,225.00
6605	Oper Equip under $7	7,822.12	7,034.62
	Construction		
7000	Capital Outlay	4,684,918.00	1,224,903.87
	Books/Publication/Membership/Training		
8851	Books	750.00	200.00
8852	Membership	500.00	175.00
8853	Training	5,000.00	1,500.00
	Travel		
9101	Travel Per Diem	25,000	8,000
9102	Travel Mileage	3,500.00	300.00
	Expenditure Total	**22,672,492.37**	**17,752,514.43**
	Revenue		
223001	Intragovernmental	113,007.00	156,766.50
223002	Ambulance Service Fees	14,273,780.37	216,029.77
223003	Contracted EMS Services	90,000.00	1,225.32
223004	Miscellaneous Revenue	51,500.00	26,608.49
223005	Balance Forward	450,000.00	450,000.00
223006	General Fund	7,694,205.00	7,694,205.00
	Revenue Totals	**22,672,492.37**	**8,544,835.08**

Figure 9-2 Sample operational budget. (*continued*)

deposited. Types of expenses and revenues are discussed further later in this chapter. Examples of accounts include the following:

- **General fund**: The dollars contributed to the department from the controlling government entity (city or county). It can also be a catch-all account for items that do not have their own, more specific, account

- Special revenue fund: An account, established by the government, to collect proceeds that will be used for a specific project

- Debt service fund: An account used to pay principal and interest on general long-term debt

- Capital project fund: An account to cover major capital acquisitions or construction

- Internal service fund: An account to cover services provided to other departments within the government (government organizations)

These are just a few examples of the elements that the EMS officer may be working with when creating or reviewing an operational budget. Every organization will be different, whether public or private, and creating a budget that meets the needs of the organization and is structured using accepted accounting principles must be a priority for any organizational leader.

Unlike an operational budget, a **capital budget** includes only outlays for capital purchases such as equipment, EMS stations, and ambulance units, and is included within the master budget. **Figure 9-3** provides an example capital budget plan for a 5-year period.

The master budget is where all budgetary activities for the entire organization are represented. It includes all revenue sources and expenses for every division (e.g., administrative, operations, sales, marketing, logistics, public education, and dispatch). In a large organization, the master budget is constructed by the finance team. In a smaller organization, it may be created by an individual who has been assigned to work with the department's budget on a regular basis and has experience with the budget process, compliance regulations, and budget audits. This individual would also require training to meet the demands of working with a master budget.

Several types of budgets are available to organizations depending on the details involved and the specific means in which the budget will be used. Some examples of budget types are as follows:

- Static or **fixed budget**: Once approved, this budget cannot be changed. Thus funds earmarked for one line item cannot be used for a different line item if organizational needs change during the fiscal year. Typically a static budget is used for one-year budget cycles. Operational budgets are usually static budgets.

- Flexible budget: In a flexible budget, expenses are adjusted as a result of variance between actual budget output and revenue.

- **Zero-based budget**: This type of budget does not include roll-over amounts from the previous budget cycle, so it always starts with a zero balance. All activities are analyzed before placing them into the budget for the upcoming year, and only those items that add value to the organization are included. Although this approach has the advantage of allowing managers to

EMS Operations Capital Improvement Plan	FY 14–15	FY 15–16	FY 16–17	FY 17–18	FY 18–19	FY 19–20
Station Replacement						
Station 1	0	$700,000	0	0	0	0
Station 2	0		0	$765,000	0	0
Station 5	0		0	0	0	$795,000
CIP Total	**0**	**$700,000**	**0**	**$765,000**	**0**	**$795,000**

Capital Equipment Replacement Plan	FY 14–15	FY 15–16	FY 16–17	FY 17–18	FY 18–19	FY 19–20
Equipment Replacement						
Portable Radios	$ 250,000.00	$ 165,000.00	$ 165,000.00	$ 165,000.00	$ 18,000.00	$ 18,000.00
Cardiac Monitors	$ 150,000.00	$ 150,000.00	$ –	$ 100,000.00	$ –	$ –
Ambulance Unit	$ 300,000.00	$ 300,000.00	$ 300,000.00	$ 300,000.00	$ 300,000.00	$ 300,000.00
Staff Vehicles	$ 41,000.00	$ –	$ 85,000.00	$ 85,000.00	$ 50,000.00	$ –
Mobile Computers	$ 85,000.00	$ 85,000.00	$ 40,000.00	$ 40,000.00	$ 40,000.00	$ 40,000.00
Capital Equipment Total	**$ 826,000.00**	**$ 700,000.00**	**$ 590,000.00**	**$ 690,000.00**	**$ 408,000.00**	**$ 358,000.00**
Total EMS Capital Improvement and Outlay	**$ 826,000.00**	**1,400,000**	**590,000**	**1,455,000**	**408,000**	**1,153,000**

Figure 9-3 Sample capital budget.

thoroughly analyze revenue and expenses, it may be very time consuming because managers are essentially constructing a budget from scratch (zero) as opposed to having a budget with the expenses already included and simply making adjustments for the following year.

- **Incremental budget**: To construct an incremental budget, the leadership team uses data (also called *actuals*) from the previous year and makes minor adjustments to create the upcoming year's budget. Although this type of budget has the advantage of considering the past year's performance, it may hamper forecasting because managers may depend too heavily on past performance rather than assessing current economic conditions and the current economic performance of the organization.

Incremental and zero-based budget activities can be used to create an operational budget. As an EMS officer, it is important to determine which budgeting approach is appropriate when creating a budget for your functional workgroup's operational budget. Will you be required to start from zero, or will you use an incremental approach and rely on historical data from the previous year's budget as a starting point to meet the possible financial demands for the upcoming year?

Expenses

Expenses can fall into several categories. The focus here is on expenses that support the operational and administrative aspects of the organization. In a line-item budget, expenses are listed, one per line, followed by the dollar amount budgeted for that item. In creating a budget, especially one based on the previous year's budget, you must review these expenses and determine whether they add value to the unit and whether there is a more cost-effective way of achieving the same outcome.

As an EMS officer, you must be prepared to justify new expenses during the budget preparation period. The goal of every financial management plan is to minimize expenses and maximize revenues. However, this poses a challenge to those personnel responsible for managing budgets. This section summarizes some of the common expenses that the EMS officer will likely be responsible for managing.

Salaries and Benefits

Salaries and benefits will probably be the organization's greatest expense. These expenditures may be difficult to forecast because of the continuously changing business environment, the need to replace employees with those who earn a higher or lower salary, merit promotions, and other factors. The most common reasons for budget variance in the salary/benefit category include the following:

- New hire. When the organization approves the hiring of new personnel, those employees' salaries are only one of the additional expenses incurred. The added expenses of replacing an employee are often termed the *cost of turnover*. Employment training, supplies and equipment to perform the job, required tests, physical examinations, background checks, and other additional criteria must be met prior to hiring a particular individual—and they all cost money. Although the numbers vary among organizations, the estimated cost for an organization to hire a prehospital EMS provider ranges from $15,000 to $25,000, not including the person's salary. Another rule of thumb is that it costs 25 percent of the annual salary to replace the lost employee.

- Incentives and bonuses. Many organizations offer incentives and bonuses to their employees. For example, incentives may be awarded for work performance, filling an interim supervisor role, having certifications beyond what the position requires, being physically fit, participating in committees, and so on. Although incentives and bonuses play an important role in improving employee morale, they can incur significant expense.

- Insurance and related benefits. The organization is responsible for providing insurance to its employees, which can cost the organization $10,000 or more per employee, depending on the insurance. Although the employee often pays for a portion of the insurance, the employer is responsible for covering a set amount of that expense. Insurance benefits may include medical, vision, and dental insurance; life insurance; and workers' compensation.

- FICA: Both employees and employers are required to make contributions to the Federal Insurance Contributions Act (FICA) tax, which subsidizes federal benefits programs such as Medicare and Social Security.

- Overtime. Overtime expenses are a significant contributor to the organization's bottom line. Organizational leaders must make every effort to routinely evaluate the organization's staffing levels to ensure that overtime hours are kept to a minimum. They must also determine why overtime is occurring, and implement a plan to address the root cause of the overtime and reduce overtime expense across the organization.

- Retirement. Employer contributions to a 401k or defined benefit contributions are another significant expense. Additionally, when an employee retires, the organization may continue to offer medical insurance and provide a payout to include accrued sick leave, accrued personal leave, bonuses, and other retirement compensation. These expenses must be factored in when evaluating the organization's financial stability.

Fleet Services

Fleet services are critical value-added components for any EMS organization. Without working ambulances, the organization would be unable to respond to calls and to transport the sick or injured to the hospital. Service delivery would be severely affected, and the delay in responding to 911 calls would expose the organization to criminal or civil liability.

To keep the fleet on track, the organization must have a unit replacement plan in place that identifies which ambulances may need to be replaced soon. A replacement plan should include certain markers that indicate to the organization's fleet manager and leadership team that a unit should be considered for surplus—for example, mileage exceeding a predetermined threshold, a history of significant repairs, the balance between how much time the unit is out of service due to mechanical issues versus in service, and the point at which the cost of maintaining a unit exceeds the benefit of having the unit. A 3-year historical analysis of preventive maintenance, oil, fuel, windshield wiper, and tire costs will provide key information and enable managers to budget for replacement units appropriately.

Purchasing new ambulances may take some time if the organization requires that units meet certain specifications. In addition, you will need to go through your organization's designated purchasing process, including the process for selecting a vendor if there is no current purchasing contract for ambulances in place. Necessary steps may include obtaining quotes from vendors; completing the material requisition paperwork; and obtaining approval to proceed with the purchase from a member of the leadership team, city, county, or township, and perhaps the city, county, or township's elected board. (See the "Purchasing" section later in this chapter.)

Replacing an ambulance is expensive, so organizations must have a system in place to reduce wear and tear on their existing units. Examples include rotating ambulances between areas with high call volumes and areas with lower call volumes, increasing the number of ambulances to share the response load, and designating ambulances that respond only to nonemergency requests for service, thereby leaving the emergency ambulances available for emergency calls. Ambulance crew members should take special care of the vehicles and report any potential issues as soon as they arise, even if it means switching to a different vehicle mid-shift. They should also be well informed about the schedule for preventive maintenance.

Over time and with the purchase of new ambulances, the organization may begin to accumulate a surplus of ambulances, which can provide some support for the front-line units and increase the organization's capabilities during peak times and natural disasters. Every effort must be made to extend the life of each ambulance, which will not only improve the EMS organization's ability to meet its service demands, but also benefit its bottom line. Beware of creating excessive ambulance surplus, however. The reserve numbers should be calculated based on deployment, maintenance schedules, and a contingency factor for surge or loss of units (mechanical or accident). For example, the threshold set for backup units may be half the number of front-line units (e.g., 30 front-line units and 15 backup units). Older units beyond the 50 percent backup/front-line ratio can be disposed of. It is important not to incur unnecessary costs by repairing older units just for the sake of having extra units; of course, you also do not want a situation in which there are no units available to respond to the scene of an emergency.

Medical Supplies

Medical providers need equipment and supplies to render care to the sick and injured. As the EMS officer, however, you must identify and track the supplies that are really needed and being used. Having a warehouse full of medical supplies that are rarely used is expensive and a poor use of the organization's money. Excess inventory of items that have expiration dates must be avoided. Implementing a tracking system for the items that are regularly used helps avoid waste, is cost-effective, and improves overall patient care.

Many EMS tools are available for purchase, but as an EMS officer managing a budget, you must determine which are nice to have and which are truly needed. Consider creating and implementing a research and development committee comprising EMS field providers and managers. This committee's primary responsibilities would be to evaluate EMS supplies and equipment before they are purchased. Its work will serve multiple purposes. First, ensuring that supplies and equipment are researched and tested by the organization's committee will improve buy-in from the employees. Second, the committee should produce sufficient information to determine whether the medical supplies or equipment are truly worth buying. Managers can offer a financial perspective that may not be as obvious to field providers but may improve the overall return on investment for equipment and supplies ultimately purchased. For any EMS organization, supplies and equipment will be an ongoing expense that must be managed effectively to avoid overspending.

If a cache of extra equipment and supplies will be needed to stock a mass-casualty unit, it is imperative that an organizational member be assigned to rotate the stock. This practice will ensure that supplies are available in case of a disaster and that the supplies are not expired and can be used to meet the needs at hand.

Training

All EMS providers within the organization must be well trained to provide patient care in an emergency event. Regardless of the training content and the medium used to deliver the training (e.g., in-class instruction, web-based training), the training will be an expense. Training expenses include course materials, medical protocols, instructors, equipment, recertification costs, and overtime pay.

As an EMS officer, you may be asked to manage training for the organization. Knowing that you will need to budget for training sessions, you must take the time to identify which courses will offer the greatest added value to your prehospital providers. Once you have identified the best training courses for your employees, you can then determine which ones fit into the training budget.

Capital Replacement and Capital Improvement

Expenses related to capital replacement and capital improvement are vital to every organization. As an EMS officer, you cannot become complacent about the organization's strategic plan. Indeed, that plan must include the items essential to ensure that the EMS organization exceeds its service delivery expectations. To do so, the organization must have a plan to replace or improve items that support the organization's EMS operations. Capital items are those items that cost more than a specific limit set by the organization (e.g., $500, $750) and have a life expectancy greater than 1 year (e.g., ambulances, station renovations, and cardiac monitors). These items are expensive, and the organization must plan and budget for their purchase and replacement. Items may break when least expected, and all items have a limited life expectancy. You must be ready to replace or repair these items before they stop working. Many organizations have an **asset** management team that maintains a list of all capital items; this team can help you budget for capital-related expenses.

Support Services

Although your main budgeting priority as an EMS officer is items that sustain EMS operations (e.g., personnel, ambulances, equipment, stations, training), you should also take the time to review the master budget and learn which other items are listed there. Examples include dispatch center operations; maintenance of a distribution center for storing operational and administrative items; personnel uniforms and protective equipment; office supplies to support day-to-day administrative tasks; and station supplies such as bed linens and pillows, pots and pans, toilet paper, and cleaning supplies.

Unfunded Mandates

Mandates are statutes or regulations imposed by the federal, state, or local government. When they are not funded through government allocations, they pose a significant challenge for any manager overseeing a budget. Examples of potential unfunded mandates include health insurance, retirement plans, medical equipment, and salaries. These unfunded mandates require that organizational leaders thoroughly assess their budgets to identify both value-added items and nonessential items that can be eliminated. Leaders may have to forego some of the current budgeted items, preferably the nonessential items, to ensure that the organization has sufficient financial resources to cover any unfunded mandates. Managing unfunded mandates is a serious challenge, especially during difficult economic times. Every manager must stay informed about current and future unfunded mandates that may affect the organization.

Revenue

Knowing the sources of the organization's revenue is critical for those personnel who are responsible for managing a budget. Efforts aimed at identifying and measuring these revenue streams will not only provide the information necessary to create an accurate budget, but also bring to light historical trends for forecasting revenues. As an EMS officer, you must become thoroughly familiar with the rules and policies pertaining to each revenue line item. These revenue streams are used to support the organization's strategic plan and ensure that the organization remains fiscally viable. Although every organization is different and revenue streams will vary, capitalizing on

Managerial Leadership **BRIEFCASE**

Central Supply Location

Maintaining a centralized headquarters and distribution center can benefit the organization in many ways. Most notably, using a central location as a depot can prevent ambulance crews and supply delivery clerks from having to travel great distances to deliver supplies. Organizations with multiple offices may find their employees spending much of their time on the road, which is wasteful if it can be avoided. Travel time impacts fuel expenses, risk of vehicle accidents, productivity, and available office support. The goal of a central office and distribution center is to meet the organization's demands as efficiently and effectively as possible. Keep in mind, however, that a centralized office requires all the ambulances to travel to central supply to restock, which may ultimately cost more in fuel and personnel time (and take units out of their service area) than a decentralized approach. Many organizations, in addition to having a central distribution center, also use a delivery system where supplies are delivered to the stations. Depending on the organization and how far each station is from the distribution center, such a delivery system can ensure that the crews and stations have the necessary tools to conduct day-to-day operations without putting a strain on the EMS response system. Ultimately, this approach may prove to be the most beneficial if the organization has set station locations. What is best will depend on the organization, its demographics, and the service area.

every opportunity to generate revenue for the organization must be a priority for the organization's leadership and its members.

Medical Transport Fees and Reimbursement

EMS organizations receive more revenues from medical transport fees than from any other source. Consequently, it is important that the billing and reimbursement process for transport services be efficient and move smoothly. Each EMS organization should ensure that it has a system in place that supports expeditious billing for transport. The efficiency of this system relies on all employees thoroughly understanding the importance of accurate and complete documentation of all pertinent patient information—not just the information necessary for the patient's care, but also the information required for billing. Required billing information includes the following items for the patient:

- Name
- Social Security number
- Insurance information
- Treatment modalities
- Medicare information
- Service level provided (BLS, ALS 1, or ALS 2)

Incomplete or inaccurate billing information can delay the billing and payment process. When the information is complete, the next priority is to have a process in place that limits the number of steps between when the information is captured and when a bill is generated. Just as prehospital providers hand off the patient care report to the emergency staff upon arrival at the hospital, so the process of submitting billing information should be straightforward.

An EMS organization may opt to contract with an EMS billing company rather than handle billing as part of its own operations. The billing process is critical because it involves continuous oversight of monies collected for services provided. The collection business is complex, and whoever is overseeing this process must understand the rules governing collection, documentation, compliance requirements, and appropriate coding of patient care for reimbursement. This area, like patient care, has no room for error, and every effort must be made to collect monies for services rendered.

Four parties may be billed by the EMS organization: Medicare, Medicaid, commercial insurance, and self-pay customers. Medicare will pay the federally mandated reimbursement limit or the department's fee, whichever is lower, as long as the ambulance transport was reasonable and medically necessary. Medicaid has a state-mandated reimbursement limit that is lower than the Medicare limit. Commercial insurance will pay 100 percent of their coverage amount (not the bill), minus any co-pays or deductibles. Self-pay is payment by the individual who received the service; it is used when the customer (patient) is uninsured or when his or her insurance does not cover EMS transport. The reimbursement rate for self-pay is very low, making forecasting revenue from user fees a bit challenging.

Consider the following example of a transport forecast analysis:

West Reed EMS Department transported 47,723 patients last year, and the organization is looking to increase its transport fees. The service level mix is as follows:

- BLS: 24%
- ALS 1: 74%
- ALS 2: 2%

Payment sources are broken out into the following classes:

- Medicare: 56%
- Medicaid: 13%
- Commercial pay: 15%
- Self-pay: 16%

After reviewing the data, the department decides to increase its transport fees as noted in **Table 9-2**. In addition to the increase in user fees, the West Reed EMS department will also use the department's historical mature charge mix (i.e., the number of accounts that were paid during the previous calendar year), the organization's transport volume, the service level transport mix (BLS, ALS 1, and ALS 2), and potential adjustments to Medicare allowable charges to calculate the department's revenue forecast. When taking all of these elements into consideration, the West Reed EMS Department forecasts a potential increase in revenue by approximately $4.5 million over the next 5 years. When forecasting revenue, one must always take into account any potential impact that may affect the projections; for example, potential healthcare reform, a decrease in the number of transports for a given year, or a change in community demographics.

The EMS officer must know how medical transport billing fees are established for the organization. Transport fees are charged to cover the expenses of transporting a patient to an emergency

Table 9-2 West Reed EMS Transport Fee Increase		
Service Level	**Current Charges**	**Recommendation**
Mileage	$9.18	$13.00
BLS	$501.00	$800.00
ALS 1	$541.00	$800.00
ALS 2	$627.00	$800.00
Oxygen	$25.00	$30.00
Lift assist	—	$50.00
Medical nontransport	—	$50.00

department or other medical facility. As an EMS officer, you should research the transport fees charged by other EMS agencies in the area, to ensure that your organization does not price itself out of the market. Although transport fees are set by the organization, the reimbursement level is determined by Medicare, Medicaid, and insurance companies. Because these fees are typically paid by Medicare, Medicaid, self-pay, or the patient's insurance, EMS agencies must have a process in place for prehospital providers to capture as much of the patient's personal and insurance information as possible. This will ensure that the billing agency or the organization's billing department has all the information necessary to receive reimbursement for the services delivered.

Compliance

Ensuring that the organization is compliant and up-to-date with billing requirements is extremely important. Regardless whether the organization does its own billing "in-house" or contracts with a billing company, being compliant with laws must be a top priority. The organization must have a plan in place that ensures the following activities:

- The organization must assign someone within the organization to ensure that compliance is being monitored throughout the billing system. This individual must receive the necessary training to meet this requirement and should be someone of high ranking authority. Even if the organization outsources billing, this individual can routinely ask the billing company's compliance officer for information about their compliance status and inquire about any billing concerns.
- If the billing is done internally, the employees must be familiar with the coding process and the laws applicable to patient billing activities. Continuous training is a priority, and routine evaluations of the employee's patient coding success rate is paramount to ensure the customers are appropriately charged for the EMS service delivery.
- Ensure that there are security and privacy controls in place to protect health information.
- Ensure that a secure method for payment is in place.
- If the billing is done in-house, the billing system should include routine internal audits by members of the organization and independent audits conducted by external billing auditors. This will ensure that any non-compliant activity is identified and corrected immediately. If the billing is done by a third party, the organization's compliance officer must request information as to the outcome of such audits.
- Ensure that policies and procedures are routinely updated and shared with the staff.

Whether an organization should conduct its billing in-house or through a billing company is a decision for the senior leadership team, as there are numerous pros and cons for either option. The one constant is that compliance must be at the forefront and the employees must be well trained. EMS service delivery billing, as with other facets of EMS service delivery, must adhere to the laws, rules, policies, and regulations set in place to prevent any variation from the accepted billing practices. An audit from the Center for Medicare and Medicaid Services (CMS) could occur at any time.

Donations

Some organizations accept monetary or equipment donations from community members, vendors, or private business. Monetary donations provide a source of revenue for the organization, and equipment donations reduce the organization's expenses.

Community Education

Organizations may generate revenue by providing safety classes for members of the community. For example, the department may offer cardiopulmonary resuscitation (CPR), first responder, bloodborne pathogen, or water safety training, as well as other safety classes for the community, taught by members of the organization. Offering community training classes can certainly provide an additional source of revenue, even as it strengthens relations between the organization and its customers.

Selling Equipment

After an organization has determined that a piece of equipment is no longer being used or is ready for surplus, the department may choose to sell it. Depending on its policy on selling equipment, the organization may choose to conduct an auction, or it may hire an auctioneer to sell the equipment (more likely with capital items). Although using an auctioneer requires payment of a fee, the organization will receive the majority of the money from the items sold.

Strategic Partnership

Some organizations also generate revenue by entering into automatic-aid agreements with other EMS providers. This arrangement is likely to be made if an emergency service department knows it cannot provide an adequate response to a certain area and, therefore, must seek an alternative for delivering the necessary service. The compensation for these agreements can be either monetary or an exchange of services that benefits each department. For example, both departments may agree to cover response areas in each other's district, thereby reducing the expense of placing a station and an additional unit there. Alternatively, an agency might offer to provide dispatch services for another department, with the second department then allowing co-habitation of crews in its station.

Subscriptions

Subscriptions are a revenue-generating mechanism similar to monthly insurance payments. A household essentially subscribes to EMS coverage throughout the year. Such a subscription program is designed to assist community members by paying for the portion of EMS delivery not paid by the user's insurance or by reducing their user fees compared to nonsubscribers who request services. For example, suppose a household pays $50 for an annual EMS subscription. If any members of that household then require EMS assistance, the subscription may be used to pay some of the out-of-pocket expense for the customer, the service delivery fee, or related expenses not covered by insurance. Subscription details are dependent on the department. Subscriptions offered to community members are voluntary, and the benefits vary with each department. Each state has its own insurance laws, and any organization contemplating a subscription program must research existing statutes and not violate insurance rules and regulations. It is ideal when subscription programs are not considered insurance programs.

Mobile Integrated Healthcare

As EMS organizations continue to expand services to better serve their community and realign resources with the requests for medical care, some organizations turn to mobile integrated healthcare community paramedicine (MIH-CP) to serve this purpose. MIH-CP services could generate revenue for an EMS organization; however, a funding source for the program must be available. Currently, the primary funding source for patient transports is the Centers for Medicare and Medicaid Services (CMS). Therefore, in order for EMS organizations to get reimbursed for services outside the EMS transport user fee, legislative changes need to occur to recognize MIH-CP services as reimbursable for healthcare provided by EMS providers.

There are, however, other viable options for obtaining funding for such a service, such as partnering with healthcare organizations. For example, a hospital is impacted by 30-day readmission penalties; therefore, some hospital organizations are already working with local EMS providers to ensure that patients are well informed of their treatment regimen assigned by their physician and are abiding by physician orders at home to prevent readmission. This is done by having designated EMS units make these routine visits to patients identified by the hospitals as candidates for readmission. Alternatively, the EMS organization may evaluate the regular users of the 911 system to request transport and begin to work with these patients to determine what can be done preemptively so an EMS emergency response is not needed.

Although MIH-CP does face some funding challenges, there is no doubt that it can be a beneficial service for the community and reduce the cost of healthcare by realigning the resources with specific patient needs. Once the necessary legislation is passed, MIH-CP will prove to be an additional funding source for EMS organizations.

Property Taxes

If the organization is a government enterprise, monies received from tax dollars will help support its operational budget. Ad valorem taxes are property taxes based on the value of real estate or personal property. These taxes are calculated using the millage rate—the tax rate per $1000 of taxable value. The millage rate is set by local government officials and will typically be adjusted only if there is significant drop in tax revenue. Depending on the enterprise, unused funds may have to be returned to a general fund if not used during the budget's fiscal year. Revenues collected through other streams may be kept for future expenses.

EMS Response Contracts

Response contracts with cities, townships, corporations, or government agencies are another important revenue source for EMS organizations. For example, a city, township, county, or federal government establishment may not offer EMS delivery to its residents or visitors and must contract with an EMS provider for such services. The contract may be with either a private EMS company or a city, township, or county EMS provider.

The process of establishing a contract for EMS delivery starts with a request for proposal (RFP), followed by a bidding process. The contract is then awarded to an EMS agency that is able to meet the organization's requirements, as stated in the RFP, and stay within the budgetary parameters. Once awarded, the contract will include a scope of work stating what is expected as far as performance and meeting specific benchmarks, the contract payment schedule, required training for EMS providers, health requirements for EMS providers, management and personnel requirements, hours of operation, and other aspects of EMS delivery. The contract includes a start and contract termination date and may vary in terms of the period of time covered. Once the contract expires, the customer may agree to renew the contract or it may start the RFP process anew.

An EMS response contract will often include a statement regarding the cancellation of the contract by either party, which may require a 30-day notice. For example, a contract could be canceled if the provider does not meet the requirements stated within the contract. As the EMS officer, you must ensure that you are familiar with the contract and know which requirements it includes.

Medical Unit Stand-By

EMS organizations can earn additional revenue by offering medical unit stand-by services during mass gatherings such as the following:

- High school, college, and professional football games
- Running or bike races
- County or town fairs
- Presidential and other dignitary visits
- Professional boat races
- Air shows

These events can be managed similar to EMS response contracts if the stand-by units will be required for an extended period of time or on a recurring basis. For example, if medical coverage is requested every year during Major League Baseball spring training, the organization might establish a contract with the baseball team that will go into effect on the first day of spring training and terminate at the end of the last game. Such a contract will include the length of the contract and an agreed amount for the medical coverage that will, at a minimum, cover all expenses and the expected coverage time during every game. The contract must also include all the standard information in an EMS response contract.

If a contract is not an option or the event is a one-time occasion, the organization must have a set medical coverage fee that is applicable for all stand-by services. For example, this rate could range from $75 to $100 per hour for one paramedic and one EMT. Medical coverage events are great opportunities not only to generate additional revenue, but also to promote the organization by speaking with those at the event, displaying the ambulance unit for all to see, and providing brochures or other items that promote safety. The organization must take advantage of these opportunities and see them not just as a potential revenue stream, but also as a means to promote and continue to build the organization's brand.

Grants

With limited funding sources, EMS organizations must continue to seek alternate ways to generate revenue or means of reducing expenses. Grants can serve as an alternative to reducing operational expenses. Grants are available to provide assistance to those organizations that require additional funding to provide life safety services. The grant award may be used to purchase medical equipment, ambulance units, training, or fitness equipment, or to fund EMS community programs. The grant award will likely be dependent on the population being served, the economic conditions, and the true need for the award. Grants may cover 100 percent of an expense, or may stipulate an 80/20 or 50/50 arrangement, in which the organization is reimbursed 80 percent (or 50 percent) of the expense and is expected to cover the other 20 percent (or 50 percent).

If the organization does not have a grant writing officer, someone must be assigned to research and monitor grant opportunities and complete and submit grant applications. Grants

Managerial Leadership **BRIEFCASE**

Unit Hour Utilization

EMS, like many other business organizations, must operate in a lean environment, making every attempt to reduce spending and operate as efficiently as possible. Some organizations calculate their unit hour utilization (UHU) to help determine the efficiency of their EMS responses. Analyzing the UHU can identify which ambulance units are under-utilized, moderately utilized, or performing at maximum utilization, thus assisting the EMS officer in adjusting the organization's EMS service delivery response. The following steps can be used to determine the organization's utilization rates:

1. Take the number of activities completed by the unit (e.g., 10 runs)
2. Take the number of hours the unit was in service for the shift (e.g., 24 hours)
3. Divide the number of activities by the hours in service (e.g., 10 ÷ 24 = 0.4)

The higher the number, the greater the utilization is for the unit, meaning the more productive the unit is for that time. Optimal utilization would be 0.55 to 0.45, average utilization would be 0.35 to 0.25, and poor utilization would be 0.15 to 0.01. These values do not paint the whole picture, however. The UHU is influenced by response requirements, the response area (i.e., rural, urban, or suburban), transport times to the hospital, hospital turn-around times, and other circumstance that may cause a variation in determining true utilization of a unit.

may be found through online searches. Many grants are offered through state and federal government, and it may take patience to find a grant that would meet your needs. When applying for a grant, the application may be lengthy and require detailed information about the project, the estimated amount of funding needed, the organization, and detailed justification as to the need for the project, how the project will be used and benefit the community and the organization, and the current status of the project. An update on the project outcome may be required 1 year post-implementation. In addition, a detailed report must be provided to the grant officials verifying that the purchase has occurred and that the grant funds have been used as required by the grant rules for the requested project.

After submitting a grant application, it may take weeks or even months to find out whether the organization has been awarded the funds. Do not delay in submitting your application.

Purchasing

The purchasing process varies significantly depending on the item being purchased, the reason for the purchase, and whether the organization is private or government-based. Familiarity with the purchasing process in your organization allows you to expedite the purchasing process and ensure that all the necessary purchasing documents are completed appropriately prior to submission to the purchasing department.

Capital Items

When contemplating the purchase of capital items, the buyer will most likely be required to obtain three price quotes. If only two quotes are available, the purchaser must include a letter explaining why three quotes were not available. If the organization has a preferred vendor or a state-contracted vendor, quotes may not be needed because the vendor will have already been approved by the organization or a state agency. If only one vendor sells the item—for example, only one training center in the area offering paramedic training, or a piece of equipment that is manufactured and sold exclusively by a specific vendor—the purchaser must include a letter stating that this vendor is the sole source for that item. Capital purchases typically require a signature from a senior leader of the organization (e.g., a county or city manager; an elected city, county, or town board member; or a chief financial officer). As an EMS officer, you must become familiar with both your organization's and your state's purchasing rules. Although private EMS organizations may not require three formal quotes or an RFP for capital projects, it is always good management practice to ensure that the organizational leaders are making prudent financial decisions, being fiscally responsible, and seeking the best product or service.

Request for Proposal

An RFP is a solicitation document, on behalf of an organization, requesting a bidding process for a purchase of significant value. The RFP process entails completing an application that includes the specifications of the product or service the organization is seeking to purchase; for example, the construction of a new EMS station, a station alerting system, new electronic patient care report writing software, or billing services.

Within a government agency, the individual responsible for the project must thoroughly complete the necessary documentation required as part of the RFP application, then send it to the purchasing department. As part of the application process, the organization will need to establish an RFP review committee, preferably with an odd number of members to prevent a tie during a vote, to assist in the review of the vendor proposals and selection of a vendor. The RFP will then require approval from the city, town, or county board of elected officials and, once approved, must be posted so all potential vendors have an opportunity to bid on the RFP. An RFP is typically posted on the department's website, and there is a set time period during which vendors can meet with organization representatives to ask questions about any of the requirements or specifications. Once the posting expires, the vendors can present their product or service to the RFP committee. After a selection has been made, any vendor choosing to dispute the process will have a predetermined amount of time to do so. The RFP process is designed to ensure that purchases meet the required specifications and that the organization's purchasing process remains fair and transparent.

Purchase Orders

Organizations use purchase orders as a mechanism to authorize vendors to invoice them for materials or services ordered. A purchase order is issued by the organization's purchasing department or the individual responsible for purchasing within the organization. It is important that proper documentation be kept and filed after the purchase has been made and a copy of the purchase order be provided to the vendor. This will ensure that the purchase is properly aligned with the materials or service being delivered. If a change is subsequently requested, the individual submitting the purchase order must create a change order request (a department-specific form) that identifies the reason for changing the order, the new items being purchased, the dollar amount, and the previous purchase order number.

Every organization will have an expense threshold that will require approval from a chief executive officer, chief, city or county manager, or local government board to complete a purchase.

Emergency Purchasing Process

Some organizations have an emergency purchase order system. Emergency purchase orders are to be used only when an item is needed to prevent an imminent threat to life or property or a disruption of essential services—for example, when an EMS station has experienced a roof collapse and employees need to be relocated until repairs are made or EMS crews are assigned to a prolonged event and will need to be fed. Although most of the same steps used for nonemergency purchases will apply, the process is rearranged, allowing the documentation for an emergency purchase order to be produced after the purchase to prevent delays in obtaining the item.

When immediate purchase of supplies or contractual services is necessary because of certain conditions, organizational leaders may have the authority to execute emergency purchases. To do so, they must adhere to the organization's policies and procedures, which may include the following elements:

- Authorization: Depending on the dollar amount of the purchase, it may require the approval of the chief executive officer, department chief, town or county manager, or senior elected official.
- Procedure: When an emergency exists, a requisition (purchasing authorization form) with an explanation of the nature of the emergency must be submitted (electronically or via fax) to the department responsible for processing purchases. The purchasing department may obtain additional price quotes prior to issuing a purchase order number, depending on the dollar amount needed for the purchase, if time permits.
- Request for an emergency purchase during nonbusiness hours: If an emergency purchase order is required during nonbusiness hours (i.e., nights, weekends, or holidays), the department may have to use purchasing cards (credit cards) to make the necessary purchases. If the amount required exceeds the limit on the purchase cards, a senior-level officer must make the necessary arrangements to complete the purchase by working with the vendor.

Emergency purchases should be made only during a narrowly defined set of emergency conditions because they can become costly. During emergency situations, when decisions are made quickly, very little thought may be given to the amount spent. When making an emergency purchase, it is essential to obtain the items needed to mitigate the crisis, while still making every attempt to be fiscally responsible.

Material Requisitions

Material requisitions are documents used to notify the purchasing department of goods or services needed to conduct business. These planned activities require specific requests for purchase and, depending on the dollar amount, will need approval from the chief executive officer, chief of the department, or city or county manager. The material requisition should answer the following questions:

- Who needs the items being requested for purchase?
- What is being requested for purchase?
- Where will the goods or services be delivered?

The material requisition form may require the following information (depending on the organization):

- Date of request
- Department or requester name
- Required delivery date

- Delivery location
- Vendor information
- Funding information for the purchase
- Description and specification of goods or services
- Quantity of units
- Unit or service price
- Justification for requesting the purchase
- Approval signature

Vouchers

Organizations may use a voucher system when conducting business with vendors. A voucher is an internal document used to obtain the necessary approvals prior to authorization of a specific transaction, such as a purchase or a service provided by a vendor. For example, the organization may have a contract with an EMS training facility (not affiliated with the organization) where department employees may go for EMT or paramedic recertification training. However, prior to attending the recertification course, the employee will need to obtain a voucher from his or her training division as verification that the employee is authorized to attend the training. The employee will then give the voucher to the vendor (training center representative) confirming that the department has agreed to pay for the employee's training. Another example is that new employees may receive vouchers from the human resources department prior to attending their new hire physical. The potential employee will give the voucher to the medical representative as an authorization that the department will pay for the employee's physical.

Prior to implementing a voucher system, a formal agreement between both parties conducting business must be in place, confirming that the vendor will accept the vouchers as authorization for a specific product or service. When the specific transaction is completed, the vendor will then include the voucher when submitting the invoice for payment.

Credit

A credit is created when the organization purchases goods or services (e.g., medical equipment, ambulance units, station construction) from a vendor and has overpaid. Depending on the organization's accounting rules, the organization may opt to get reimbursed or use the credit to purchase additional equipment or services from the vendor. A vendor may also agree to grant a line of credit to an organization to allow the organization to make purchases and pay at a later time. Even with the established line of credit, the organization must use the appropriate purchasing methods for this type of transaction and assign a purchase order number or other indication of which line-item in the budget will be used to pay for the purchases.

Credit Cards

A credit card, also referred to as a purchasing card, is provided to those individuals who have been authorized to make business purchases. Purchasing cards are usually supplied to individuals who may be in a position where a purchase is needed immediately. The purchases may be for station repairs, administrative and operational supplies, training conference tuition, travel expenses, professional journal subscriptions, or other expenses. The purchasing card will have the person's or organization's name on it and will have a pre-determined set limit. The cards are not meant to replace any of the other purchasing methods, but can be used when more formal purchasing methods are not required.

If your organization is tax exempt, you must ensure that no taxes are applied to the purchase made with the purchasing card. Save all sales receipts and match them with the monthly card statements. When reconciling the expense report, provide justification for the purchase, as it must be approved by a senior leadership member.

The purchasing card must be used for business transactions only and not for personal purchases. Purchasing card users must be familiar with the organization's purchasing policies.

Cash

Some organizations may choose to use cash for certain purchases. Having cash available to make purchases does have advantages; for example, when a transaction accepts only cash, when making a small purchase that does not require any formal paperwork, or reimbursing an employee for making a company purchase with his or her own money. Organizations may use petty cash funds for necessary, non-reoccurring, on-the-spot purchases. Petty cash can be used for necessary purchases below a set dollar amount, determined by senior leadership, and do not require a purchase order or a formal bidding process. Working with cash may pose some challenges because it may be difficult to keep track of the expenditures. When using cash for any transaction you should obtain approval prior to making the transaction, get a receipt for the purchase, and report the expenditure to the purchasing and/or finance department.

WRAP-UP

Concept Review

- As an EMS officer, you must focus on your organization's financial management objectives to ensure that your organization or division stays on track and within its budget.
- A financial management plan conveys the big picture of the organization's strategic and financial goals and can be useful when deciding what to include in the organization's budget.
- The basic steps in the budgetary process are as follows:
  - Identification of the organization's (unit's) needs and required resources
  - Budget request preparation

- Review and approval of the budget request
- Adoption of the approved budget
- Administration of the approved budget
- As an EMS manager, you are most likely to create an operational budget and a capital budget.
- Be prepared to justify any new expenses requested during the budget preparation period. The goal of every financial management plan is to minimize expenses and maximize revenues.
- The most common expenses for an EMS organization include the following items:
  - Salaries and benefits
  - Fleet services
  - Medical supplies
  - Training
  - Capital replacement and capital improvement
  - Support services
  - Unfunded mandates
- Efforts to identify and measure an organization's revenue sources will not only provide the information necessary to create an accurate budget, but also illuminate historical trends for forecasting revenue.
- The most common sources of revenue for an EMS organization are as follows:
  - Medical transport fees
  - Property taxes
  - EMS response contracts
  - Medical unit stand-by
  - Grants

- The purchasing process varies significantly depending on the item being purchased, the reason for the purchase, and whether the organization is private or government-based.

Managerial Terms

Asset A resource that can benefit the organization.

Budget A detailed financial plan that includes lists of income sources, expenses, and other categories, and a specific amount of money assigned to each line item.

Budget variance A difference between a budgeted amount and the actual amount.

Budget worksheet An itemized list of expenses and revenue sources.

Capital budget A budget that covers only outlays for capital purchases, such as equipment, EMS stations, and ambulances.

Demand analysis An evaluation of what customers are willing to pay for a product or service.

Financial management objectives A set of activities used to ensure that the organization is meeting revenue and expense forecasts, and its operations are supporting the organization's strategic goals.

Financial management plan A plan used to ensure that the organization can sustain its daily operations, achieve its revenue forecasts, meet its financial obligations, and fulfill its strategic goals by planning, organizing, directing, controlling, and coordinating.

Fiscal year The year for which a budget is meant to be used; also called a budget year.

Fixed budget A budget that covers one year. Some adjustment may be made to this budget, but it typically remains unchanged throughout the year.

Fixed cost A cost that is independent of how much the item is used (e.g., building rental).

Forecasting The process of predicting future outcomes or trends.

General fund The dollars contributed to the department from the controlling government entity (city or county). Or, a catch-all account for items that do not have their own, more specific accounts.

Incremental budget A budget that is based on data from previous budgets, with only minor adjustments being made from one budget to the next.

Line-item budget A budget that groups specific financial activities by description and funding account.

Master budget The budget that covers the entire organization. It includes all funding sources and expenses of every division (e.g., administrative, operations, sales, marketing, logistics, public education, and dispatch).

Operational budget A budget with a predetermined target for revenues and expenses for a specific period for the organization/section. It usually covers one year.

Variable cost A cost that depends on the output or use of a resource.

Zero-based budget A budget created by starting at zero dollars for each line item and developing a dollar amount without any preconceptions.

Case Review: Adapting to a Revenue Shortfall

The Underwood EMS Department was bracing for a significant shortfall in revenues for the upcoming budget cycle and needed to evaluate the organization's strategic plan as well as its proposed budget. The anticipated decline in revenues was due, in part, to a decrease in property values in the area and local government officials' decision not to increase the millage. There were also decreases in other revenue-generating activities. The managing EMS officer acknowledged that something needed to be done to ensure the organization would remain viable and to prevent employee layoffs.

The managing EMS officer, with other members of the leadership team, began to dissect the organization's master budget and determine which purchases could be deferred to future budgets. Also, the team addressed the realignment of service delivery to better match the customers' needs. For example, if a customer made an appointment to be transported to a doctor's office for a scheduled appointment, in the past the department would routinely send an advanced life support (ALS) ambulance staffed with two paramedics and a complement of ALS equipment. This level of resources was actually unnecessary for transportation of a stable individual to a scheduled appointment, and using an ALS unit was more expensive than providing a non-stretcher ambulatory service van with a nonmedical driver to provide the same service. The leadership team also reviewed employee salaries and benefits, overtime pay, acting pay (i.e., the pay of those individuals working out of their assigned job classification), and the organization's incentive costs because these line items represented the greatest expense.

The leadership team was committed to ensuring the organization operated in a lean state while continuing to provide quality service; it was also conscious of the need to support employee morale. During the review of the organization's financial data, the EMS officer identified that reducing overtime costs could result in significant savings. In its current scheduling arrangement, the Underwood EMS Department averaged between 5 and 10 open paramedic slots during three 24-hour shifts. The EMS officer, upon conducting an internal assessment, noted that the organization routinely filled all of the open paramedic slots with another paramedic, even though sometimes those slots could have been filled by emergency medical technicians. The vacancies in question already had an assigned paramedic to the unit, so that the second paramedic served as an extra ALS provider. Having two paramedics on board every ALS unit had been the organization's staffing profile for years. The leadership team acknowledged that the proposed new staffing profile would yield a significant cost savings and began working to make the transition. All of the department's initial-response ALS transport units would eventually be staffed by one paramedic and one EMT.

Although the initiative in this case would contribute to significant cost savings for the organization, the leadership team needed to find a way to introduce the plan without creating pushback from the paramedics, who would no longer have the opportunity to work overtime on a regular basis. The field crews, managers suspected, would see this initiative as diminishing their opportunities to make extra money. Prior to rolling out the initiative, the leadership team met with the field district supervisors as well as union representatives to share the plan and to explain why this plan was so important and how it would benefit the entire organization. These conversations created an opportunity to seek feedback and buy-in from employees and supported open lines of communication between the field providers and the leadership team. The district supervisors could address any questions posed by field personnel when making station visits, and union leadership representatives could reach out to their members and do the same. This was only one cost-saving initiative taken by the Underwood EMS Department, but it was a step in the right direction, reducing waste, avoiding layoffs, and ensuring that the organization would remain in operation for future EMS delivery.

Case Discussion

By readjusting the staffing profile on all ALS initial-response units, the organization not only saved money by minimizing the higher-paid paramedics' overtime costs, but began operating in a lean environment without jeopardizing patient care. It took a threat of potential financial crisis to encourage organizational leaders to thoroughly review the organization's budget and take a hard look at the organization's current strategic plan. Many organizational leaders will attest that it is easy to become complacent and to continue to do business as usual without truly scrutinizing the organization's operating processes and systems on a regular basis. As an EMS officer, you should not wait for an impending financial, operational, or natural crisis to conduct an organizational risk assessment and evaluate the organization's strategic plan.

Case Review: Replacing Outdated Equipment

The Shelby EMS Department consisted of 25 front-line ALS transport ambulances and needed to find a way to replace some of its capital equipment. The department had experienced a decline in revenues as a result of low transport volume, a decrease in the forecasted revenue collections, and stagnant property taxes leading to a decrease in the general fund. As a result of the diminished revenue stream, the department had no choice but to postpone the purchase of capital equipment until economic conditions improved. Nevertheless, it was faced with a difficult decision regarding upgrades to the organization's cardiac monitors. The department had a total of 35 cardiac monitors (25 front-line and 10 backup units) that were between 10 and 15 years old, and some were constantly out of service and in need of repair. To make matters worse, the department was notified that the cardiac monitor model would no longer be sold by the vendor, warranties would not be extended, and repairs would be done only if parts were available. The department needed to come up with a plan to replace the aging cardiac monitors before several of them began to fail at the same time.

Considering that the department did not have sufficient funds to purchase 25 new heart monitors at $30,000 each (a total of $750,000), the EMS officer contacted the vendor for ideas and suggestions. The vendor provided a list of state and federal grant opportunities that would prove invaluable for the organization; the vendor also referred the EMS officer to a grant specialist who worked for the vendor and specialized in cardiac monitor grants. Some of the grants would pay for 100 percent of the cost; others, considered matching grants, would cover half the funding (i.e., the organization would be responsible for 50 percent of the cost of the equipment and would be reimbursed for the other 50 percent). Still others offered 80/20 funding, wherein the organization would be reimbursed for 80 percent of the purchase price of the equipment.

Ultimately, the department was awarded an 80/20 federal matching grant, with which it purchased 29 cardiac monitors. The total cost for all 29 cardiac monitors was $870,000; however, the organization was reimbursed $696,000 and had to pay only $174,000 from its own funds.

Case Discussion

As a managing EMS officer, it is important to maintain positive professional working relationships with colleagues and vendors. This approach will prove beneficial when information is required on specific EMS equipment or other related service delivery topics. In this case, although the organization's leadership was aware of grant opportunities, it was the collaborative effort between the vendor's grant writing professional and the Shelby EMS Department's leadership team that made the submission of the grant possible.

Every organization must have a capital improvement plan. In this case, although the outcome was favorable, an alternative outcome could have posed some significant patient care challenges. Upon initial purchase of capital equipment, a department must immediately begin planning for its replacement. The life expectancy of a piece of equipment may be longer than expected due to advanced technology, minimal wear and tear, and preventive maintenance; however, having a capital improvement plan in place may serve as a trigger to begin addressing the aging units and preventing procrastination. Without such a plan, if a decision is made to delay capital purchases due to budgetary constraints, you might find yourself without working equipment and without the means to meet your customers' needs. By making incremental but consistent capital improvements, you can achieve the desired results and not fall behind.

Management of Emergency Medical Services (FESHE) Correlation Guide

Management of Emergency Medical Services (FESHE) Course Outcomes	Corresponding Chapter(s)	Corresponding Page(s)
1. Discuss the basic philosophy, organization and operation of injury prevention and risk-reduction programs.	8	222–227, 243, 245
2. Compare and contrast management and leadership.	2	23–35
3. Provide practical examples of the principles of customer service in EMS.	6	171–195
4. Apply the technique for conducting an effective performance appraisal.	4	101–103
5. Identify strategies to optimize reimbursement for EMS services.	9	277–279
6. Apply quality improvement techniques to various aspects of EMS operations.	5	123–165
7. Define due process and apply the principles of a progressive disciplinary program.	3	73–75
8. Define ethical behaviors and the decision-making strategies when faced with an ethical dilemma.	2	42

After-action report A document created after an incident, often including a snapshot summary of the incident, the goals and objectives in managing the incident, performance outcomes, lessons learned, and actions taken to better prepare for future crisis situations.

Asset A resource that can benefit the organization.

Balance scorecard A management tool that focuses on aligning key business practices and processes with the vision, mission, and strategy of the organization.

Benchmarking The process of comparing one's business processes, practices, and metrics to those of industry leaders.

Big picture The overall structure, composition, and direction of an organization.

Brand An organization's reputation among actual and potential customers as determined by the organization's quality of goods and services and the market's perceptions of the organization.

Budget A detailed financial plan that includes lists of income sources, expenses, and other categories, and a specific amount of money assigned to each line item.

Budget variance A difference between a budgeted amount and the actual amount.

Budget worksheet An itemized list of expenses and revenue sources.

Capital budget A budget that covers only outlays for capital purchases, such as equipment, EMS stations, and ambulances.

Coaching A method of directing, instructing, and training a person or group of people with the aim to achieve some goal or develop specific skills.

Continuous quality improvement (CQI) A management process activity to make immediate or ongoing improvements to organizational processes or systems. The improvements are made by applying quality improvement tools. Also called *continuous process improvement.*

Control limit chart A chart with upper and lower limit specifications for a process or system.

Crew resource management (CRM) A multidisciplinary management system with the primary goal of improving safety and efficiency by focusing on leadership, communication, situational awareness, teamwork, decision making, and use of all resources available to meet the goal.

Crisis A situation that poses a serious threat to a single customer, a community, or the organization and its stakeholders.

Crisis management plan A plan that includes key activities necessary for managing a current organizational threat or crisis, customers, and the community. An incident action plan may be included within a crisis management plan.

Crisis review audits Inspections of the organization's current operational risks, processes, systems, weaknesses, and threats.

Decoding How the receiver interprets the message.

295

Demand analysis An evaluation of what customers are willing to pay for a product or service.

Due process The opportunity for an individual to know the charges and have evidence considered prior to disciplinary action.

Encoding How the sender formats the message.

Equipped for business A concept indicating that an organization has all the necessary plans and resources to function effectively and efficiently.

External customers Individuals to whom an organization provides goods and services, and who do not work for the organization.

Feedback The response from the receiver to the sender based on the message received.

Finance/administrative section chief (FSC) The individual responsible for addressing and managing administrative and financial requests during a crisis incident.

Financial management objectives A set of activities used to ensure that the organization is meeting revenue and expense forecasts, and its operations are supporting the organization's strategic goals.

Financial management plan A plan used to ensure that the organization can sustain its daily operations, achieve its revenue forecasts, meet its financial obligations, and fulfill its strategic goals by planning, organizing, directing, controlling, and coordinating.

Fiscal year The year for which a budget is meant to be used; also called a budget year.

Five business priorities (5 BPs) The foundation for any organization and a roadmap for all EMS officers. The five business priorities

are people, strategic objectives, financial management objectives, learning objectives, and a culture of quality.

Fixed budget A budget that covers one year. Some adjustment may be made to this budget, but it typically remains unchanged throughout the year.

Fixed cost A cost that is independent of how much the item is used (e.g., building rental).

Forecasting The process of predicting future outcomes or trends.

Functional-level strategic plan A plan created by and for members working in a division of an organization.

General fund The dollars contributed to the department from the controlling government entity (city or county). Or, a catch-all account for items that do not have their own, more specific accounts.

Goals Set targets (short or long term) that organizational members attempt to achieve.

Histogram A group of vertical bar graphs illustrating data points and the frequency of each data point.

Incident action plan (IAP) The formal documentation of activities pertaining to incident goals, objectives, strategies, tactics, and other pertinent information specific to an incident.

Incident command system (ICS) A system implemented to manage disasters and crisis incidents in which section chiefs report to the incident commander.

Incident commander (IC) The individual responsible for developing the incident objectives and for all aspects of implementing the crisis management plan.

Incremental budget A budget that is based on data from previous budgets, with only minor adjustments being made from one budget to the next.

Internal customers Individuals who work for an organization and depend on the organization's support to serve the external customer properly.

Key performance indicators (KPIs) Specific performance measures essential to the sustainability of an organization's strategic goals.

Language barrier Use of a particular language or technical terminology with which the receiver of a message is not familiar.

Lean A quality program focused on eliminating waste.

Line-item budget A budget that groups specific financial activities by description and funding account.

Logistics section chief (LSC) The individual responsible for providing necessary resources to assist in mitigating a crisis.

Managerial leader An individual who combines both the manager's and the leader's skills.

Master budget The budget that covers the entire organization. It includes all funding sources and expenses of every division (e.g., administrative, operations, sales, marketing, logistics, public education, and dispatch).

Mean The sum of a set of values divided by the number of values; the average.

Median The midpoint in a series of values.

Medium The format through which the sender is trying to communicate.

Mentoring A developmental relationship between a more experienced person (a mentor) and a less experienced person (a mentee).

Message What the sender is trying to communicate.

Mission statement A statement that identifies what you are doing now as an organization—that is, the purpose of the organization.

Mode The value that occurs most often in a data set.

National Incident Management System (NIMS) A Department of Homeland Security system designed to enable federal, state, and local governments and private-sector and nongovernmental organizations to effectively and efficiently prepare for, prevent, respond to, and recover from domestic incidents, regardless of their cause, size, or complexity.

Noise Any internal or external element that affects the message being received as the sender intended.

Norms Attitudes and behaviors that the organization or individuals within the organization see as normal.

Objectives Instructions used to support a goal. Objectives must be specific and measurable.

Operational budget A budget with a predetermined target for revenues and expenses for a specific period for the organization/section. It usually covers one year.

Operations section chief (OSC) The individual responsible for the operational management of a crisis and the development of the strategy and tactics used to mitigate the crisis.

Organizational (or corporate) strategic plan The overall strategy that is created to meet and exceed an organization's overall mission.

Organizational behavior The way people behave within an organization.

Organizational culture The behavior of the organization's members as a result of the organization's norms, values, and beliefs.

Organizational silos Groups of individuals within an organization assigned to work in a specific division or department—for example, logistics division, EMS division, finance division.

Organizational spokes Components of an organization that support and add value to the organization (the five business priorities) while keeping it moving on the right path.

Pareto chart A graphical bar view, where bars are in descending order.

Personal barrier A breakdown in communication based on the sender's or receiver's poor communication.

Physical barrier Any environmental factor (including distance) that disrupts the communication process.

Pie chart A circular graph divided into sections, where specific data are assigned to each section.

Plan–do–check–act (PDCA) A quality management program used to control and manage continuous improvement.

Planning section chief (PSC) The individual responsible for capturing and analyzing scene data that are then used to plan the response to a crisis event.

Process A set of steps or actions to achieve an end result.

Process barrier A breakdown of communication based on failure of part of the communication process.

Process flow chart A diagram or algorithm that displays each step in a process.

Project charter A document, commonly prepared by a senior leadership team member or the project manager, that contains information about how a project will be managed.

Public information officer (PIO) The individual responsible for disseminating information about a crisis incident to the news media, to incident personnel, and to the community.

Quality Meeting or exceeding customer expectations by delivering goods or services consistently with minimal to no variation from the expected outcome.

Quality assurance (QA) A quality management process established to monitor (audit) organizational standards and detect any variations from the organization's goods or services delivery desired outcomes.

Quality control (QC) A quality management process intended to ensure that necessary procedures are in place to support a quality outcome.

Quality management program A program that consists of methods used to achieve quality outcomes. Such programs include management activities and methodologies to support continuous quality improvement. Also called *quality methodology program.*

Quality planning A component of quality management that involves creating a plan to improve organizational performance outcomes.

Range The difference between the highest and lowest numbers in a set of values.

Receiver The person with whom the sender is trying to communicate.

Recognition primed decision making A method of rapidly solving problems by implementing a solution that has been previously used in similar situations.

Risks Processes, systems, stakeholder activities, and other business activities that may turn into crises if not monitored or managed appropriately.

Safety officer (SO) The individual responsible for the safety of on-scene personnel.

Scatter plot A graph in which individual data points are plotted in two dimensions to show their relationship.

Scope creep A phenomenon that occurs when the project objectives are not met because the project has grown beyond the desired outcome. It commonly results from a lack of clearly defined objectives, poor communication among the project manager and the team members, and absence of a check system that alerts the team that they have deviated from the initial intent of the project.

Semantic barrier Use of confusing wording or sentence structure that keeps the receiver from understanding the message.

Sender The person who is trying to communicate.

Six Sigma A quality management program focused on achieving near-perfect outcomes.

Stakeholders Individuals or groups that have a professional or financial investment in something, such as an organization or business. There can be both internal and external stakeholders.

Standard deviation The amount of variation or distance from the mean.

Strategic plan An organizational plan designed to clearly and concisely communicate how an organization will achieve its desired future organizational goals.

Strategy The approach taken to achieve a goal.

SWOT analysis A brainstorming tool used to analyze information about an organization's current and potential future state by evaluating internal and external business activities; its components are strengths, weaknesses, opportunities, and threats.

System A group of interrelated components working together to ensure a specific outcome.

Tactics A set of actions or processes used to achieve the organization's strategic plan.

Total quality A commitment to creating a culture of quality across all levels of the organization, ensuring that the goods and service meet or exceed customer expectations and that continuous improvement is at the center of every quality initiative.

Trend A movement of a series of data points in a specific direction over time.

Unified command Use of an incident command system in which each agency involved works together and shares command authority as one command center.

Value stream mapping (VSM) A methodical process, pertaining to the flow of organizational activities, that identifies the analysis and elements included in each of the activities that make up the process.

Values Ideas that reflect what the organization or individuals within the organization believe is right or wrong, good or bad.

Variable cost A cost that depends on the output or use of a resource.

Variation A value or data point that differs from the mean.

Vertical snapshot A look at the basic elements of an organization, from top to bottom.

Vision statement A statement that identifies where the organization should be in the future. It serves as the compass of the organization.

Zero-based budget A budget created by starting at zero dollars for each line item and developing a dollar amount without any preconceptions.

Index

Note: Page numbers followed by *f* indicate figures; page numbers followed by *t* indicate tables; and page numbers followed by *b* indicate box.